The Great Plague Scare of 1720

From 1720 to 1722, the French region of Provence and surrounding areas experienced one of the last major epidemics of plague to strike Western Europe. The Plague of Provence was a major disaster that left in its wake as many as 126,000 deaths, as well as new understandings about the nature of contagion and the best ways to manage its threat. In this transnational study, Cindy Ermus focuses on the social, commercial, and diplomatic impact of the epidemic beyond French borders, examining reactions to this public health crisis from Italy to Great Britain to Spain and the overseas colonies. She reveals how a crisis in one part of the globe can transcend geographic boundaries and influence society, politics, and public health policy in regions far from the epicenter of disaster.

CINDY ERMUS is Assistant Professor of History at the University of Texas at San Antonio.

GLOBAL HEALTH HISTORIES

Series Editor:

Sanjoy Bhattacharya, University of York

Global Health Histories aims to publish outstanding and innovative scholarship on the history of public health, medicine and science worldwide. By studying the many ways in which the impact of ideas of health and well-being on society were measured and described in different global, international, regional, national and local contexts, books in the series reconceptualise the nature of empire, the nation state, extra-state actors and different forms of globalisation. The series showcases new approaches to writing about the connected histories of health and medicine, humanitarianism, and global economic and social development.

The Great Plague Scare of 1720

Disaster and Diplomacy in the Eighteenth-Century Atlantic World

CINDY ERMUS

University of Texas at San Antonio

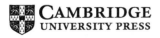

CAMBRIDGE
UNIVERSITY PRESS

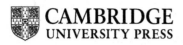

Shaftesbury Road, Cambridge CB2 8EA, United Kingdom

One Liberty Plaza, 20th Floor, New York, NY 10006, USA

477 Williamstown Road, Port Melbourne, VIC 3207, Australia

314–321, 3rd Floor, Plot 3, Splendor Forum, Jasola District Centre, New Delhi – 110025, India

103 Penang Road, #05–06/07, Visioncrest Commercial, Singapore 238467

Cambridge University Press is part of Cambridge University Press & Assessment, a department of the University of Cambridge.

We share the University's mission to contribute to society through the pursuit of education, learning and research at the highest international levels of excellence.

www.cambridge.org
Information on this title: www.cambridge.org/9781108747349

DOI: 10.1017/9781108784733

First published 2023
First paperback edition 2025

A catalogue record for this publication is available from the British Library

Library of Congress Cataloging-in-Publication data
Names: Ermus, Cindy, 1979– author.
Title: The Great Plague scare of 1720 : disaster and diplomacy in the eighteenth-century Atlantic world / Cindy Ermus, University of Lethbridge, Alberta.
Description: Cambridge, United Kingdom ; New York, NY : Cambridge University Press, 2023. | Includes bibliographical references and index.
Identifiers: LCCN 2022026117 | ISBN 9781108489546 (hardback) | ISBN 9781108784733 (ebook)
Subjects: LCSH: Plague – Europe – History – 18th century. | Plague of Provence, France, 1720–1722. | Epidemics – Europe – History – 18th century. | Disasters – Social aspects – Europe – History – 18th century. | Disasters – Social aspects.
Classification: LCC RC178.A1 E76 2023 | DDC 614.5/732094–dc23/eng/20220610
LC record available at https://lccn.loc.gov/2022026117

ISBN   978-1-108-48954-6   Hardback
ISBN   978-1-108-74734-9   Paperback

For Arlo, who showed me the meaning of life

Contents

Acknowledgments

A lot has happened in the ten years since I began research for this project. I earned my PhD; I moved to beautiful Canada for my first job as an assistant professor; I later accepted a new position back in the US; I married the love of my life; I had my sweet son. In that time, and in those travels, so many people have been part of the journey. Some have only been there a short time, while others have been there all along. All have helped, in their own ways, to make this book – this part of me – possible.

Taking it back to the beginning of my career as a historian, I would like to thank the faculty and staff in the Department of History at Florida International University, especially Joseph Patrouch, Darden Pyron, Felice Lifshitz, Howard Rock, and so many others, who were among the first to encourage me to further my studies, and who helped to stir in me a fervent, life-long passion for history. I would also like to thank my mentors and teachers at the Department of History and the Institute on Napoleon and the French Revolution at Florida State University. Above all, I would like to thank my advisor and friend Darrin McMahon, whose expertise, patience, humor, dedication, and invaluable mentorship helped shape me as a scholar. He gets credit for encouraging me to pursue my interests in the history of disasters, and, years later, for agreeing to be the reader at my wedding! I could not have asked for a more inspiring and dedicated mentor, and for that, I am truly grateful. I would also like to give special thanks to Rafe Blau-farb. To say that I might not have completed this study without him is not an overstatement, since he helped direct me toward a topic on the 1720 plague. For his continuing support through the years, I owe him a debt of gratitude.

I am grateful to all the programs and institutions that helped fund the research for this project, beginning with National Endowment for the Humanities, and the Institute on Napoleon and the French Revolution at Florida State University. Financial support also came from the Florida extension of the McKnight Foundation (FEF), which funded my graduate education through a generous doctoral fellowship and helped fund my research abroad. The people at FEF, including Dr. Lawrence Morehouse, Mr. Charles Jackson, and the rest of the McKnight family, are doing amazing things to help increase the number of underrepresented minorities in academia, and I am proud to be part of the family. I am also indebted to the University of Lethbridge for generously funding multiple summers' worth of research for the completion of this project.

As isolating as it may seem at times, the life of the mind depends on the work of many. I would like to thank all archivists and librarians around the globe for helping to make the pursuit and creation of knowledge possible. In particular, I must thank the staff of the institutions that I visited throughout the course of my research for their hard work and assistance. Many of the archives in which I had the privilege of conducting research are severely underfunded, yet their knowledgeable and dedicated personnel help to make archival research a pleasure and a privilege. My thanks go to the staff at the Archives nationales de France in Paris, the Archives nationales d'outre-mer in Aix-en-Provence, the archives at the Ministère de la Défense at Vincennes, the Bibliothèque nationale de France, the Archives départementales des Bouches-du-Rhône in both Aix-en-Provence and Marseille, the Archives municipales de Marseille, the Archives historiques de la Chambre de Commerce et d'Industrie Marseille-Provence, the Archivo Histórico Nacional in Madrid, the Archivo Municipal de Cádiz, the Archivo Provincial de Cádiz, the Archivo General de Indias in beautiful Seville, the Biblioteca Nacional de España, the Archivio di Stato di Genova, the Archivio di Stato di Roma, the Archivio di Stato di Venezia, the Arquivo Nacional da Torre do Tombo in Lisbon, the Arquivo Municipal de Lisboa, the Biblioteca Nacional de Portugal, the British Library, the National Archives of the United Kingdom, the UK Parliamentary Archives, and the US Library of Congress. I met some incredible people in each of these places (and even scored a couple of informative tours of the grounds!), each of whom helped to make my time abroad as memorable as it was fruitful. A sincere thanks, *merci, gracias, grazie, obrigada*.

I would also like to thank the many individuals who, in a variety of different ways, helped me along throughout the process of writing this book. A sincere thanks to Junko Takeda for her insight and for sharing her dissertation with me all those years ago; to Claire Edington, Libby Neidenbach, and Sarah Ghabrial for the adventures in the south of France; to Ann Carmichael, David K. Smith, and Arad Gigi for willingly and happily sharing their expertise; special thanks to biologist Boris Schmid of the University of Oslo for generously sharing his insight; to Suman Seth for recommending this particular press and series in the first place; to Javier Bobillo Blanco, who went out of his way to make sure I received my digital files after I left Madrid; and to Pedro Pinto, who was, and continues to be, an incredible resource for research in Portugal. *Muito obrigada por toda sua ajuda.* Special thanks to my colleagues, both past and present, for their friendship and support. For example, my big move to Canada might have proved more challenging without the help of Sheila McManus, who hosted me on Thanksgiving Days and gave me all too many rides to or from the airport. Thank you. Also Kristine Alexander, Christopher Burton, Catherine Clinton, Wing Chung Ng, Catherine Komisaruk, Anne Hardgrove, and others for their mentorship and support. A sincere thanks, too, to my students through the years for always inspiring me, teaching me, and keeping me young; to Lucy Rhymer and the team at Cambridge University Press, who have been an absolute pleasure to work with; to the anonymous readers whose feedback helped shape this manuscript; and to Fritz Davis, Malick Ghachem, Jacob Steere-Williams, Lori Jones, Mary Ashburn Miller, Meghan Roberts, Michael Bustamante, Scott Gabriel Knowles, Jane Maienschein, and so many others who have shown genuine interest in my work and/or invited me to discuss my research at their institutions. In this context, I must give very special thanks to Monica Green for her support, and for her invaluable insight, which has been instrumental in helping me understand the ongoing genetic plague research.

I must also express my sincere gratitude to my amazing friends and family for always being there for me, for letting me vent, and for being such wonderful company through it all. Among them (in no particular order), Gabriel Ortega; Lauren White; Maria Yaima Carmona; Camilo "Woody" Suarez-Bitar; Mathew Masters; Christopher Wilhelm; Justin Black; Madisen Rard; Elliott Florence; Bryan Banks (my *Age of Revolutions compadre*); Sergio Suarez; Johanna Herrera; Jessica Jassal; my nephew George; Maria Pelaez; the late, great Rangy Pelaez; the entire Gibson clan (with special thanks to Martha Sue and Benny Gibson for their love and support); Jessica Eise, Rebecca Bria,

Valeria Meiller, and Sarah Lasley for their company during the final stretch of writing this book; *a todos mis familiares en Cuba*; and to all of those I may be leaving out, but who have nevertheless brought me joy and comfort when I needed it – thank you.

I owe the greatest debt of gratitude to those who have been closest to me in the process of writing this book – those who have brought me the greatest happiness and with whom I have created the most precious memories. Inevitably, this is the part where I cry, so here goes. Thank you, Ashley Ermus, George Ermus, Christopher Aaden Valcarcel, and Ellison Marie Livesey, for your love and support, for making me smile, and for keeping me sane. Thanks, too, to my parents, Elsa and Jorge Ermus – and here I will switch to Spanish: *Gracias, mamá y papa, por tu cariño, tus consejos, por apoyarme, por siempre inspirarme, y por los muchos sacrificios que han hecho para que sus hijos puedan vivir en un país donde pueden decir, pensar, escribir, y vivir como deseen.* I am also more grateful than I could put into words for my husband, Abraham Gibson, who has supported me throughout the entire process of writing this book with his love, his patience, his humor, and his kindness, which knows no bounds. Thank you, Abe, for being my rock. Finally, I thank my son, Arlo, to whom I dedicate this book. Nothing I can say could possibly describe the joy that you have brought to my life. Thank you, my son, for your unconditional love, for your smile, for your laughter, and for just being you.

Abbreviations

AC	Actas Capitulares (AMC & AMU)
ACCIM	Archives historiques de la Chambre de Commerce et d'Industrie Marseille-Provence, Marseille
ADBRM	Archives départementales des Bouches-du-Rhône, Marseille
AE	Affaires étrangères (AN)
AGI	Archivo General de Indias, Seville
AHN	Archivo Histórico Nacional de España
AMC	Archivo Municipal de Cádiz
AMM	Archives municipales de Marseille
AMU	Archivo Municipal de Murcia
AN	Archives nationales de France, Paris
ANOM	Archives nationales d'outre-mer, Aix-en-Provence
ARV	Archivo General del Reino de Valencia
ASG	Archivio di Stato di Genova
ASR	Archivio di Stato di Roma
ASV	Archivio di Stato di Venezia
BL	British Library, London
BNF	Bibliothèque nationale de France, Paris
BNP	Biblioteca Nacional de Portugal
JHL	*Journal of the House of Lords*
MAR	Fonds de la Marine (AN)
MNE	Ministério dos Negócios Estrangeiros
PNAS	*Proceedings of the National Academy of Sciences*
Sanità	Antichi regimi, Provveditori e Sopraprovveditori alla sanità (ASV)
SP	State Papers Foreign (TNA)
TdT	Arquivo Nacional Torre do Tombo
TNA	The National Archives of the United Kingdom, London

Introduction

"You have seen earthquakes, but tell me, young lady, have you ever had the plague? ... If you had," said the old woman, "you would admit that it is far worse than an earthquake."

Voltaire[1]

From 1720 until 1722, the French city of Marseille, one of eighteenth-century Europe's most important port cities, suffered an epidemic of plague that, as the traditional story goes, arrived at its port on the *Grand Saint-Antoine*, a trade ship that had journeyed for a year in the Levant. Caused by the bacillus *Yersinia pestis*, the epidemic of 1720 claimed approximately 45,000 lives in Marseille alone, reportedly about half of the city's population. From there, it spread throughout the French region of Provence and surrounding areas, ultimately taking as many as 126,000 lives. It is for this reason that I refer to this epidemic, traditionally known as the Plague of Marseille, as the Plague of Provence throughout this book. Referring to it as the Plague of Marseille not only erases the experiences of those who endured the epidemic well beyond the region's primary port city, but it was in towns and villages like Aix-en-Provence, Arles, Salon, Toulon, Avignon, and so many others that the largest number of lives were collectively lost to this public health disaster. Moreover, much like the Great Lisbon Earthquake or Hurricane Katrina in New Orleans, the plague of 1720 has left an indelible mark on the social fabric of these areas, becoming part of the collective memory no less than it has in Marseille.[2] As French historian Paul Gaffarel and the Marquis de Duranty wrote in their early-twentieth-century history of the outbreak: "The plague

---

[1] Old woman to Cunegonde in *Candide*. Voltaire, *Candide, ou l'Optimisme* (Paris: Larousse, 1991), 63.

[2] The 1720 outbreak is also referred to as the plague of Provence in numerous contemporary documents.

1

which ravaged the south of France, and especially Marseille, in 1720 and 1722, left deep traces in the popular memory. It was, in truth, a national catastrophe."[3]

Marseille's history as a port of entry for contagion is well known, as is the story of this outbreak – the last major wave of bubonic plague to strike the city and surrounding areas. What is not well known is the impact that the Plague of Provence had *beyond* French borders. To be clear, the infection never left southeastern France, yet all of Europe, the Mediterranean, the Atlantic, and parts of Asia (including the Spanish Philippines) mobilized against its threat, and experienced its social, commercial, and diplomatic repercussions. Accordingly, rather than discuss only what took place in France, this book looks across national boundaries to identify and analyze the ramifications of the epidemic beyond Gallic borders. It is a transnational, transoceanic history that looks at some of the foremost port towns of the early modern world in order to begin to shed light on the influence of this event abroad. Cities explored here include Genoa, London, and Cádiz – the official capital for the Spanish monopoly over the Indies market, and thus eighteenth-century Spain's most important seaport – as well as some of the principal colonial ports in the Americas. These ports were not only major hubs for commercial activity in the first half of the eighteenth century but also shared inextricably close links with one another.

In the early modern world (roughly 1500–1800), port cities served as focal points for the expansion of the commercial community of the Atlantic and the world, essentially serving to unite disparate segments of the globe through the interchange of peoples, information, and commodities.[4] Conducting research in more than twenty archives across Western Europe, I traced a vast network of communication regarding the Plague of Provence – what I term an "invisible commonwealth" – that circled the globe. In many ways, this invisible commonwealth functioned like

---

[3] Paul Gaffarel and the Marquis de Duranty, *La Peste de 1720 a Marseille et en France, d'après des documents inédits* (Paris: Perrin et Cie, 1911), v.

[4] These bustling commercial hubs also serve as ports of entry for disease epidemics that traverse the oceans, carried by humans or by animal vectors that stow away in the cargo and eventually come ashore to proliferate among unsuspecting coastal populations. Port cities' locations along coasts and major waterways put them in another vulnerable position as they are exposed to the dangers of natural hazards such as hurricanes and tsunamis. It is the very commercial and dynamic nature of seaports that renders them susceptible to such threats.

a separate, autonomous community or detached state where consuls, ambassadors, public health officers, and others exchanged and spread information, and worked to shape responses to the public health crisis on the ground in their respective regions. They discussed, for example, precautions and measures taken against the plague in France and throughout Europe, or debated the effectiveness of quarantine in preventing the spread of plague. They also exchanged stories – their own and those of others – about arrests, forced searches of vessels and people, ship-burnings, quarantines, and even executions, almost always in port cities, as people attempted to travel or conduct business while the plague raged in southern France. Essentially, what emerges from archival documents at this time is a network of interconnected port cities that increasingly represented a global community – a series of settlements that while geographically distant, functioned together in many ways. Each port discussed in this book was a significant trading hub, all of which were connected by their close commercial and diplomatic ties to one another, and all responded to the Plague of Provence in unique ways and for unique motives. For this reason, each book chapter focuses on a different port city or region. Taken together, chapters cover the years from the 1713 Peace of Utrecht through roughly 1750 – a traditionally understudied period of the eighteenth century, since the great majority of historical literature typically ends in 1720 or begins with the Seven Years' War.[5] Fundamentally, however, this book explores a moment in history; the Plague of Provence is representative of important shifts that were taking place by the eighteenth century both in approaches to the handling of disease and disasters and in the ways in which these were understood.

The First Modern Disaster

Among different types of disasters, disease epidemics hold a special status, particularly in regard to vulnerability.[6] One could argue that

---

[5] This was true in 1996 when Peter Campbell referred to the period between the Regency and 1750 as an "important but neglected period of French history," and it remains true today. Peter R. Campbell, *Power and Politics in Old Regime France, 1720–1745* (London: Routledge, 1996), 1.

[6] Here I refer to vulnerability as defined by the United Nations Office for Disaster Risk Reduction (UNDRR): "The conditions determined by physical,

they are, in some ways, the ultimate disaster. One rarely sees disease coming. Its general unpredictability and invisibility make it impossible to seek safer grounds. Once established, an epidemic can spread quickly and extensively, and can potentially strike down large portions of a population in a relatively short time. It can change an entire society's behavior, isolating individuals, separating loved ones, or even pitting family members against one another. For these reasons and more, the panic and anxiety triggered by the threat of disease is uniquely terrifying. It is a fear of the unknown induced by an invisible killer. Yet, like other disasters, infectious disease outbreaks are fundamentally environmental – from their origins to their transport to their transmission – and can be as revealing as they are destructive, "laying bare underlying power structures; the strengths or vulnerabilities of existing resources and infrastructures; and the values, prejudices, and belief systems of an affected population."[7] Consequently, this study makes the case that epidemics and pandemics *are* disasters. By examining the 1720 Plague of Provence through the lens of disaster studies, this book offers a new perspective of epidemic disease that breaks from traditional histories of medicine.[8]

---

social, economic, and environmental factors or processes which increase the susceptibility of an individual, a community, assets, or systems to the impacts of hazards." A "hazard," in turn, is "a process, phenomenon, or human activity that may cause loss of life, injury, or other health impacts, property damage, social and economic disruption, or environmental degradation." United Nations Office for Disaster Risk Reduction, www.undrr.org/terminology.

[7] Cindy Ermus, "Memory and the Representation of Public Health Crises: Remembering the Plague of Provence in the Tricentennial," *Environmental History* 26, no. 4 (October 2021): 778.

[8] Disaster may be broadly defined as "a serious disruption of the functioning of a community or a society involving widespread human, material, economic, or environmental losses and impacts, which exceeds the ability of the affected community or society to cope using its own resources" (UNDRR). However, I invite the reader to consult Andy Horowitz' incisive discussion of the term in the introduction to his book *Katrina: A History*. The section offers insight into the ways in which historians (and other scholars) of disaster think about, and struggle to define, this loaded, complex, and oft-misunderstood word. Andy Horowitz, *Katrina: A History, 1915–2015* (Cambridge, MA: Harvard University Press, 2020), 12–16. For a foundational text that has helped to shape the field of historical disaster studies over the past twenty years, see also Ted Steinberg, *Acts of God: The Unnatural History of Natural Disaster in America* (New York: Oxford University Press, 2000).

Although, as historian Cynthia Kierner has noted, historians have generally regarded the 1755 Great Lisbon Earthquake as the first modern disaster,[9] the extent, duration, and influence across time and space of the Great Plague of Provence render it more deserving of this designation. The Plague of Provence has often been seen as the closing of a chapter in Europe – the last of a long series of medieval outbreaks of bubonic plague.[10] Yet, it signified a beginning in many ways. It is true that it represents one of the final assaults of the Black Death that had been plaguing Europe since the middle of the fourteenth century – outbreaks that were traditionally perceived as horrific reminders of God's anger. By 1720, however, understandings of disaster and contagion, and ideas about how to best manage these, were very much in flux. The so-called Scientific Revolution and Enlightenment Era had ushered in new empirical and mechanistic ways of understanding disasters and the environment, slowly moving away from strictly religious or astrological explanations. Epidemics were now described not only in terms of divine vengeance or celestial movements or prodigies, but increasingly as products of commercial activity.[11] Ideas about contagion, too – about the possibility that disease resulted from contact with an infective agent (there were many hypotheses about what these agents could be) – were in development. From 1720, the Plague of Provence inspired an outpouring of literature and debates that sought to explain the nature of contagion in new, more rational ways. Not until the Great Lisbon Earthquake of 1755 did another disaster cause quite as much distress and intellectual inquiry in Europe and the Atlantic as the Plague of Provence.

The 1720 plague also marked a major shift in parts of Europe from local- or municipal-level disaster management toward "disaster centralism," a term I have coined to refer to the centralization of disaster and crisis management that developed, most notably, in the eighteenth

[9] Cynthia A. Kierner, *Inventing Disaster: The Culture of Calamity from the Jamestown Colony to the Johnstown Flood* (Chapel Hill: University of North Carolina Press, 2019), 4.

[10] There is evidence, including reports of higher death rates at some points between 1720 and 1722, that there were also cases of pneumonic, and perhaps septicemic, plague during the Plague of Provence.

[11] Daniel Gordon, "Confrontations with the Plague in Eighteenth-Century France," in *Dreadful Visitations: Confronting Natural Catastrophe in the Age of Enlightenment,* edited by Alessa Johns (New York: Routledge, 1999), 5.

century. This premise forms the central argument in this book. Prior to the Plague of Provence, crisis management took place primarily at the municipal or local level, with few, if any, expectations on the part of the people for the government in a far-flung capital to step in and offer relief. This began to change over the seventeenth century, and the Provençal plague represented the first, most prominent opportunity to advance the power of the state in the name of public health. At this time, the monarchs of Western Europe's emerging nation states – including France, Great Britain, and Spain – all ruling from a recognized capital, stepped in to manage the crisis, at once replacing the authority of local officials.

The development of disaster centralism over the past 300 years has been neither neat nor continuous. Local customs and responses, changes in administration, revolutions, and other factors have continually influenced approaches to the handling of disasters and crises. Yet the centralization of disaster management that is evident across parts of Europe during the Plague of Provence marked a significant shift that is discernible in our approach to disaster relief today. Consider, for example, centralized agencies such as the US Department of Health and Human Services or the Federal Emergency Management Agency, the UK Health Security Agency, the Public Health Agency of Canada, *Santé Publique France*, or Spain's *Ministerio de Sanidad* (which can trace its origins to the *Junta de Sanidad* created in response to the Plague of Provence in 1720). Indeed, scholars across disciplines have noted that, as historian Frank Uekötter phrased it, "When a natural disaster strikes nowadays, government aid is hailed as something akin to a birth right in Western democracies."[12] Existing literature has typically traced the origins of this centralized disaster management to the development of modern welfare states in the nineteenth to twentieth centuries,[13] yet, as this book demonstrates, this history – the history of disaster centralism – began much earlier. In the eighteenth century as today, disasters served as tools of statecraft, and proved useful to the centralizing state. In 1720, it was the Crown – in Paris,

---

[12] Frank Uekötter, "It's the Entanglements, Stupid," *Journal for the History of Environment and Society* 5, Special issue on "COVID-19 and Environmental History" (2020): 106.

[13] For example, "[S]ince the late nineteenth century, it was the nation-state that galvanised everyone's attention in the wake of a disaster, more precisely the

Madrid, London, and beyond – that called for measures to prevent the spread of the Provençal plague into their own regions. Some of the measures enacted at this time from the capitals of these kingdoms included (but were not limited to): amplified surveillance and police presence in ports and along borders; the enactment of controversial vessel searches and quarantines, and directions for carrying them out; the restriction or prohibition of movement across borders or in areas suspected of infection and the use of health certificates; the establishment of military cordons; the deployment to the provinces of royal representatives charged with reporting back to the Crown; and, notably, the founding of centralized public health agencies that remain to this day (albeit under new structures and with new names).

Public health and disaster management were essential to the centralizing state of the eighteenth century. Throughout the Plague of Provence, monarchs across Europe employed plague-time measures to achieve various political and commercial objectives. Among these, the threat of plague served as a pretext to clamp down on smuggling (as we see in Chapters 3 and 5); to deliberately consolidate monarchical power and reign in defiant portions of the population (as we see in Chapters 4 and 5); to outmaneuver, or improve one's place among, commercial competitors (as seen throughout this book); or merely in retaliation for perceived transgressions, such as the imposition of quarantines, embargoes, and/or vessel searches (as evident in Chapters 2 through 4). Commercial interests and diplomatic relationships drove responses to the plague no less than did concerns over public health.

Focusing on this one major crisis, then, has allowed me to explore these dynamics and developments, and to identify the numerous ways in which a disaster in one place has the potential to influence ideas, power structures, trade, diplomacy, public health policy, and local practices in different parts of the globe. By decentering the site of disaster, I demonstrate that catastrophes are not merely localized events. History is rarely monolithic or confined – the influence of an

---

resourceful, interventionist nation-states that Charles Maier has described as Leviathan 2.0 (Maier, 2012). Disaster relief has been a test for national governments ever since, and they are widely expected to be caring and generous. Few things are more corrosive to the legitimacy of political power than a botched response to a disaster, and ambitious politicians saw an opportunity." Uekötter, "It's the Entanglements," 106.

event in one place can spread like seismic waves. The goal here has been to follow those waves across national boundaries to explore how they manifested themselves abroad, and how local historical contexts in turn informed how the threat of plague was experienced far beyond ground zero. In the end, the 1720 Plague of Provence emerges as a complex, influential event with ramifications that extended well beyond France and well beyond 1722, despite the disease never crossing Gallic borders. As historians Lynn Hunt and Jack Censer have observed, "French events were not just French."[14]

The Chapters

In this book, I explore how the Plague of Provence was experienced not only in France but in regions far from where the epidemic unfolded. The chapters therefore proceed geographically in order of distance from Provence, as they trace the outbreak's ramifications to some of the most active port cities of the eighteenth-century Atlantic world. Chapter 1 lays the groundwork for the rest of the book by addressing the emergence of plague in the port city of Marseille and its spread into southeastern France. It tells the story of the *Grand Saint-Antoine*, the infamous vessel that allegedly transported the plague to France from the Levant in 1720. It then situates this traditional narrative within the context of recent genetic studies that call its accuracy into question. Although the science has not yet been able to disprove the accepted *historical* explanation for the outbreak – which is to say that the pathogen arrived on the ill-fated vessel – it has offered a valuable opportunity to revisit traditional understandings of disease as a product of the "orient," and to examine and appreciate the influence of new technologies – in this case, genomic DNA analysis – on historical research and our interpretations of archival documents. The chapter

---

[14] Although the authors were writing about the French Revolution and Napoleon, the statement applies just as well to the earlier eighteenth century. The longer quote is as follows: "Scholars are now showing that revolutionary ideas circulated globally before 1789 and that events in the Atlantic world, in particular, reverberated across many different borders ... French events were not just French." Lynn Hunt and Jack R. Censer, "Think Globally, Act Historically: Teaching the French Revolution and Napoleon," *Age of Revolutions* (December 11, 2017), https://ageofrevolutions.com/2017/12/11/think-globally-act-historically-teaching-the-french-revolution-and-napoleon.

moves on to discuss civil and religious responses to the epidemic and what I argue was the implementation of disaster centralism in France, as authorities in Paris stepped in to mitigate the threat of infection from Provence before it spread any further.

Chapter 2 travels from the coasts of Provence to the Italian peninsula with a focus on the port city of Genoa, considered by some to be *l'état le plus exposé*, or "the most exposed" to the threat of plague by its proximity to Marseille. The Genoese port stands out as among the most frequently mentioned in contemporary plague-related documents across Europe as region after region mobilized against the threat of infection from France. The chapter begins with a brief introduction to Genoa's place as a maritime capital and port of entry for contagion. It discusses the city's rich history of quarantine and public health and examines the arrival of news that plague was in France. Here, I ask why it took roughly two months for the rest of Europe to begin learning about the outbreak. The fact that the number of plague cases began to rise more rapidly in the month of July forms only part of the answer. More significantly, from the earliest documented deaths in May through the end of the epidemic, Marseillais officials, merchants, and others (initially including public health officers) perpetuated a campaign of misinformation meant to protect the livelihood of this wealthy and bustling ancient port city. Claims that the disease was merely a malignant fever, or that the outbreak had ended or was under control (when, in fact, it had not and was not), caused confusion in the first months of the outbreak. Nevertheless, the inevitable truth that plague was in France began to arrive in cities across Europe via envoys, ambassadors, and especially via consuls who reported back to their respective states from Marseille, Aix, Toulon, and other areas. From there, word traveled rapidly as these accounts were copied or repeated in letters and printed in newspapers across Europe and the colonies, creating an invisible commonwealth based in contemporary communication networks. The chapter then examines responses to the Plague of Provence in Genoa and Italy and how they influenced, and were influenced by, Italian trade and diplomacy. Here, and throughout the rest of the book, it becomes clear that reactions to the plague in France cannot be looked at in isolation. Officials across Europe looked to other states as they contemplated how to handle the threat of plague from France. In some cases, more rigorous public health measures were implemented to protect commercial relationships by adhering to certain standards and/or by helping a port city to appear both safe and competent. In others, measures against another region were imposed in kind as retaliation, resulting in instances of what we may refer to as tit-for-tat public health diplomacy. In disease and disaster management, then, public safety is seldom the only, or even primary, consideration.

Chapter 3 moves north from Genoa to the port city of London, where the Plague of Provence caused waves of fear, opposition, and intellectual inquiry. Taking place against the backdrop of the recent South Sea Bubble, the epidemic in France became a major topic of discussion among politicians, journalists, scholars, physicians, grocers, merchants, and others as they protested perceived infringements on their civil liberties and freedoms or debated the nature of contagion and the usefulness of quarantine. When London received word of the outbreak in Marseille, the city experienced a series of protests against a possible embargo with "despotic France" and a toughening of quarantine regulations under the Quarantine Act of 1721. Merchants, grocers, and other groups in the city were especially resistant to measures that would in any way impede their industry. In 1720, just as plague cases emerged in the south of France, the bursting of the South Sea Bubble unleashed waves of anxiety and suspicion. Passionate attacks against the perceived injustices of the Crown as it attempted to enact quarantines and impede illicit commerce were filled with accusations that government authorities and "South Sea scheme men" meant to take away the inviolable rights of the people under the pretext of a foreign plague. Meanwhile, debates between contagionists and anti-contagionists about the transmission, or lack thereof, of infectious disease also erupted with special force in the wake of the 1720 plague in Provence. This chapter explores these reactions, placing them in the larger historical context of early-eighteenth-century politics and diplomacy and considers the various factors that came into play as England designed its new emergency public health policy.

From London, we travel south to the ancient port city of Cádiz, the Gateway to the Indies after it replaced Seville as the point of departure for the Americas in 1717.[15] Chapter 4 explores reactions to the threat, and the centralization of disaster management, during the reign of Spain's first Bourbon monarch, Philip V. It also examines the 1720

---

[15] This occurred with the formal move of the *Casa de la Contratación de las Indias* from the inland river port of Seville to the Atlantic port of Cádiz.

plague's long-term influence on Spain's public health policy. What emerges in this chapter is an understanding of how Spanish authorities exploited the epidemic by ignoring the terms of treaties and tightening control over Spain's borders, people, and commercial activities. Ultimately, they hoped to reap the advantages of excluding their primary competitors – France and Great Britain – from the hypercompetitive arena of Atlantic commerce. When official news of the plague in Marseille reached Madrid, the Spanish Crown introduced regulations and supervisory committees that sought to extend the state's control over commercial activities, both domestic and international, and that meant to exclude its greatest competitors from its commercial market. Trading restrictions were implemented against Great Britain, for example, which had refused to return the recently acquired territory of Gibraltar to Spain. Britain, in turn, responded by issuing similar restrictions against Spain – and Portugal was drawn into the dispute, used as a Spanish pawn to further hurt English interests in the Iberian Atlantic and Mediterranean. Strict new regulations also included, among others, the issuing of health permits for vessels (*patentes sanitarias de barcos*), new guidelines for navigation and fishing, the construction of new *lazarets* or *lazarettos* (maritime quarantine stations), and the creation of a new police force for customs (*Policía Sanitaria en Aduanas*). Notably, news of the outbreak in France also spurred the creation of Spain's first Supreme Committee of Health (*Junta Suprema de Sanidad*) in 1720 – the Crown's first administrative body dedicated solely to the management and protection of public health for the entire kingdom. Even after Spanish ports finally reopened to all French merchants in 1724, certain controls remained, including the Spanish right of *fondeo* searches – a significant and persistent point of contention for foreign merchants dealing with Spain. Much of the new centralized system for disease prevention in Spain followed from reactions to the plague in Provence and remained into the following century, resulting in major changes in the management of both public health and customs inspections.

The final chapter transports the reader across the Atlantic Basin to explore how the Great Plague Scare unfolded in the entangled colonial empires of France and Spain. Despite their intwined histories in the early-eighteenth-century Atlantic, few works in the English language have focused on Franco-Spanish colonial relations. Chapter 5 describes the orders coming from the metropoles for dealing with the threat of plague and analyzes how those on the ground – the people, as well as colonial authorities – ultimately responded. In the end, it answers the question, what was different in the colonies? The chapter opens in Fort Royal, Martinique, at the time a wealthy French possession and a major administrative center for the French Antilles. Here, a great scandal unfolded when a French vessel arrived from the Languedocien port of Sète. What I call the Sète affair offers the opportunity to examine, in the words of one contemporary, the "esprit de sédition" (or "spirit of sedition") that endured in the French Antilles throughout the eighteenth century, well before the Age of Revolutions.[16] The chapter then transitions to plague-time violence and Franco-Spanish relations in the Caribbean, including anti-French and anti-foreign reactions to the Great Plague Scare in the Spanish colonies. As we will see, the demands of the metropole were not always in line with the needs or wants of the people in the overseas colonies. On the surface, disaster centralism during the Plague of Provence seemed to extend from Europe to the colonies, as officials in the metropole dispatched directives against the spread of plague and tried to monitor activities abroad, but on the ground, local needs and economic concerns often outweighed the demands of a far-flung ruler.

The book concludes with an epilogue that briefly summarizes some of the study's central findings and offers a few words on their significance in the present day. Each chapter in this book may be read individually, but when read together they reveal the global scope and influence of the disaster in France, and the numerous factors that come into play in the management of disasters and crises. A study like this, which seeks to elucidate how disasters were managed and understood in the eighteenth century – when society was undergoing such dramatic social, political, and intellectual transformations – can be instructive for us today as we grapple with the challenges of climate change and increasingly frequent disasters, including global pandemics, in similarly transformative times.

---

[16] François de Pas de Mazencourt, marquis de Feuquières, *gouverneur general* of Martinique to Louis-Alexandre de Bourbon, head of the Marine Council, Fort Royal, May 9, 1721, Col. F3 26, f. 472 & 472v, Archives nationales d'outre-mer (henceforward ANOM).

1 | *Plague in Provence*

Oh, Marseille, what hand has robbed you of your beauty? Where is the rival of Carthage? The sister of Athens? The shouts of joy of your pompous celebrations are replaced by grumbles of a pain that appears eternal. The foreigner, once drawn to your city walls, your beautiful skies, and the kindness of your denizens, now flees an all-consuming earth. The ships that once carried into your sumptuous markets the treasures of all the nations have abandoned your shores from which now arise only the sounds of suffering. Death is found in every row, corpses litter the streets. One only encounters men who carry in their bosom the very poison that consumes them. Their pale eyes, withered cheeks, discolored countenances, infected breath, the pain and bewilderment betrayed by their stares—all of this renders them objects of eternal pity. The husband marries his last breath with that of his dying wife. The grandfather expires surrounded by the cold bodies of his many children. Thus, lightning strikes this ancient oak, and its youths are cast away.[1]

This city seems like a desart: We see nothing in the Streets but dead and dying Persons: Ten Tumbrels will not suffice to carry them away: All

---

[1] "O! Marseille, quelle main t'a ravi ta beauté? Où est l'émule de Carthage, la soeur d'Athènes, aux cris de joie de tes fêtes pompeuses, ont succédé les plaintes d'une douleur qui semble éternelle, l'étranger qu'attiraient dans tes murs, ton beau ciel, l'aménité de tes habitans, fuit une terre dévorante, les vaisseaux qui portaient dans tes sompteux marchés les trésors des nations abbandonnent un rivage d'où s'élève une voix lamentable. La mort parcourt tous les rangs, les cadavres jonchent les rues, on ne rencontre plus que des hommes qui portent dans leur sein le poison qui les consume, leurs yeux livides, leurs joues flétries, leurs visages-décolorés, une haleine infecte, l'égarement de la douleur qu'expriment leurs regards, tout les rend les objets d'une éternelle pitié. L'époux mêle son dernier soupir au dernier de son épouse, l'ayeul expire entouré des corps glacés de ses nombreux enfans, ainsi la foudre frappe le chêne antique et ses jeunes rejettons." Anonymous, *La Fête séculaire de la peste de 1720, ou Éloge de Belsunce*, Delta 2450, 9, Archives départementales des Bouches-du-Rhône, Marseille (henceforward ADBRM). All translations throughout this book are mine unless otherwise noted.

the Burying Places of the Churches were full 15 Days ago; and several Church-yards have been made without the City, which have been likewise fill'd in two or three Days: We cannot exactly tell the Number of those who have dy'd within the Month or six Weeks; but we cannot be said to stretch beyond the Truth, if we affirm it amounts to above 40,000 ... They are now burning Clothes and Bedding, and cleansing the Streets, which 'tis hoped will render the Air less unhealthful.[2]

On May 12, 1720, the *intendants de la santé* (health officials) in Marseille wrote to the *maréchal*, Duc de Villars, at the time *gouverneur* of the region of Provence in Paris, requesting to expedite the construction of a new building for the local *Bureau de la santé* or Health Board. The structure that had stood there since 1660 was a *bureau flotant* – literally a floating office – that stood on the water near fort Saint-Jean, at the entryway to the port of Marseille. They explained that the building was "entierement pourry," entirely rotten, and that they were sometimes forced to postpone their assemblies lest they run the risk of being completely submerged. For this reason, the *intendants* wished to work with the certainty that the completion of their new bureau was underway, for there was word that plague was raging in Palestine and Syria.[3] Given their perceived urgency of the situation in the Levant, they explained that their meetings would need to occur more frequently, so they could more effectively prevent the disorders that could ensue upon an outbreak of contagion.[4] Less than two weeks later, plague appeared in the port of Marseille, reportedly arriving aboard a vessel named the *Grand Saint-Antoine*. It was to rage for two and a half years and take over 100,000 lives in the region of Provence and parts of Languedoc.

---

[2] "Marseilles, Sept. 20," *Daily Post* (London), October 13, 1720, issue 323. Almost one month later, an account printed in a London newspaper changed the number of tumbrels: "27 tumbrels are not sufficient to carry off the dead." "Paris October 26: Extract of a Letter of the 12th Instant from Martigues a Small City Situated Between Avignon, Aix and Marseilles," *Evening Post* (London), October 18–20, 1720, issue 1751. All spellings in passages that I have not translated are as they appear in the original.

[3] "Car nous aprenons, Mgr., que la peste fait des grands ravages dans la Palestine, et la Sirie, le dangér destre submergés dans le Bureau flotant qui est entierement pourry, nous force quelque fois de différer nos assemblees." "Livres des copies des lettres éscrittes par messieurs les intendants de la santé de Marseille," May 12, 1720, 200 E 166, ADBRM.

[4] Ibid.

This chapter tells the story of the Plague of Provence as it unfolded in southeastern France. It begins with a detailed narrative of the appearance of plague as described in archival documents from across the Atlantic world. Rather than rely on the now classic secondary sources on the topic, namely those of Charles Carrière and colleagues, Jean-Noël Biraben, Daniel Panzac, Françoise Hildesheimer, and others, or on printed primary sources written decades after the epidemic, this chapter describes the appearance of plague in the port of Marseille as the people on the ground portrayed it in their personal correspondence, official documents and reports, and eyewitness diaries and memoirs.[5] I then complicate these traditional narratives by introducing recent, and ongoing, genetic evidence that may tell a very different story. This ongoing research challenges the persistent narrative of the *Grand Saint-Antoine* – long unquestioned and oft repeated in historical documents across the globe – and makes it seem more like what I refer to as "epidemiological scapegoating" than an accurate description of events. Using contemporary eyewitness accounts and government records detailing the official response to the outbreak, the chapter then moves on to describe the events that unfolded after the appearance of plague in May 1720, again giving voice to the officials who managed the disaster, whether from Paris or within Provence, as well as those at ground zero – victims, physicians, priests, and others – who experienced, and in many cases lived through, the disaster.

This retelling of the Great Plague of Marseille chronicles the chaos and destruction that ensued almost immediately upon the anchoring of the *Grand Saint-Antoine* (whether or not the bacteria actually arrived on the ship), and the comprehensive system of plague management enacted in its wake. Government responses to the epidemic of 1720 were completely in line with the French Crown's centralizing objectives. As this chapter will argue, the rise of the French state over the

---

[5] For example: Charles Carrière, Marcel Courdurié, and Ferréol Rebuffat, *Marseille ville morte: la peste de 1720* (Marseille: M. Garçon, 1968); Jean-Noël Biraben, *Les hommes et la peste en France et dans les pays européens et méditerranéens*, vols 1 & 2 (Paris: Mouton & Co., 1975); Françoise Hildesheimer, *La terreur et la pitié: L'Ancien Régime à l'épreuve de la peste* (Paris: Éditions Publisud, 1990); Françoise Hildesheimer, *Le Bureau de la santé de Marseille sous l'ancien régime* (Marseille: Fédération historique de Provence, 1980); Daniel Panzac, *Quarantaines et lazarets: l'Europe et la peste d'Orient, XVIIᵉ–XXᵉ siècles* (Aix-en-Provence: Édisud, 1986).

seventeenth century, combined with the aggressive centralizing initiatives of Louis XIV that transformed France into a "mature monarchical state,"[6] allowed for an explicitly involved administration to express
its authority and control during the emergency in Provence – a case
of what I term "disaster centralism" in the eighteenth century. Later
chapters will demonstrate that responses to the Provençal plague came
from the capitals of emerging nation states all over Europe, despite
the fact that the infection never spread beyond southeastern France.
Each responded with extraordinary force to the French outbreak as a
means to not only fend off the infection, but also to impose a variety
of measures that would *advance* the very processes of administrative
centralization and control that were already underway.

Disaster centralism, or the centralization of disaster management,
was a major part of state formation, and the Plague of Provence
represents one of the earliest, most pronounced instances of such a
rigorous, large-scale, transnational, centralized response to disaster.
In France, this happened at a time during which the people looked
increasingly to the central government to assist in various aspects of
their everyday lives, including criminal justice, infrastructure, and
social welfare, which for centuries had rested in the hands of local,
often ecclesiastical, authorities. In many ways, then, the management
of the Provençal plague symbolized a break from the past, marked in
part by augmented communication between the Crown and provincial
officials that represents an early example of the more comprehensive
state-centralized responses to disasters that we see all over the globe
today.

A Port of Entry for Contagion?: Plague Appears in Southern France

The *Grand Saint-Antoine*, a large vessel constructed in Holland,
departed from Marseille for Syria on July 22, 1719. For nearly a year,
it journeyed in the Levant amassing cargoes of rich fabrics and other
valuable goods.[7] Among these were silks and bales of cotton – about
100,000 *écus* worth of merchandise (or between 300,000 and 600,000

---

[6] James B. Collins, *The State in Early Modern France* (New York: Cambridge
University Press, 2009), xiii.
[7] Biraben, *Les hommes* ... vol. 1, 231.

livres tournois in 1720) – most of which belonged to Jean-Baptiste Estelle, *premier échevin* of Marseille (premier municipal magistrate) and part owner of the *Grand Saint-Antoine*.[8] The merchandise was bound for sale at the popular *foire de Beaucaire* scheduled to open on July 22, 1720.[9] This tax-free trade fair was held annually from the thirteenth to the nineteenth century in the Languedocien town of the same name, situated on the Rhône River directly across from Tarascon. It began each year on the feast day of Saint Mary Magdalene and lasted for at least three days thereafter.[10] By the seventeenth century, it had become one of the most important trade fairs of the Mediterranean.[11] Traders and businessmen from Europe, Africa, and Asia sought to participate in the event, not least of whom were those of Marseille.[12] The *foire de Beaucaire* would therefore feature prominently in the story of the Provençal plague's origins.

The ship arrived back in Marseille on May 25, 1720, but not before making some fateful stops along the way. Beginning with the death on April 5 of a Turkish passenger who had boarded at Tripoli two days earlier, seven to eight men, including the ship's surgeon, are said to have died with buboes aboard the vessel on its route from Tripoli to Livorno, where the captain, Jean-Baptiste Chataud, made an emergency stop before heading back to Marseille.[13] Despite the deaths on board, doctors in Livorno (who allegedly may not have inspected the bodies

---

[8] Biraben, *Les hommes ...* vol. 1, 231. Monique Lucenet, *Les grandes pestes en France* (Paris: Aubier, 1985), 219.

[9] "Copie d'une lettre écrite par Mr. Reymond, médecin de Marseille, le 21 août 1720, touchant l'origine, les progrès, et l'état du mal contagieux qu'il y'a a Marseille," 1F 80/37, ADBRM. Panzac, *Quarantaines et lazarets*, 81.

[10] Hector Rivoire, "Notice sur la Foire de Beaucaire," *Mémoires de l'Académie Royale du Gard* (Nimes: C. Durand-Belle, 1844), 158.

[11] Brian Fitzpatrick, *Catholic Royalism in the Department of the Gard, 1814–1852* (Cambridge: Cambridge University Press, 1983), 6.

[12] "There is in France no commercial affair more useful or more enjoyable than that of the annual fair at Beaucaire on the feast day of St. Mary Magdalene ... During the fair, an infinite abundance of fine merchandise arrives via the convenience of the Rhone. Not only do the French arrive here from the most remote parts of the kingdom, but also the Africans, Greeks, and peoples of Asia. Nothing is more beautiful than the diversity of foreigners, and as peace fosters trade, it can be said that Beaucaire is extremely prosperous." Anonymous, *La Foire de Beaucaire: Nouvelle Historique et Galante* (Amsterdam: Paul Marret, 1708), 9–10.

[13] "Copie d'une lettre écrite par Mr. Reymond ...," 1F 80/37, ADBRM. Biraben, *Les hommes ...* vol. 1, 233.

themselves) declared the illness a case of pestilential fever rather than plague.[14] As a result, health authorities in the port city allowed the ship to depart for Marseille with a *patente nette*, or certificate of health, that declared it free from infection.[15] Meanwhile, the ship's captain, reportedly in a hurry to transport the valuable cargo to Provence in time for the trade fair, was happy to depart.[16] Yet on the journey from Livorno to Marseille, three more are said to have perished in the same manner.[17]

---

[14] "Relation de ce qui s'est passé à Marseille pendant la peste de 1720 de son principe, des effets qu'elle à produit, de ses suites et se sa fin," *Relation de la peste arrivée à Marseille l'an 1720 écrite le 20 octobre 1754, copiée sur un manuscrit de [?] Mr. Pierre Honoré Roux, mon pere ancien, 1er échevin de Marseille qui fus témoin oculaire de la peste*, 1, 1F 80/39, ADBRM. Lucenet, *Les grandes pestes*, 220.

Here is a letter written from one of the doctors in Livorno to the governor of the city, as transcribed in Jean-Pierre Filippini, *Il Porto di Livorno e la Toscana, 1676–1814*, vol. 2 (Naples: Edizioni Scientifiche Italiane, 1998), 198:

Al signor Governatore di Livorno. (ASL, Sanità, 78, c. 234). Livorno adì 17 maggio 1720

Io infrascritto medico della Sanità ho visitato al moletto nø tre cadaveri di tre persone della nave Il Grand S. Antonio, capitano Giovan Battista Chataud di Marsilia venuta di Seida etc.

Una delle quali persone riferisce il detto capitano esser morta doppo quattordici giorni di male e le due altre doppo cinque giorni onde dai sintomi che ho potuto ricavare dal detto capitano, che erano congiunti con detto male e dalla recognizione che ho fatta di detti cadaveri, quali ho trovati tutti ricoperti di macchie livide, giudico esser morte tutte le dette tre persone di febbre maligna pestilenziale. E in fede

C. Marcellino Ittieri medico della Sanità.

Pestilential fever was considered different from the plague in certain particulars. The fever, for example, was generally less violent. See seventeenth-century physician, Thomas Sydenham's relevant discussion in: Thomas Sydenham, *The Works of Thomas Sydenham, M.D., on Acute and Chronic Diseases: With Their Histories and Modes of Cure* (Philadelphia: Benjamin & Thomas Kite, 1809), 52–7. In eighteenth-century discussions on the subject of pestilential and malignant fevers and plague, he was considered an important source and often referenced.

[15] As mentioned in Chapter 2, the decision to let the ship depart for Marseille later hurt the credibility of Tuscan and Livornese officials, whom some blamed for the epidemic for their failure to immediately isolate the vessel. Captain Chataud, meanwhile, was later imprisoned at the Château d'If (later made famous by Alexandre Dumas in his novel *The Count of Monte Cristo*).

[16] Letter from the *intendants de la santé* in Marseille to the Duc d'Orléans in Paris, July 9, 1720, "Livre des copies des léttres Escrittes par messieurs les Intendants de la santé de Marseille commencé le 4 May 1713," 200 E 166, f. 67, ADBRM.

[17] "Copie d'une lettre écrite par Mr. Reymond ...," 1F 80/37, ADBRM.

Upon arrival at the port, the ship nevertheless endured an unusual, and unusually short, quarantine considering the deaths that had taken place on board. For one, as a result of its health inspection certificate, local authorities decided to have the ship undergo its quarantine at the usual island of Pomègues, in the Frioul archipelago just off the coast of Marseille, rather than at the island of Jarre, further away in the Riou archipelago, where it would have immediately been sent if it had been deemed a danger to public health (and where the doomed vessel was later burned and sunken on September 26, 1720). Moreover, on June 3, after only a few days in quarantine, the ship was authorized to unload part of its cargo and drop off its remaining passengers at the lazaret. As the story goes, Estelle, Marseille's *premier échevin* had used his influence to arrange for the premature unloading of his cargo of imported silks and bales of cotton into the city's warehouses – later reported to be infected with the plague – so that they could be sold soon thereafter at the *foirede Beaucaire*.[18] By June 14, only twenty days after the arrival of the *Grand Saint-Antoine* at port, passengers were authorized to depart the lazaret.[19] Meanwhile, more were falling victim to the illness. Several porters who had reportedly handled the ship's merchandise became ill, developing buboes in the groin and perishing within two to three days.[20] At this time, a local surgeon was called on board to inspect the bodies and determine the cause of death. Only then was the ship redirected to the island of Jarre.[21] But it was too late – plague had arrived in Marseille.

...

This is the story that has been repeated in accounts across the globe since the earliest days of the outbreak. There is, in fact, a remarkable amount of consistency among archival sources, which agree that the plague arrived on the ill-fated *Grand Saint-Antoine*. Contemporary

---

[18] Panzac, *Quarantaines et lazarets*, 81. Danièle Larcena et al., *La Muraille de la peste* (Vaucluse: Les Alpes de Lumière, 1993), 21.

[19] Biraben, *Les hommes ...* vol. 1, 232.

[20] "Relation de ce qui s'est passé à Marseille pendant la peste de 1720 de son principe ...," I, 1F 80/39, ADBRM.

[21] It was not until around July 15 that the order to remove the ship to Jarre was executed. See: "Relation de ce qui s'est passé à Marseille pendant la peste de 1720 de son principe ...," I, 1F 80/39, ADBRM. Lucenet, *Les grandes pestes,* 220.

testimonies from both Livorno and Marseille also support claims that there had indeed been deaths on board the vessel during its journey, and that porters fell ill and died quickly soon after the ship arrived in Marseille. The health *intendants* at the opening of this chapter also alluded to reports of plague in Palestine and Syria only days prior to the arrival of the ship in the city. All of this seems to support traditional explanations for the emergence of plague in Provence.

But what if the plague did not actually arrive on the notorious vessel? What if this outbreak came not from far-flung lands in the Levant but from within Europe itself? This is the question that both geneticists and historians of plague have been tackling in recent years. To be clear, there is no doubt that the ship existed, that it traveled where it was documented to have traveled, or that it docked at port in Marseille despite having carried persons infected with a deadly illness, as countless contemporary sources acknowledge; but recent genetic studies have brought the question of this epidemic's origins to the fore, potentially challenging the traditionally accepted, heretofore unquestioned story of the *Grand Saint-Antoine*, and raising important new questions about the influence of modern science and technology on the practice of history and vice versa.

Plague is caused by the bacillus *Yersinia pestis*, a bacterium discovered independently but almost simultaneously by Alexandre Yersin and Kitasato Shibasaburō in 1894 during the third plague pandemic. The bubonic form is communicated from rodents to humans through the bites of infected fleas.[22] The plague survived in the medieval to early modern periods in Europe much as it does today, namely, through flea-borne transmissions among populations of rodent species,[23] which can include not only the notorious

---

[22] Recent scientific research has introduced the possibility that human ectoparasites (including body lice and human fleas) had a role to play in transmission of the disease, as well. See: Katharine R. Dean et al., "Human Ectoparasites and the Spread of Plague in Europe during the Second Pandemic," *Proceedings of the National Academy of Sciences* (henceforward *PNAS*) 115, no. 6 (2018): 1304–9. However, the reader should be aware of the study's limitations. See: Sang Woo Park et al., "Human Ectoparasite Transmission of the Plague During the Second Pandemic Is Only Weakly Supported by Proposed Mathematical Models," *PNAS* 115, no. 34 (2018): E7892–3; Katharine R. Dean et al., "Reply to Park et al.: Human Ectoparasite Transmission of Plague During the Second Pandemic Is Still Plausible," *PNAS* 115, no. 34 (2018): E7894–5.

[23] Ann G. Carmichael, "Plague Persistence in Western Europe: A Hypothesis," *The Medieval Globe* 1, no. 1 (2014): 157.

domestic black rat (*Rattus rattus*) – long believed to have served as the primary reservoir host for plague – but also gerbils, marmots, ground squirrels, wood rats, chipmunks, deer mice, voles, prairie dogs (in North America), and other animals such as rabbits and cats.[24] It is therefore not too difficult to imagine that any time plague has entered Europe – whether during the first or second plague pandemics (and genetic studies have looked at DNA samples from both),[25] or during other, smaller introductions of plague – it could have survived in remote populations of animals like these for years after an outbreak subsided within the human population. In 2016, for example, historian Ann Carmichael looked at primarily sixteenth-century documentary sources to suggest that plague could have persisted in the southern Alpine region of Europe, perhaps among populations of the Alpine marmot (*Marmota marmota*).[26] Others, meanwhile, have suggested that it could have resided in rodent populations in England and the Low Countries.[27] Paleogenetic studies have yet to pinpoint these,

---

[24] Which is to say, a wildlife (rather than an urban) reservoir. A "reservoir" in this context may be defined as "one or more epidemiologically connected populations or environments in which the pathogen can be permanently maintained and from which infection is transmitted to the defined target population." Daniel T. Haydon, S. Cleaveland, L. H. Taylor, and M. K. Laurenson, "Identifying Reservoirs of Infection: A Conceptual and Practical Challenge," *Emerging Infectious Diseases* 8, no. 12 (December 2002): 1468.
   The word "permanently" in this definition is relative, as in some instances it can mean a few years, while in others a few decades or centuries. Boris V. Schmid, "Re: On 1720 Plague," personal email communication, July 29, 2021. Cited with permission from the author.

[25] The first plague pandemic, also known as the Plague of Justinian, lasted from the sixth to eighth century CE, while the second pandemic began with the Black Death of the fourteenth century and lasted through the early nineteenth century. The third plague pandemic began in mid-nineteenth-century China and lasted through the early to mid-twentieth century. For possible thirteenth-century epidemiological origins of the Black Death, see: Monica Green, "The Four Black Deaths," *American Historical Review* 125, no. 5 (December 2020): 1601–31. For more on the three pandemics, see chapter 3 in Frank M. Snowden, *Epidemics and Society: From the Black Death to the Present* (New Haven: Yale University Press, 2019).

[26] Carmichael, "Plague Persistence," 162.

[27] Bas den Hond, "Plague Bug May Have Lurked in Medieval England Between Outbreaks," *Earth & Space Science News* 98 (May 8, 2017), https://doi.org/10.1029/2017EO073063. Another study recently argued for central Germany. Philip Slavin, "Out of the West: Formation of a Permanent Plague Reservoir in South-Central Germany (1349–1356) and Its Implications," *Past & Present* 252, no. 1 (August 2021): 3–51.

or any other plague foci, or reservoirs, in Europe with any certainty, but they, too, have begun to cast doubt on the idea – widespread in Europe by the eighteenth century – that plague was strictly an eastern import, which calls the story of the Provençal plague's *Grand Saint-Antoine* origins into question.

Advances in DNA sequencing technologies have allowed for the genomic recovery of pathogens found in human skeletons. By successfully sequencing plague DNA from bones or teeth found in plague pits across Eurasia, scientists have been able to learn a great deal about the pathogen, including what other strains it most resembles, and thus where it might have come from. In recent years, this has led to a surge of research on, and debates about, the spread of plague in Europe during both the "first plague pandemic" of the sixth to eighth centuries and the "second pandemic" of the fourteenth through early nineteenth centuries. Since the studies are very much ongoing, however, there remains little consensus on some major questions. Most notably, for our purposes, several concurrent studies have arrived at different conclusions about the source of plague in Europe after the introductions of the mid-fourteenth century (the Black Death). In 2015, the findings of Boris Schmid and colleagues "strongly suggest[ed] that the bacterium was continuously reimported into Europe [from possible rodent reservoirs in Asia] during the second plague pandemic," which is to say, from the Black Death until the early nineteenth century, while a study by Kirsten Bos and colleagues months later suggested that an unidentified, now-extinct plague reservoir established during the Black Death in Europe may have been responsible for the resurgences of plague throughout the second pandemic, including that of Provence.[28]

While disagreements remain about whether or not the 1720 plague was imported into France from the Levant, there is a growing consensus among these genetic studies that plague reservoirs may indeed have been established in parts of Europe and/or western Asia after the initial arrival of plague that caused the fourteenth-century Black Death, and

---

[28] Boris V. Schmid et al., "Climate-Driven Introduction of the Black Death and Successive Plague Reintroductions into Europe," *PNAS* 112, no. 10 (March 2015): 3020–5. Kirsten I. Bos et al., "Eighteenth-Century *Yersinia pestis* Genomes Reveal the Long-Term Persistence of an Historical Plague Focus," *eLife* (2016), doi: 10.7554/eLife.12994.

that at least some subsequent outbreaks of the second pandemic came from these reservoirs. For example, a study by Maria Spyrou, Marcel Keller, and colleagues, first published in November 2018, analyzed the genomes of post-Black Death outbreaks from Central and Western Europe and found evidence for "the local diversification of an extinct *Y. pestis* lineage between the late-14th and 18th centuries that may have resided in more than one disease reservoir." The researchers suggested that at least some post-Black Death outbreaks may have emerged from one of these disease foci, but they stopped short of asserting definitively that the outbreaks of 1665 London or 1720 Marseille were among these: "given that both Marseille and London were among the main maritime trade centres in Europe during that time, it [remains] plausible that introduction of the disease in these areas occurred via ships."[29] In December of 2018, the evidence from a different study by Namouchi et al. again pointed to repeated introductions of plague in European ports throughout the Middle Ages "by means of fur trade routes, as well as the recirculation of plague within the human population via trade routes and human movement," and supported the idea that the 1720 plague in Provence had "an extra-Western European source."[30] In agreement with other studies, including that of Spyrou, findings by Karen Giffin and colleagues indicate a shared ancestry between reconstructed plague genomes from *l'Observance* plague pit in Marseille (dated 1722) and those of the New Churchyard (or Bedlam) burial ground in London (in use from the sixteenth to eighteenth century), among others; but they, too, suggested that, "As both London and Marseille were connected to a vast system of trade networks in the Mediterranean and beyond, many candidate plague source locations exist in areas underexplored from the vantage point of ancient DNA."[31] As of yet, in other words, no

---

[29] Maria A. Spyrou and Marcel Keller et al., "A Phylogeography of the Second Plague Pandemic Revealed Through the Analysis of Historical *Y. pestis* Genomes," *Nature Communications* 10, no. 4470 (2019), doi: 10.1038/s41467-019-12154-0.

[30] Amine Namouchi et al., "Integrative Approach Using *Yersinia pestis* Genomes to Revisit the Historical Landscape of Plague during the Medieval Period," *Proceedings of the National Academy of Sciences* 115, no. 50 (December 2018): 11790 & 11794.

[31] Karen Giffin et al., "A Treponemal Genome from an Historic Plague Victim Supports a Recent Emergence of Yaws and Its Presence in 15th-Century Europe," *Scientific Reports* 10, no. 9499 (2020): 6.

aDNA (ancient DNA) sequences exist for plague victims in the Levant or North Africa where reports of plague were frequent throughout the early modern period and into the nineteenth century. For our purposes, this is significant, because as long as we have no aDNA samples from the eastern Mediterranean, the importation of plague from this region in 1720 cannot be ruled out.

Meanwhile, a different study by Meriam Guellil and colleagues highlighted the importance of western and central Asia and the regions surrounding the Black Sea in plague pandemics of the past.[32] The results, based on a synthesis "of historical sources and phylogeny," point to the existence of a plague reservoir outside of Europe, "specifically in Western Asia or the Black Sea region," that would have been responsible for the post-Black Death plague lineage. From this reservoir, plague may have been introduced into Western and Eastern Europe and western Asia "in multiple waves." Rather than challenge the traditional narrative of the *Grand Saint-Antoine*, then, this study – like those of Schmid and colleagues and Bos and co-authors) – highlights the importance of the Caucasus and western Asia as possible locations for these yet-to-be-identified plague foci. It also reminds the reader yet again that "more data from other regions of the world, which remained affected by plague beyond the outbreak of Marseille *l'Observance* in 1720, are needed to gain insights into the global diversity of lineages during the Second Plague Pandemic."[33]

Finally, a 2021 study by Andaine Seguin-Orlando and colleagues that focused on the Italian plagues of the seventeenth century

---

[32] Meriam Guellil et al., "A Genomic and Historical Synthesis of Plague in 18th-Century Eurasia," *Proceedings of the National Academy of Sciences* 117, no. 45 (November 2020): 28328–35.

[33] Guellil et al., "A Genomic and Historical Synthesis," 28332–3. For a discussion on the recent research, see also: Paul Slack, "Perceptions of Plague in Eighteenth-Century Europe," *Economic History Review* (April 2021): 1–19.

In 2021, Bramanti et al. cited Guellil et al. (2020) when they asserted that "for two locations (Pestbacken, Sweden 1710 [PEB10] and Marseille, France 1722 [OBS]), an origin from the Ottoman Empire is historically and archaeologically well supported." In this study, the authors concluded that *Y. pestis* was most likely introduced in Europe "from Asia several times during the second plague pandemic." Barbara Bramanti et al., "Assessing the Origins of the European Plagues Following the Black Death: A Synthesis of Genomic, Historical, and Ecological Information," *Proceedings of the National Academy of Sciences* 118, no. 36 (August 2021): 2–3.

nevertheless contributed to the question of the *Grand Saint-Antoine*. Building on the work of earlier studies, the authors point out that the "genome characterization" of plague strains from the epidemic waves of the second pandemic following the Black Death "[has] been found to form at least two main phylogenetic groups, potentially indicative of different origins from strains descending from the Black Death and either surviving in Europe (Bos et al., 2016) or in nearby foci (Guellil et al., 2020)." The first cluster "grouped together strains retrieved from individuals buried during the late 15th to the mid-17th century CE in Italy, Switzerland, and Germany," while the second of these phylogenetic clusters "included strains stretched throughout the Caucasus and Europe and spanning the mid-15th to the late 18th century CE."[34] For our purposes, this includes the 1720 Marseille strain (from *l'Observance* burial pit) and those that are related to it, including London's New Churchyard, Sweden's Pestbacken, Germany's Ellwangen, and others that are located across, and on the outskirts of Europe. The geographic placement of these aDNA sequences is potentially telling, and could suggest that those of the first cluster, which is grouped closely around Germany and the Alps, came from a nearby, domestic plague reservoir/s; while those of the second cluster – which are much more spread out, include numerous port cities, and in some cases are associated with origin narratives – were imported from an external reservoir.[35] Again, without aDNA samples from other parts of the world, it will be difficult if not impossible to know for certain.

There are nevertheless several takeaways from the preceding summary regarding the origins of the Great Plague of Provence. First, and most fundamentally, traditional European understandings of plague as strictly an oriental evil that was continually imported from the East through commerce are no longer tenable. Mounting genetic evidence supports the existence of plague reservoirs in Europe and on the outskirts that were responsible for at least some of the post-Black Death outbreaks of the second pandemic. While this evidence has not yet been able to disprove the historical narrative of the *Grand Saint-Antoine*

---

[34] Andaine Seguin-Orlando et al., "No Particular Genomic Features Underpin the Dramatic Economic Consequences of 17th-Century Plague Epidemics in Italy," *iScience* 24 (April 23, 2021): 6.

[35] Boris V. Schmid, "Re: On 1720 Plague," personal email communication, July 29, 2021. Cited with permission from the author.

with any certainty, there is nevertheless reason to question the story's veracity. By searching for the origins of European plague outbreaks during the second pandemic, these paleogenetic studies have directed attention to long-standing orientalist narratives that linked disease with understandings of Asia and Africa as unclean, uncivilized, and inept in matters of public health – what historian Nükhet Varlık has termed "epidemiological orientalism." Here, the orient is seen "as the site of disease and [is] made into Europe's epidemiological 'Other.'"[36] Consequently, plague – at times referred to in Spanish and French archival documents as "peste Levantina/e" (Levantine plague or scourge) – is seen as its product. If paleogenetic evidence could disprove the accuracy of the *Grand Saint-Antoine* account – and it very well may – its consistency and ubiquity across historical records would make it a prime example of this kind of misdirected epidemiological scapegoating. According to Varlık, moreover, "Historical data collected from the Ottoman archives do not indicate a major outbreak of plague in the eastern Mediterranean – the alleged origin of the outbreak – preceding or contemporary with the Plague of Marseille."[37] While this contradicts reports in France of plague in Palestine and Syria days before the arrival of the *Grand Saint-Antoine* (see this chapter's introductory paragraph), it seems likely that Ottoman officials at this time would have documented any epidemics within the Empire or in neighboring regions.[38] Whatever the origins of the Plague of Provence, however, we now know of other plague outbreaks that may have seeded from

---

[36] Nükhet Varlık, "Introduction," in *Plague and Contagion in the Islamic Mediterranean: New Histories of Disease in Ottoman Society*, edited by Nükhet Varlık (Kalamazoo: ARC Humanities Press, 2017), xiii.

[37] Nükhet Varlık, "Rethinking the History of Plague in the Time of COVID-19," *Centaurus* 62, no. 2 (May 2020): n10.

[38] In 2014, historian Nükhet Varlık pointed out that, "There was no systematic recording of plagues in the Ottoman empire before the eighteenth century." More recently, however, she has found that "the empire's tenacious record-keeping bureaucracy ... left behind an extraordinary body of documentation to track recurrent plague epidemics in this part of the world over six hundred years." For the former, see: Nükhet Varlık, "New Science and Old Sources: Why the Ottoman Experience of Plague Matters," *The Medieval Globe* 1, no. 1 (2014): 206. For the latter, see: Nükhet Varlık, "New Questions for Studying Plague in Ottoman History," *TRAFO – Blog for Transregional Research* (June 29, 2021), https://trafo.hypotheses.org/29284.

European foci. Essentially, the marriage of paleogenetic and historical research is causing scholars across disciplines to rethink what we
thought we knew about plague.

Although it remains possible, based on the evidence currently available, that the 1720 plague was imported from the eastern Mediterranean, there exist other potential explanations for the outbreak that
do not necessarily implicate the *Grand Saint-Antoine*. According, for
example, to Pichatty de Croissainte (lawyer, king's prosecutor, and
"Conseil orateur de la Communauté"), who in 1721 published his
*Concise Journal on the Events in the City of Marseille Since it Became
Afflicted with the Contagion*, at least four other ships from the eastern
Mediterranean (from Sidon and Alexandretta or İskenderun) arrived
after the *Grand Saint-Antoine* in Marseille's lazaret in May and June
1720 with *patentes brutes*, or foul bills of health. Several porters died
soon thereafter without the telltale "marks of contagion" – the buboes,
or swollen lymph nodes at the armpits and/or groins; the *charbons*, or
ulcers on the surface of the skin; or the gangrene in one's extremities
(the symptom that inspired the name "Black Death" centuries later).
The cadavers were quickly interred in quicklime (calcium oxide) and
their clothing burned.[39] Infections nevertheless continued through
June, then accelerated rapidly in July. If this account is accurate,[40]
then it is possible that the plague was introduced not from the *Grand
Saint-Antoine*, but from any of the other ships that arrived with foul
bills of health around the same time (Croissainte mentions those of
captains Aillaud, Gabriel, Gueymart, and others).[41]

A multiple-introductions theory is therefore also possible, in which
there were at least two arrivals of plague in 1720, with one on the

---

[39] Nicolas Pichatty de Croissainte, *Journal abregé de ce qui s'est passé en la
ville de Marseille, depuis qu'elle est affligée de la contagion, tiré du Mémorial
de la Chambre du Conseil de l'Hôtel de Ville; tenu par le Sieur Pichatty de
Croissainte Conseil & Orateur de la Communauté, et Procureur du Roy de la
Police* (Paris: Jacques Josse, 1721), 2–5.

[40] The source originated from local authority and was aimed primarily at
justifying the actions of the city's *échevins*. Anonymous, "Musée d'Histoire de
Marseille—Chroniques de la peste: 1720," *Musées Méditerranée: Association
pour la conservation et la valorisation des collections publiques de France,
Région Sud Provence-Alpes-Côte d'Azur* (2019), www.musees-mediterranee
.org/portail/index.php?menu=1&num_musee=68.

[41] Croissainte, *Journal abregé*, 3–5.

Grand Saint-Antoine, and the other on one of the other vessels, or born of a local plague reservoir in July just before infections accelerated. The genetic evidence has not yet answered these questions, and the historical evidence – namely, eyewitness accounts and essentially all other archival records – insists that it arrived on May 25, 1720 on the *Grand Saint-Antoine.* For now, then, we can rely only on the evidence available and choose not to ignore the historical record.[42] Although conclusive evidence that the 1720 outbreak came from within Europe does not yet exist, I deliberately refer to the plague's "emergence" or "appearance" throughout this study, rather than its "arrival," in order to reflect ongoing uncertainty about the epidemic's origins. What follows now is a history of the days and weeks after the arrival of the *Grand Saint-Antoine* in Marseille on May 25, 1720, and the unfolding of a major public health crisis in Europe.

"Les funestes ravages de la contagion"[43]: Plague Spreads in Provence

Immediately upon the notorious ship's docking at Pomègues, the number of infections began to rise, slowly at first, then gaining momentum with the wetter and warmer July summer weather. The precise sequence of infections and deaths at this early point varies somewhat from source to source. In his *Concise Journal on the Events in the City of Marseille,* Pichatty de Croissainte laid out the first suspected cases of

---

[42] As biologist Boris Schmid has observed: "Much of the reconstruction of how plague spread through Europe is based on historical records, yet we have the curious situation that for the Plague of Marseille in 1720, some of us have put very little weight on historical records that are pointing to multiple plague-infected ships coming from the Middle East at the start of plague outbreak, in favor for a putative reservoir of plague in Europe, location unknown … [T]o me that seems to put too much weight on the geographic location from where aDNA samples [have been] recovered … and too little credit for the historical records." Boris V. Schmid, "Re: New piece on Black Death introduction today in *PNAS*," Medmed-L electronic mailing list, November 27, 2018, https://lists.asu.edu/cgi-bin/wa?A0=medmed-l. Cited with permission from the author.

[43] "Les échevins et deputez du commerce de la Ville de Marseille à Monseigneur Le Duc d'Orléans," *Chambre du Commerce de Marseille, 1721–1722,* January 19, 1721, f. 3v, Affaires étrangères (henceforward AE), BIII, 42, Les Archives nationales de France (henceforth AN).

plague in Marseille beginning with two sailors who died on board the *Grand Saint-Antoine* after its arrival at port (this is also where he listed the ships that arrived with the *patentes brutes* from the eastern Mediterranean in late May and June).[44] Another account, this one written three decades later, reported the deaths of a father and son "bearing the marks of contagion" a few days after the earlier deaths of the porters in late May.[45] Historians Jean-Noël Biraben and Monique Lucenet, too, describe some of the deaths that took place in the earlier phase of the outbreak, including one on June 20 on rue Belle-Table in Marseille, a small street near the port, where a woman quickly succumbed to an infection that bore the signs of bubonic plague.[46] From Paris, English diplomat Sir Robert Sutton wrote Secretary James Craggs in London:

The Court has received the melancholy news of a pestilential distemper being crept into Marseilles by the infection of some bales of cotton brought from Sidon by a vessel which belonging to some *échevins* of the town, was favoured by shortening the usual quarantaine. Those who open'd the bales were struck with the plague and died suddenly, since which about 24 persons are dead in one street and others in the neighbourhood.[47]

And in a letter to Dr. Bellier of Carpentras written some weeks after the appearance of the first cases in late May, Dr. Reymond of Marseille, an eyewitness, offered a more detailed account of developments in July:

One young boy—a fifteen-year-old whose father had items from the cargo in his home—was attacked first, and he died with the symptoms described above [Reymond had earlier described the victims' chest pains, vomiting, and buboes in the groin area, and claimed that they perished within two days]. The physician and surgeon who had attended him advanced the report of the boy's death to the consuls [Reymond's term for local officials]. After this, the evil seemed to stop, but no sooner than we sang victory, after eight days, that is to say on 24 July, after the frightful thunders and excessive rain and winds that were felt here, the street to which [some] contrabandists from the infirmary had

---

[44] Croissainte, *Journal abregé*, 1–19 (for events from late May through July).
[45] "Relation de ce qui s'est passé à Marseille pendant la peste de 1720 de son principe ...," II, 1F 80/39, ADBRM.
[46] Biraben, *Les hommes* ... vol. 1, 232. Lucenet, *Les grandes pestes*, 221.
[47] Robert Sutton to James Craggs, secretary of state, Paris, August 7, 1720, State Papers Foreign (henceforward SP) 78/168, France, The National Archives of the United Kingdom (henceforward TNA).

moved was the first to be taken by this evil, because in two days, ten people died with buboes, and they perished not in two days, but quite suddenly, or at most, in one day. Since that time, this street, which was once bustling with people, has become deserted by the mortality of its inhabitants, and if anyone was spared death, it was through flight, thereby innocently taking the infection with them.[48]

While there is thus some uncertainty about the number of deaths in those earlier weeks from late May through June, we know that infections began to climb rapidly in July, and that the disease spread outward from the areas near the port with great virulence. To a growing number of physicians and other eyewitnesses, the signs of plague became undeniable. On July 9, 1720, for example, after examining a fourteen-year-old victim on rue Jean-Galant, doctors Charles and Jean-André Peyssonnel, father and son, identified the illness as plague.[49] Over the course of the summer, more physicians who inspected the bodies of victims would reach the same conclusion and inform the *échevins* of the city.[50]

---

[48] "Copie d'une lettre écrite par Mr. Reymond …," 1F 80/37, ADBRM. "Un jeune garçon aagé de 15 ans dont le pere avoit une de ces pieces dans la maison en fut attaqué le premier, et il mourut avec les symptomes de cy dessus, le raport du genre de sa mort fut posteé aux Consuls par le Medecin et Chirurgien qui l'avoit assisté et visité. Le mal ne s'etendit pas alors, car il parut assoupy ou éteint et on commencois a chanter victoire, mais huit jours aprés, c'est a dire vers 24 juillet aprés les tonnerres effroyables la pluye abondante et les vents de bise qui s'étoient fait sentir icy, la rue ou s'etoit retiré les Contrebandeurs des Infirmeries se trouva la premiere a être prise de ce mal, car dans deux jours il y mourut dix personnes avec des charbons et des bubons, non point dans deux jours mais subitement ou tout au plus dans un jour. Depuis ce temps cette rüe qui etoit des plus fournie de petit peuple est devenüe deserte par la mortalité de ses habitants, et s'il y a quelqu'un qui ait pu se garantir de la mort, ce n'a été qu'en fuyant et emportant avec foy."
The storm that Reymond alludes to here is described in a separate document as follows: "On the night of the 21st and 22nd [of July], there was a furious storm consisting of rain, hail, lightning and thunder, so frightful that no one could not recall a storm so terrible. The lightning struck a thousand times around the city, as if to rouse the inhabitants. The storm not only threatened them, but it seems it was a fatal omen of the misfortunes that were to come soon thereafter." "Relation de ce qui s'est passé à Marseille pendant la peste de 1720 de son principe …," II, 1F 80/39, ADBRM.

[49] Croissainte, *Journal abregé*, 7–8. Biraben, *Les hommes* … vol. 1, 232. The elder Peyssonnel succumbed to the plague later in 1720.

[50] On July 18, for example, Dr. Sicard reports to officials the presence of plague on rue de l'Escale. Jamel El Hadj, "Les chirurgiens et l'organisation sanitaire contre la peste à Marseille, 17e–18e siècles" (PhD diss., EHESS, 2014), 116. Biraben, *Les hommes* … vol. 1, 235.

Yet from the appearance of the earliest cases, local officials, including members of Marseille's *Bureau de la santé*,[51] adopted a policy of denial, rejecting that the illness was plague, despite evidence to the contrary in reports from local doctors. With the *foire de Beaucaire* opening in late July, the unloading of the ship's lucrative cargo seemed to take precedence over any risk of infection in the city. What ensued was a major campaign of misinformation that would persist in one form or another for the duration of the epidemic. One eyewitness described the apparent indifference of municipal officials during the crucial early days of the outbreak:

On 26 July, on the feast of Ste. Anne, a doctor told the *échevins* of the city that he had found on the rue de l'Escale and surrounding suburbs – places where one usually finds the warehouses for the contraband from the infirmaries – various sick persons and dead bodies bearing the veritable marks of plague. He added that it appeared that the same disease was moving from one house to another, and should be considered dangerous, as it will have unfortunate consequences. The *échevins* replied that they would send a surgeon to the scene, but they did not make a big deal of the doctor's declaration, claiming that he was just a young doctor. Nevertheless, the more prudent and sensible people began to gather their belongings and resolved to withdraw to the country, after which one saw many people of distinction leaving the city; an infinite number of bourgeois, as well as those who imitated them, which caused a great movement of people in all parts of the city; and in three or four days, thirty or forty thousand people left.[52]

---

[51] It is worth noting that Marseille's *Bureau de la santé*, established in 1640 and situated at the entrance to the port, was primarily composed of sixteen *intendants de la santé* who were selected from among the principal merchants of the city, and were rotated annually. These men, chosen to direct plague prevention in Marseille, were not doctors but merchants who had financial interests and personal connections to the broader merchant community of the Mediterranean. Junko Thérèse Takeda, *Between Crown and Commerce: Marseille and the Early Modern Mediterranean* (Baltimore: Johns Hopkins University Press, 2011), 122.

[52] "Relation de ce qui s'est passé à Marseille pendant la peste de 1720 de son principe ...," II, 1F 80/39, ADBRM.

The exact number of those who fled in the early days of infection, before the city was completely isolated, is unknown. Nevertheless, the mass exodus that followed may help to explain why reportedly about half the population of Marseille succumbed to the plague rather than an even larger proportion: a considerable number of the other half managed to get away, thanks in part to the local officials who reportedly did little in the earliest phase of the outbreak to prevent its spread from the streets near the port.

Fearing the consequences that a plague epidemic could have for Marseillais commerce, the city's *échevins* and the *Bureau de la santé* sent letters in July 1720 to the regent, Philippe d'Orléans, in Paris, as well as to the *officiers conservateurs* of health in ports all over Europe stating that local authorities had managed to contain the disease.[53] Even through the month of August, Marseillais administrators were reporting to the regent that the local distemper was not plague but merely a malignant fever that, in any case, was under control. In this time, some locals, including Dr. Reymond, expressed concern about such a mishandling of information. He wrote:

The interests of the consuls lie in concealing the cause of this evil, because they can be accused of having introduced it, or of not having taken just and appropriate measures in a suitable amount of time to stop the progress and communication of the illness. To this day [August 21, 1720], they declare that it is only a verminous, putrid, or at most, a malignant fever, that they attribute to the bad alimentation of the poor during the spring … But there are a great many people of all sorts of conditions affected by the evil.[54]

Marseillais officials allegedly went as far as paying doctors to corroborate their claims that the illness was only a fever. On August 12, 1720, the regent sent three medical practitioners to Marseille from Montpellier – doctors François Chicoyneau and François Verny (sometimes Verni or Verney), and surgeon Jean Soulier (or Soullier) – to investigate the epidemic that by then was killing as many as 400 people per day.[55] Despite the virulence of the disease and the rising

---

[53] Takeda, *Between Crown and Commerce*, 126.
[54] "Copie d'une lettre écrite par Mr. Reymond …," 1F 80/37, ADBRM. "Les consuls dont l'interét est de cacher le nom du mal, parce que l'on peut les accuser de l'avoir introduit, ou de n'avoir pas pris a tems de justes et sages mesures pour en empecher le progrés et la communication, ont fait publier jusqu'a present que ce n'etoit qu'une fievre vermineuse, putride, ou tout au plus maligne, qu'ils attribuent aux mauvais aliments dont les pauvres gens s'etoient nourris pendant le printemps … Mais on n'a que trop veu de gens de toutes sortes de conditions, envelopes dans le mal … ce que ce mal a de particulier, c'est d'attaquer plus souvent les enfans et les femmes, et parmi elles, celles qui sont enceintes sont dans un grand danger, et on n'a point vu de ces dernieres sans faire des fausses couches, et mourir bientôt aprés."
[55] "Chicoyneau, Verny, Soullier, Pons, Boyer, médecins," *Honoraires (y compris ceux des apothicaires)*, GG362, Archives municipales de Marseille (henceforward AMM).

number of deaths, however, the physicians did not initially declare plague. The aforementioned Dr. Reymond, who accompanied them on their visit, reported as follows:

I have no doubt that you have heard of the arrival of Mr. Chicoyneau and Mr. Verny, doctors from Montpellier, in the company of a surgeon [Soulier] from the same town, who by order of the Regent, have come to learn about the state and nature of the illness that reigns here, and to report back to him. From the moment they arrived, the governors and consuls assigned Mr. Montagner and myself to accompany these men on their visits to the sick and to the hospitals, and to assist them in the opening of the corpses. We were occupied with the examinations for two days, after which the gentlemen from Montpellier wished to say nothing more about the disease, except that it was a pestilential and contagious malignant fever, and I believe that they gave this name to the disease only to please the Consuls, one of whom happened to have an interest in the said vessel and is accused moreover of having favored its entry into the infirmaries [a likely reference to Estelle]. But you may judge for yourself what we should call this illness, and if it deserves the name of plague, based on the following information. I cannot, Sir, call it anything but plague for three reasons: its brevity, its contagious nature, and its symptoms. For one, it kills quickly and without notice ... Secondly, it is highly contagious ...[56]

Mixed messages outside of Marseille, about both the nature of the epidemic and whether it was abating, reveal that local attempts to obscure the truth of plague initially caused significant confusion in the rest of Europe. Throughout the month of August, Robert Sutton reported from Paris about the rumors of an epidemic in the south. On

---

[56] "Copie d'une lettre écrite par Mr. Reymond ...," 1F 80/37, ADBRM.

The physicians of Montpellier were handsomely paid. According to one contemporary payment registry, in September 1720 alone, Chicoyneau and Verny earned 2,000 *livres* each, and Soulier earned 3,000 *livres*, at a time when standard pay was closer to 1,000 *livres* a month for doctors and 500 *livres* a month for surgeons (Laurence Brockliss and Colin Jones, *The Medical World of Early Modern France* [Oxford: Clarendon Press, 1997], 354–5). In January 1721, the *échevins* of Marseille paid them 1,000 *livres* each, and on the 24th, the *échevins* of Aix-en-Provence paid each of the three physicians another 1,500 *livres*. In May 1721, they saw 1,500 *livres* each from the *échevins* of Aix, and in June, the *échevins* of Marseille paid Chicoyneau and Verny 3,000 *livres* each, and another 2,000 to Soulier. "Chicoyneau, Verny, Soullier, Pons, Boyer, médecins," *Honoraires (y compris ceux des apothicaires)*, GG362, AMM.

August 10, for example, he wrote, "I have nothing new to acquaint you with by this occasion except the advice which the Duke Regent has received by a courier from Marseille that the distemper which was at first judged to be the plague is only a malignant and contagious fever, which is allready much abated."[57] By the 15th, he related that, "The plague abates so much at Marseilles that it is hoped it will soon be quite extinguished," and a week later reported once more, "The inclos'd copy of a letter from Aix will give you an account of the precautions used to prevent the spreading of the plague at Marseille which succeeded so well that it is said to be wholly extinguished. The feaver which reigned there and in the neighborhood among the common people is much abated."[58] It was not until August 28, 1720 that Sutton expressed explicit knowledge that a plague outbreak in Marseille – far from abating – was in fact only beginning. He wrote, "The distemper which lately broke out at Marseilles is the plague and now rages more than ever, having spread itself into the neighboring country beyond the line, which was drawn to prevent it."[59] By August, "the plague in Marseilles [could] no longer be conceal'd," and efforts to disguise the gravity of the situation ultimately proved futile.[60] Officials across Europe quickly enacted strict measures to protect against what they determined, through communications with their consuls and other representatives on the ground, to be an outbreak of plague in Marseille.[61]

Why were local authorities not forthright, even as more and more people lay dying? To begin with, it is possible that officials, including Estelle, simply did not believe that they were witnessing the beginnings

---

[57] Robert Sutton to Secretary Craggs, Paris, August 10, 1720, SP 78/168, France, TNA.

[58] Robert Sutton to Secretary Craggs, Paris, August 15, 1720, SP 78/168, France, TNA. Robert Sutton to Secretary Craggs, Paris, August 21, 1720, SP 78/168, France, TNA.

[59] Robert Sutton to Secretary Craggs, Paris, August 28, 1720, SP 78/168, France, TNA.

[60] "Paris, Sept. 11," *Weekly Packet* (London), September 3–10, 1720, issue 427. For more on the campaign of misinformation undertaken in Marseille, see the section on "Conflicting Narratives and the Invisible Commonwealth: How News of Plague was Received in Genoa and Europe" in Chapter 2.

[61] These reactions to the crisis across Europe and the overseas colonies are covered in the rest of this book.

of a major outbreak of bubonic plague the likes of which, by 1720, France had not seen in generations. Beginning with the Black Death, recurrences of plague continued in Europe almost uninterruptedly, with over 6,000 documented outbreaks, through the eighteenth century – what is now known as the second plague pandemic. By the seventeenth century, however, larger outbreaks had begun to slow down enough that by 1720, the last time France had seen a resurgence of plague was in 1668–1670.[62] For years, the plague was instead understood as a disease of the orient – a Turkish or Levantine plight – constantly raging in foreign lands, but seldom entering the ports of Europe. For many in the eighteenth century, then, plague had started to become a distant memory, both a thing of the past and an oriental affliction. And despite the city's long history as a port of entry for disease, as well as contemporary understandings that the plague always loomed in nations commercially close to France, this was no less the case for many in Marseille.[63]

It is also worth noting that not all of those who contracted the plague bore the notorious "marks of contagion," which is to say, the buboes or the *charbons* as described earlier. Instead, contemporary accounts tell of some who perished quickly and without these telltale signs, which could indicate the presence of septicemic or pneumonic plague.[64] The former is an infection of the blood that is especially lethal and can result in rashes on the skin. Like the bubonic form, it is spread through the bites of infected fleas and is not transmissible from person to person except by direct contact with contaminated fluid or tissue. Pneumonic plague, meanwhile, infects the lungs and results either when a person

---

[62] Brockliss and Jones, *The Medical World*, 353. Biraben, *Les hommes ...* vol. 1, 118. This epidemic was less widespread than the more significant reappearance of 1650–1653.

[63] As historian Charles Carrière and co-authors noted, "Non, vraiment, en ce mois de mai 1720, Marseille ne pense pas à la peste." Carrière et al., *Marseille ville morte*, 50.

[64] It is also possible to contract pharyngeal plague (or plague pharyngitis) – a rare condition that may result from the inhalation of respiratory droplets or from the ingestion of infected meat. In fact, Michelle Ziegler has argued that manifestations of plague should be understood by their method of transmission. Accordingly, traditional understandings of plague as occurring in any of three forms – bubonic, pneumonic, or septicemic – should be revised to include a fourth gastrointestinal form. Michelle Ziegler, "The Black Death and the Future of Plague," *The Medieval Globe* 1, no. 1 (2014): 259–83.

inhales infectious droplets in the air or when the bacteria in bubonic or septicemic cases spreads to the lungs. In any case, neither the septicemic nor the pneumonic form of plague – both highly virulent – necessarily exhibit the usual "marks of contagion." While it is difficult to know for certain, historical descriptions of symptoms, as well as contemporary depictions (see, for example, the work of contemporary artist Michel Serre), indicate that not all of those who died of plague in Provence shared the symptoms of bubonic plague, which may have confused some in the earliest weeks of the epidemic.[65]

Yet, even as the presence of a plague epidemic in southeastern France became irrefutable, Marseillais officials and traders continued to deny that the disease was the evil they most feared. For this reason, a more likely explanation for the denials of leaders and merchants was their city's commercial distinction. Founded by the Greek Phocaeans from Asia Minor in the sixth century BCE, the ancient city of Massilia, as it was once known, has served as an important commercial port for millennia.[66] By the seventeenth century, Marseille was one of the most important port cities in the Atlantic and Mediterranean worlds with a complete monopoly over France's trade with the Levant. The Edict of 1669 that recognized this distinction also established it as a duty-free port, removing the twenty percent customs tax on all goods filtering through the city, which other French cities still had to pay if they acquired Levantine merchandise from any port besides Marseille.[67] In

---

[65] In her article on the 1720 plague for the Edward Worth Library, Dr. Elizabethanne Boran wrote: "[I]t is clear that [the plague's] spread beyond Marseille owed more to human-to-human transmission, rather than adventurous rats. The virulence and spread of the Marseille plague strongly suggests that by the time it reached Aix-en-Provence it had mutated into pneumonic plague, which was far more lethal and which was spread by human-to-human transmission." Elizabethanne Boran, "The 1720 Marseille Plague," *Edward Worth Library* (2020), https://edwardworthlibrary.ie/exhibitions-at-the-worth/smaller-exhibitions/1720-at-the-edward-worth-library.

[66] Some believe that the city was founded by the Phoenicians around the eighth century BCE, but evidence suggests that the city was founded earlier, around 600 BCE by the Phocaeans, after they suffered major losses in a great sea battle against the allied Etruscans and Carthaginians over the territory of Alalia (around 540 BCE), in modern-day Aléria in Corsica.

[67] Gaston Rambert, *Histoire du commerce de Marseille*, tome 5, *De 1660 à 1789* (Paris: Librairie Plon, 1957), 11–12. Junko Thérèse Takeda, "Between Conquest and Plague: Marseillais Civic Humanism in the Age of Absolutism, 1660–1725" (PhD diss., Stanford University, 2006), 57.

obliging French traders and those of other European countries to purchase Levantine merchandise from Marseille for a better price, the city could potentially serve as "a massive depot for international trade."[68] Also under this edict, quarantines were made compulsory in Marseille, and in 1668, construction of the city's new lazaret, the *Nouvelles Infirmeries*, was completed.[69] These changes in effect launched a century of unparalleled commercial growth in the port. They also revealed the French Crown's aspirations to achieve superiority on the increasingly competitive stage of European commerce.

By the beginning of the eighteenth century, at the dawn of the War of the Spanish Succession that was to gain for France a series of new privileges in the Spanish Indies, Marseille had also become a principal point of departure for cities all over the New World, including the lucrative ports of Peru and Chile via Cape Horn.[70] It was a major depot for the trade that all of France, and especially the city itself, increasingly relied on for both goods and bullion. It is no wonder then that when plague emerged in 1720, local leaders worked to protect their livelihood by containing the news.

Despite some initial success in obscuring the truth outside of Provence, on the local level it was much more difficult to conceal. As the number of deaths quickly mounted, numerous families began fleeing the city as early as June and July, and word quickly spread into neighboring towns. On July 31, 1720, the *parlement* of Aix-en-Provence issued an *arrêt* (or decree) that suspended all commerce and communications between Marseille and the rest of Provence under pain of death. (Soon thereafter, in fact, four people were hanged for attempting to flee Marseille for Aix.[71]) One contemporary related, "Despite the artifice of the *échevins* of Marseille, and their persistence in hiding the evil, [the *parlement* of Aix] recognized in a few days that the city was undeniably infected." The *arrêt* of July 31 served to inform other areas of Provence about the infection and was later referenced in a letter from the *parlement* of Aix to Versailles when they wrote, "How many citizens that single *arrêt* saved in Provence! How

---

[68] Takeda, "Between Conquest and Plague," 84.
[69] Ibid., 204.
[70] For more on these privileges, see Chapters 3 and 4 on London and Cádiz, respectively.
[71] "Paris, Sept. 11," *Weekly Packet* (London), September 3–10, 1720, issue 427.

many subjects were conserved for your majesty!"[72] The decree, however, was not enough to save the town. In October 1720, the comte de
Pertuis related to the governor of Genoa: "I wish, dear neighbor, that
I had good news to share with you about Provence ... The poor town
of Aix begins to suffer from it[;] they do not say it is plague, but the
people there drop like flies."[73] Other cities followed with their own
decrees until "even the smallest villages closed their doors, the roads
carefully guarded, and all Provence was mobilized and alarmed."[74]
Outside of Provence, too, towns began taking measures in an attempt
to halt the spread of infection. The *parlement* at Toulouse, for example, forbade anyone leaving Marseille from entering the province of
Languedoc on pain of death.[75] Like Aix-en-Provence, however, towns
across southeastern France – including Arles, Salon, Toulon, Saint-
Rémy-de-Provence, Carpentras, Sisteron, Avignon, Orange, Gevau-
dan, La Canourgue in Languedoc, as well as parts of Auvergne, le
Comtat, the Dauphiné, and others – eventually suffered the effects
of the epidemic, until nearly all of Provence and its outskirts were
infected.[76]

---

[72] Louis-François Jauffret, ed. *Pièces historiques sur la peste de Marseille et
d'une partie de la Provence, en 1720, 1721 et 1722, trouvées dans les archives
de l'hôtel de ville, dans celles de la préfecture, au bureau de l'administration
sanitaire et dans le cabinet des manuscrits de la bibliothèque de Marseille,
publiées en 1820 à l'occasion de l'année séculaire de la peste; avec le Portrait
de Mr. de Belsunce et un fac simile de son écriture*, vol. 1 (Marseille: Chez les
principaux libraires, 1820), 129–30.

[73] "Ojala querido vezino que tubiese buenas noticias que darle de Provenza:
Marcella va mucho megor por falta de gente, hay no obstante algunos que
escapan, aunque les haya prendido fuertemente el mal: La pobre villa de Aix
empieza a padecerlo, no dizen que sea peste, pero la gente muere alla de la
misma manera que como moscas." "Copia de capitulo de una carta escrita por
el Conde de Pertuis, Governador de Bellaguar, da al exmo." Sr. Baron D'huart
Governador de Genova, October 11, 1720, Estado 4837, Archivo Historico
Nacional de España (hereafter cited as AHN).

[74] Anonymous, *Discours sur ce qui s'est passé de plus considérable à Marseille
pendant la Contagion* (Marseille: Chez Jean-Antoine Mallard, 1721), 16.

[75] Toulouse was the capital of the province of Languedoc until the lines on
French maps were redrawn during the French Revolution, and the provinces
were dissolved. "Paris, Sept. 11," *Weekly Packet* (London), September 3–10,
1720, issue 427.

[76] In Arles, for example, plague was officially recognized on December 24,
1720, at a meeting of the local health office. Odile Caylux, *Arles et la peste,
1720–1721* (Aix-en-Provence: Presses Universitaires de Provence, 2009), 62.

In some areas, the disease was especially virulent. A letter from the *intendants de la santé* in Toulon reveals the severity of the epidemic in that part of the region: "The bureau of health in this city is composed of eight *intendants*, out of which two are dead, two others are sick with the contagion, a fifth has the infection in his home where he has lost three people."[77] As symptoms began appearing in new towns all over the south of France, those who did not or could not flee could only hope that it was indeed only a fever rather than the feared plague. Yet the inevitable truth followed shortly behind as the magnitude of the outbreak became more and more evident. One contemporary source in La Canourgue wrote, "[The] extraordinary Precautions [taken by local authorities] make it still fear'd that the Disease, of which several Persons have dy'd there, is *not* only a common Fever."[78]

As a result of the panic that gripped Europe, French towns as far north as Normandy, which would ultimately remain safe from contagion, nevertheless suffered the epidemic in their own way as a result of the false rumors of infection that spread from the summer of 1720 at least through 1721. In the autumn of 1720, English officials exchanged letters about reports that the plague had made it into Saint-Malo in Brittany and parts of Normandy. Owing to this area's proximity to England, the news was not taken lightly. Secretary Craggs wrote Robert Sutton in October:

Several reports have been spread here within these few days as if the plague had been brought into some of the ports on the hither side of France, amongst which that of St. Malo is particularly named. Your Excellency will be pleased to make the strictest enquiry into all accounts of that important nature and to give us the earliest notice of them.[79]

English official and member of parliament, Daniel Pulteney, followed up with this news from Paris in a letter to Secretary Craggs when he wrote:

---

[77] "Le bureau de la santé de cette ville est composé de huit intendants depuis quelque temps il en est mort deux, deux autres ont eu le mal contagieux, le cinquième la eu dans la maison et a perdu trois personnes." "Les Intendants de la Santé à Toulon," Toulon, June 2, 1721, f. 198, Fonds de la Marine (henceforward MAR) B3 275, AN.

[78] "Paris," *Daily Post* (London), June 5, 1721, issue 524. Emphasis added.

[79] Secretary Craggs to Robert Sutton, Whitehall, October 27, 1720, SP 78/169, France, TNA.

There have been reports as if the plague was at St. Malo and in some part of Normandy, near the sea; I don't find reason to believe those reports true, though they have not been altogether groundless with respect to Normandy, and I should not repeat them if I did not think that in cases of this nature, it is very excusable to have rather too much suspicion and caution than too little. By the last accounts from Provence and Dauphiny, the plague encreased.[80]

Rumors became such an issue that some towns attempted to persecute those who were suspected of spreading them. Such was the case, for instance, in Languedoc, where officials reacted to false reports with particular severity:

Tis advised from Languedoc, that the Intendant of the Province, M. de Barnages, has caused several Persons to be taken into Custody, for having spread false Rumours of the Plague's being got on this side of the River Rhone; Nevertheless the Duke de Roquelaure and General Medavi have caused Lines to be thrown up, which shut in Canorgue and several other Villages so securely, that 'tis scarce possible for any Person to come out of them, without Falling into the Hands of the Troops that guard those Lines.[81]

Accounts like these reveal the level of panic and fear that overtook both town and country during the Plague of Provence. Across France (and elsewhere in Europe, as well), those who could afford to do so fled the cities for the countryside even if there were no signs of contagion nearby. By November 1720, for example, several Lyonnaise families had already fled the town, though no cases of infection had been identified. Paris was no less anxious. Daniel Pulteney wrote from the capital in November:

Paris itself is not thought out of danger. The Regent said on this occasion that he would remain here, as the Emperour did at Vienna when the plague was there; two or three persons came here some weeks ago, from within the lines about Marseilles. The *Lieutenant de Police* has made strict search after them, but I have not heard if they have been found. I would not mention this circumstance till I had repeated assurances of the truth of it.[82]

---

[80] Daniel Pulteney (member of parliament) to Secretary Craggs, Paris, November 1, 1720, SP 78/166, France, TNA.

[81] "Paris," *Daily Post* (London), June 5, 1721, issue 524.

[82] He related further: "The accounts of the plague are very bad; they reckon it is spread about 40 leagues in compass. The people of Lyons begin to

A few weeks later, in December 1720, he reported a similar incident:

The conductors of six mules laden with muslins, embroidered petticoats, and other turkey goods from Marseilles designed, as is suspected, to be brought here for some persons of distinction, having attempted to pass the Rhone into Languedoc in a boat prepared for that purpose, and been hindered by the guards, they went into an island on the Rhone where 20 dragoons were sent to seize them. Six of the conductors were killed and three of the dragoons. The rest of the conductors were taken and are to be executed. The goods were burnt.[83]

From the moment word began to spread about the epidemic, episodes like these took place not only in France but across Europe, in regions including England, Spain, Italy, Portugal, the Dutch Republic, and others. In the wave of panic, moreover, as more and more southern French towns and villages were isolated, uninfected hinterlands were sometimes quarantined along with the diseased epicenter. The county of Avignon very nearly became one of them when officials debated isolating the entire *comte* along with infected parts in December 1720. The controversial bid was rejected on ethical grounds, however, and was not immediately put into effect.[84]

In the end, the plague took more than 100,000 lives in southern France, although there is little consensus on the precise figure. In Marseille alone, accounts report anywhere from 40,000 to upward of 80,000 deaths. To confuse matters more, deaths during the plague resulted not only from infection, of course, but from other causes, including malnutrition (owing in part to the strict quarantines and lack of food).[85] Various contemporary accounts nevertheless give

---

apprehend it very much and several familys are already retired from that city." Mr. Pulteney to Secretary Craggs, Paris, October [a mistake, should read November in the letter] 18, 1720, SP 78/166, France, TNA. For English reactions and responses to the plague in France, see Chapter 3 on London.

[83] Mr. Pulteney to Secretary Craggs, Paris, December 27, 1720, SP, 78/166, France, TNA.

[84] "The plague is got into a part of the Comte d'Avignon. The French commandant in those parts proposed the shutting up the whole Comte[;] the vice legat would not consent to it; it is thought they will shut up only the infected part." Mr. Pulteney to Secretary Craggs, Paris, December 27, 1720, SP 78/166, France, TNA.

[85] A letter from the town of Schaffhausen dated November 28, 1720. claims that there had already been 80,000 deaths in Marseille. "For tho' at Marseilles,

estimates of the number of people who fell victim to the plague. Writing in his *livre de raison* some years after the epidemic, Claude Isnard (1692–1766), *hebdomadier* and Jesuit priest at *Église Saint-Agricol* in Avignon (from 1719 to 1724),[86] recounted his experiences during the Plague of Provence:

I must not omit in the account that follows anything that concerns me, everything that took place during the time that the plague afflicted this city of Avignon, and all that took place before the disease attacked our city.

where they have lost eighty thousand Souls," *Post Boy* (London), December 1–3, 1720, issue 4893. Another account addresses famine during the plague: "The accounts from Marseilles are very melancholy. The people there are press'd between the plague and famine; it is certain that a considerable number have forced through the line or barrier which was to keep inclosed the infected district and are dispersed on this side of it; the necessity they were reduced to forced them to it." Mr. Pulteney to Secretary Craggs, Paris, September 17, 1720, SP 78/166, France, TNA. Yet another describes the kind of hardships that victims experienced while out at sea: "Another Vessel, they tell us, is driven on Shore on the Coast of Majorca, all the Seamen on board being dead of the Plague, some of which were found lying dead in their Cabbins, and some on the Decks, in a most deplorable Manner; and that the Governor of the Island had caused the Ship to be set on fire and burnt, with all the dead Bodies in it; the Priests saying the Office for Burial of the Dead on the Shore, at the Time of setting the Ship on Fire. The Condition of the poor Inhabitants of Marseilles has been particularly miserable every Way; those who have been able to [have made] their escape to Sea, having been thus reduced to the utmost Distress. They speak of another Ship from the same City, driven on Shore on the Back of Calabria, in the Kingdom of Naples, the Men belonging to which, had suffer'd inexpressible Hardships and Miseries at Sea, by Storms and Want of Provisions; that many of them being dead at Sea, the rest that were left, tho' not at all infected, were yet almost dead with Hunger and hard Labour. They remain, it seems, lock'd up in an old ruin'd Castle, where Provisions are carry'd to them by the Officers appointed, but none are permitted to visit them, neither for the Relief of their Bodies, or Comfort of their Souls; that is to say, neither Priest or Physician; and there, it is said, they are to perform a tripple Quarantine, viz. of 120 Days, by which Time, it may be supposed, some of them may die for Want of Help, whether they had the Plague or no." *Applebee's Original Weekly Journal* (London), October 22, 1720.

[86] Hebdomos, in Greek, means "seventh," hence Hebdomas or hebdomada – a seven-day cycle. The *hebdomadier* is "the one week," the "weekly." In the liturgical world, the hebdomadier is, in priestly or religious communities, the priest assigned to preside over the Eucharist and the Office for the duration of one week. As his name implies, Saint Agricol, patron saint of the city of Avignon since 1647, is invoked for rain in times of drought, as well as good weather and harvests. Notably, devotees also look to Saint Agricol for protection against bubonic plague and other calamities.

The contagion entered via Marseille in 1720 and was communicated that year and the next to several towns and villages of Provence, taking with it approximately seventy-seven thousand people [he later offers the more precise number of 76,776].[87]

However, in January 1722, months before the end of the epidemic, Cardin Lebret, intendant of Provence, reported to the controller-general of France that Provence had seen 122,469 infected individuals, 93,290 of whom perished from a total population (in the infected areas) of 292,165. According to this report, Marseille alone lost 39,115 inhabitants.[88] More recent estimates include those of historian Daniel Panzac, who estimated that out of a total of 293,113 people in 81 Provençal communities, approximately 105,417 perished from plague (50,000 in Marseille), which amounts to a mortality rate of 36 percent.[89] Meanwhile, in Comtat Venaissin (now part of Provence) the infection took 8,062 lives out of 36,641 inhabitants, and in Languedoc, 12,597 out of 75,377, at 22 percent and roughly 17 percent mortality rates, respectively. According to these figures, then, the outbreak of 1720 to 1722 took approximately 126,000 lives in Provence and Languedoc.[90]

...

Accounts of the plague describe hellish scenes of widespread grief and misery. Following a massive fire that erupted in Marseille on August 25, 1720, burning one quarter of the city after another, one observer described the dramatic spectacle that was revealed when the smoke cleared:

[87] "Livre de raison de moy, Claude Isnard, hebdomadier à Saint Agricol et prieur de Roquemartine," 24 E 11, 34, ADBRM. Isnard used local records for the information that he provides in this list.

[88] Cited in: Shelby T. McCloy, "Government Assistance During the Plague of 1720–22 in Southeastern France," *The Social Service Review* 12, no. 2 (June 1938): 301.

[89] The population of the whole of Provence was roughly 658,000 in 1700. By 1765, according to L'abbé Expilly, it totaled 698,168. In 1720, then, it was likely much larger than 293,000. See: André Bourde, "La Provence au grand siècle," in *Histoire de la Provence*, edited by Édouard Baratier (Paris: Privat, 1987), 316; l'Abbé Jean-Joseph Expilly, *Tableau de la population de la France* (Paris: 1780), 32.

[90] Panzac, *Quarantaines et lazarets*, 61.

The streets were filled with cadavers, and all the public places paved with the dead. It was then, dear God, that one could see all the horrors contained within the walls of the city—the light of day revealed a deluge of despair and desolation unleashed on the inhabitants. And if the sun's rays reached one's eyes, it was to display seven or eight thousand cadavers rotting without burial, a great number of them eaten by the dogs who nourished themselves on the human flesh.[91]

In August 1720, consular letters out of Marseille described a worsening crisis "the likes of which would make the entire world break down in tears."[92] Those who witnessed the unhappy scenes of the dead and dying and lived to write about it describe in their letters and accounts "les horreurs d'une mortalité terrible" – the horrors of a terrible death.[93] The following passage exemplifies how this "terrible death" was most commonly described in contemporary documents:

The people die within two or three days; their malady begins with headaches and vomiting, followed by a violent fever. Some have buboes or *charbons*, while those who do not have these exterior marks die more quickly than those who do [possible evidence of pneumonic or septicemic plague in Marseille], so that the number of dead could be as much as 50 persons per day, all with the same symptoms.[94]

But the situation became far worse than even this account indicates. At its height in 1720, the illness may have taken as many as 1,000 lives per day in Marseille.[95] Countless contemporary reports tell of victims abandoned by their families, left to die alone for fear of being infected, children torn from their mothers, and mounds of corpses strewn about the streets. Such scenes of desolation survive for us to this day in the artwork of the period, particularly in the paintings of Catalan-born

---

[91] "Relation de ce qui s'est passé à Marseille pendant la peste de 1720 de son principe ...," VIII, 1F 80/39, ADBRM. The fire may have accidentally resulted from one of the regular burnings that took place during the epidemic. These were meant to impede the infection through the destruction of infected cadavers, homes, and properties.

[92] "Copia de una carta escrita de Montpeller a un Capellan de Figueras," Montpellier, August 2, 1720, Estado 506, AHN.

[93] "Lettre de Mr. Villars du 6 mars 1721," 13 E 16, Family Papers, ADBRM.

[94] "Relation de ce qui s'est passé à Marseille pendant la peste de 1720 de son principe ...," III, 1F 80/39, ADBRM.

[95] Takeda, *Between Crown and Commerce*, 109.

French painter Michel Serre, who captured the tragedy of the Plague of Provence on canvas.[96]

To Dr. Reymond at least, who by August 1720 claimed to have visited about 1,000 victims in his region over a period of 20 days, the disease seemed at first to predominantly affect women and children.[97] Ultimately, however, it appeared to affect everyone, including men and the elderly. It also took clerics, physicians, galley slaves, and prisoners (who often cleared the cadavers) – that is, those who were most often exposed to it – in large numbers. In a letter to his secretary of state in 1720, George Henshaw, British consul in Genoa, reported:

By the severall advices that are come here since my last, the mortality at Marseilles was dayly greater and greater, it being said there dyed sixteen hundred in three days time, and two thousand five hundred from the 18th to the 25th: It is said also, that about fifty persons that had been condemned to the galleys had been sent ashoar [ashore] there in order to bury the dead, but since that they are all dead themselves, so that now the people that dye are tost out of the windows into the streets and lye there, unburyed, and the distemper was spread in many of the neighbourghing country houses, and several vilages, as well as Aix, so God knows where it will end.[98]

Dr. Reymond, too, described the unspeakable scenes in his letter to Dr. Bellier, where he reiterates his conviction that the blame for the calamity fell on municipal leaders:

[W]e see a family of six or seven people gone extinct in one week, and the same occurs on entire streets that the scourge has entirely depopulated. We

---

[96] For more on the art of the period, see, for example: Chapter 4 in Meredith Martin and Gillian Weiss, *The Sun King at Sea: Maritime Art and Galley Slavery in Louis XIV's France* (Los Angeles: Getty Publications, 2022); Cindy Ermus, "Memory and the Representation of Public Health Crises: Remembering the Plague of Provence in the Tricentennial," *Environmental History* 26, no. 4 (October 2021): 776–88; Meredith Martin and Gillian Weiss, "The Art of Plague and Panic: Marseille, 1720," *Platform*, April 27, 2020, www.platformspace.net/home/the-art-of-plague-and-panic-marseille-1720; Régis Bertrand, "L'iconographie de la peste de Marseille, ou la longue memoire d'une catastrophe," *Images de la Provence: Les représentations iconographiques de la fin du Moyen Age au milieu du XXe siècle, edited by Centre méridional d'histoire sociale des mentalités et des cultures* (Aix-en-Provence: Presses Universitaires de Provence, 1992).

[97] "Copie d'une lettre écrite par Mr. Reymond ...," 1F 80/37, ADBRM.

[98] George Henshaw, British consul in Genoa, to Secretary Craggs, Genoa, September 10, 1720, SP 79/13, Genoa, TNA. For more on galley slaves, see Martin and Weiss, *The Sun King at Sea*; and "The Art of Plague and Panic: Marseille, 1720."

have lost nine or ten surgeons ...; those who guard the sick die quickly, all those who collect the bodies or bury them ["corbeaux et enterremorts"] have nearly all perished, so that the sick die with no care or treatment, and the cadavers are without sepultures, exposed all around the streets, at church doors, or at the cemeteries where no there is no one to bury them. Imagine then what sad and lamentable state we find ourselves in, amidst a frightful disorder ... What is more, patients are without broth, and those in hospital have spent four days without a drop to drink ... [And] the cause of all these disorders and calamities comes only from the consuls [local leaders], who had no foresight, or who did not want to have any, so to speak, in order to conceal an evil which does them no honor, and of which one of them is perhaps the cause. The consuls—whose only interest is to conceal the name of the evil [plague] because they could be accused of having introduced it, or of not having taken just and wise measures in time to prevent its progress and communication—have thus far stated only that it is a verminous, putrid, or at most, malignant fever, which they attribute to the bad foods that nourished the poor in the spring ... but we have seen too many people of all conditions enveloped by [the present] evil.[99]

Contemporary eyewitness accounts also pointed blame at the looters, murderers, and thugs who emerged from the chaos and added to the misery. A *Declaration du Roy* of October 1720 specified the ways in which criminal cases were to be handled during the contagion, using the *Ordonnance du mois d'août 1670* as a foundation, but making adjustments for the unique circumstances.[100] Such directives were deemed particularly necessary during the plague. For one, policing and court systems proved fragile entities that could dissolve when the infection reached a town, causing magistrates to disperse, thus leaving behind potential chaos. When the plague reached Aix, for example,

---

[99] "Copie d'une lettre écrite par Mr. Reymond ...," 1F 80/37, ADBRM. Such an account – one that recognizes the failures of those in power to prevent a disaster once it occurs, or to adequately respond to it in the crucial early moments and days after it takes place or begins – could just as easily been written today. In fact, during the ongoing COVID-19 pandemic, such failures have been the focus of numerous writings and commentaries that seek to unravel the complex set of events that allowed what began as a local outbreak to evolve into a global pandemic.

[100] "Declaration du Roy, Concernant les Procés criminels, qu'il s'agira d'instruire dans les villes & lieux infectés du mal contagieux," November 18, 1720, GG426, AMM. The ordonnance of 1670 established the rules for criminal procedure that were to remain in use until the French Revolution.

the Aixois *parlement* first relocated to Saint-Rémy-de-Provence, but soon thereafter scattered in the face of the spreading infection, causing the temporary dissolution of the Provençal *parlement*.[101] Strict quarantines and regulations, moreover, had created in Marseille a "large, insolent populace ready to revolt at all times."[102]

Reports describe numerous thefts, rapes, and murders committed amid inexpressible scenes of disorder. One story stands out among the more outrageous. It took place in the early phase of contagion in Marseille, and it involved a troop of brigands who entered local homes and slaughtered a great number of people. The account represents an example of the more extreme crimes committed during the outbreak. One contemporary related the story as follows:

They have written from Marseille that affairs improved a great deal, thank God, after three captains accompanied by 1,500 navy men expelled several murderers and brigands who mercilessly killed those that contagion had spared, mostly women, after taking their jewels. The thieves entered the houses with impunity and committed the horrible carnage. Forty of these cruel monsters were hanged, and one of them, who confessed to having killed over a thousand people in barbaric ways, was broken on the wheel while still breathing. He was a swordsman [*breteur*] from Avignon named Roüane. He was in this city only to commit this horrible massacre, and thereby satisfy his execrable passion. And it is said that ever since the troops cleared the city of Marseille of this abominable excrement and washed the streets of the city by means of fountains that made to run freely, there died only twenty people in two days, rather than the seven to eight hundred that previously died in the same amount of time, so that we assumed that half of the dead were killed and slaughtered by these execrable thieves, on one of whom we found the value of 30,000 *livres* of jewels, and we hope to discover many other items in the future.[103]

---

[101] "Lettres de translation du parlement de Provence en la ville de Saint Remy," November 18, 1720, GG426, AMM. See also Takeda, *Between Crown and Commerce*, 138.

[102] "Une populace nombreuse, insolente et prete à tous moments à se revolter." Jean-Louis Guey, *Mémoires ou livre de raison d'un bourgeois de Marseille, 1674–1724* (Montpellier: Bureau des Publications de la Société pour l'étude des Langues Romanes, 1881), 39, 41, 163; cited in Alessandro Pastore, *Crimine e giustizia in tempo di peste nell'Europa moderna* (Rome: Editori Laterza, 1991), 211.

[103] "De Lyon ce 15 7tbre 1720," 1F 80/38, ADBRM.

Other reports similarly describe the breakdown of civil society brought about by a virulent and deadly disease epidemic. The following account describes events that took place around the same time, and depicts a city abandoned by local authorities, left to fend for itself – the people unable to flee upon pain of death:

The plague rages still very much at Marseilles ... All the magistrates except 5 of the *échevins* and the people of distinction retired very early and left the town without government or order, insomuch that a troop of gypsies entered the houses and plundered them, stifling those that they found sick, and numbers of dead corps were left in the streets corrupting, until the commanders and officers of the gallies, who had barricaded themselves in the port, took the courage to go out with the slaves, seized and executed the gypsies, caused the dead carcasses to be burned, cleared the streets, and establisht a better order and police. The plague has reached Aubagne, Marignane, and other villages, but 'tis assured it has not got beyond the lines, the guards shooting all those who offer to pass them.[104]

During the epidemic, the punishment for the lesser crimes of burglary or the carrying of arms could consist of banishments, lengthy prison sentences, or death. For the greater crimes of murder and rape, the punishment was more consistently execution, most often by hanging. Such was the case for Roüane and his accomplices, as described earlier, as well as for one Jacques Amy, a twenty-four-year-old hatter from Marseille who was tried and convicted for the rape of nineteen-year-old Geneviève Aymard during the epidemic. In times of health, his subsequent promise to marry the young woman may have spared him, but in August 1721, he was condemned and delivered into the hands of the *exécuteur de la haute justice*, who saw to it that Amy suffered his sentence. With cord around his neck, *en chemise*, head and feet bare, and the burning flame of a candle between his hands, he proceeded toward the scaffold through town, pleading for forgiveness from "God, king, and justice," before suffering death by hanging and strangulation.[105] During the Plague of Provence, when many blamed

---

[104] Robert Sutton to Secretary Craggs, Paris, September 26, 1720, SP 78/168, France, TNA.

[105] "Conclusion diffinitive sur le procés en crime de rapt contre Jacques Amy," August 9, 1721, GG428, AMM.

the pestilence on the depravity of sinners who had incurred God's wrath, there was little tolerance for wrongdoing.[106]

Throughout the plague outbreak, public prayers, processions, and fasts to ward off the pestilential evil were held in France, and all over the European continent. Among many others, observances for Saint Roch – not only on his feast day of August 15, but throughout the epidemic – were among the most ubiquitous. Saint Roch, who may not have ever lived, was for centuries among the most venerated saints in times of pestilence in Europe, along with Saints Sebastian and Agricola of Avignon, among others. Each of these was said to intercede for the faithful in times of pestilence, with Saints Roch and Sebastian having themselves allegedly witnessed the plague during their lives. Feasts, fasts, and other acts of worship for these patron saints of pestilence were held in the hope that they could help end the plague in France by interceding before God on behalf of sinners, thus sparing those on earth from the infection.[107] During plague years, then, feast days and churches dedicated to these saints saw an upswing of events and attendance in cities such as London, Paris, Rome, Naples, Madrid, and Lisbon.[108] Predictably, however, the most public and extravagant demonstration of piety during the Plague of Provence took place in Marseille itself.

Foremost among those who condemned the wanton ways of the Marseillais and called for public acts of contrition was Henri François Xavier de Belsunce de Castelmoron, bishop of Marseille. Upon the

---

[106] Takeda, *Between Crown and Commerce*, 145.

[107] "Foreign Affairs, Rome, August 17," *Weekly Packet* (London), September 3–10, 1720, issue 427. "Avis au public," GG325, AMM. This *Avis* for the *Fête du Glorieux St. Roch* celebrated on August 15, 1720 warned that those who failed to participate by lighting a candle at their doors in the evening would be fined: "On invite tous les Habitans de cette Ville de faire chacun à la Porte de sa maison des Feux aujourd'huy jeudy sur les huit heures du soir, tant à l'occasion de la Fête du Glorieux St. Roch, que pour purifier l'Air dans ce temps de calamité. Et on avertit que ceux qui y manqueront, seront amendés."

[108] Newspapers in Europe reported heavily on the plague, and on measures taken against it including religious celebrations, throughout the plague years. See, for instance: *London Journal*, September 3–10, 1720, issue LIX. *Daily Courant* (London), September 6, 1720, issue 5890. *Daily Post* (London), September 12, 1720, issue 296. *Daily Post* (London), August 29, 1721, issue 597. *Daily Journal* (London), September 14, 1721, issue CCII.

appearance of plague in the port, Belsunce immediately took to the task of exorcizing the infection from the city by performing public acts of devotion and organizing public masses and processions through the main avenues of the commercial capital, despite the churches being closed through the following year. On November 15, 1720, for example, he initiated a procession through the city in which he sang the *Pange lingua*, and on December 31, he closed the year with another event in which he prayed to Saint Roch for succor.[109] The danger of obliging large crowds to gather during a virulent epidemic – what may now be referred to as a super-spreader event – was not lost on contemporary critics, who condemned the frivolity and shortsightedness of these public functions. In 1720, one observer wrote:

> The distemper rages with as much violence as ever, which in all probability is owing to the error they have committed in suffering processions at so unreasonable a time. It is to be hop'd the general one, which had been put off for some days, will be entirely laid aside, and that they will reflect on the ill consequences. Ceremonies of the like nature are generally attended with, of which they had an instance here during the last plague, 10 thousand people having been carried off the day after a general procession had been made to St. Rocco, by whose intercession the plague was said to have cease'd.[110]

Religious processions and other rituals not only continued, however, but accelerated. Ecclesiastical authorities did not perceive these events as contributing to the disaster, but rather as insufficient for demonstrating to the Heavens that the city was truly repentant. As a result, these earlier religious ceremonies served only as preludes to the much larger events that would take place in the following months.

At the behest of Anne-Madeleine Rémuzat, a self-mortifying Visitationist nun who shared with the bishop her visions of the Sacred Heart, Belsunce decided against earlier plans for a major procession of holy relics, and concluded instead that the most effective method for achieving deliverance from the retributive scourge unleashed in

[109] The *Pange lingua* is a Medieval Latin hymn. D. Théophile Bérenger, O.S.B., *Journal du maitre d'hotel Mgr de Belsunce durant la peste de Marseille, 1720–1722* (Paris: Mairie de Victor Palmé, 1878), 10–12, Delta 150, ADBRM. Raymond Jonas, *France and the Cult of the Sacred Heart* (Berkeley: University of California Press, 2000), 41.

[110] Henry Davenant, British envoy extraordinary to the Italian states, to Secretary Craggs, Genoa, September 25, 1720, SP 79/12, Genoa, TNA.

Marseille was the open and comprehensive consecration of the city to the Sacred Heart of Jesus.[111] He announced his plans to publicly perform this consecration in a mandate dated October 22, 1720, and established the festival in the city's ecclesiastical calendar.[112] On November 1, 1720, All Saint's Day, Belsunce began a procession from his episcopal residence in the garb of a penitent. In an act of atonement, he "stepped barefoot onto the cold streets of plague-ridden Marseille," and headed for the *reposoir* or altar that was constructed at the intersection of the Grand Cours and the Canabière, where he proceeded to consecrate himself to the "Venerable Heart of the Savior of all men."[113] This was to be his first act in the process of dedicating the port city to the Sacred Heart – the ultimate show of devotion and utter submission to the Heavens on a municipal level.

The next major act would take place on Friday, June 20, 1721, at the *Fête du Sacré-Cœur*. The ceremony began at eight in the morning at the bishop's palace with the ringing of the *tocsin*, which was followed by a three-hour-long procession through the center of the port.[114] Here, Belsunce gave the benediction and celebrated mass in a marriage of the city's commercial and religious elements. A few months later, on November 8, 1721, another procession followed, but the persistent reappearance of plague suggested that the consecrations of November and June had failed to demonstrate to the Heavens that Marseille was truly contrite. Belsunce therefore insisted that the return of plague in 1722 resulted from the moral failings of the city's secular officials and their failure to participate in the earlier religious ceremonies of 1720.[115] Consequently, on May 28, 1722, municipal leaders, including chief officer Jean-Pierre Moustier, Balthazar Dieudé, Pierre Remusat, and Jean-Baptiste Saint-Michel, assembled at Marseille's *Hôtel de Ville* and made a solemn vow to consecrate the city to the Sacred Heart of Jesus and to oblige their successors to do the same. The following month, on June 12, the feast of the Sacred Heart, the men did just that when they joined the procession to Marseille's *Notre-Dame de la Major* cathedral, where the vow to

---

[111] Jonas, *France and the Cult*, 37–9.
[112] Takeda, *Between Crown and Commerce*, 172.
[113] Jonas, *France and the Cult*, 39.
[114] Takeda, *Between Crown and Commerce*, 173.
[115] Jonas, *France and the Cult*, 43.

the Sacred Heart was renewed with Marseille's *Grandes-Maries de la Visitation* in attendance.[116] By September 27, 1722, a *Te Deum* (hymn of praise) was sung, followed by an evening procession in recognition of the Sacred Heart for ending the plague. To many, it appeared that because the people prayed, the plague finally ceased: "Pro populo deprecatus est et plaga cessavit."[117]

The apparent success of these acts of consecration and contrition from 1720 to 1722 served to strengthen the celebration of the *Fête du Sacré-Cœur* in all of France well into the twentieth century. As historian Raymond Jonas observed:

Marseille and Belsunce appeared in sermons and print literature before and after the wars of 1870–71 and of 1914–18, by which time "Marseille at the time of the plague" could serve as an analogy for France in peril. The episodes of 1720 and 1722 were cited not only as examples of remarkable faith in desperate times but also as part of a pattern of divine appeals to France as a nation.[118]

Yet, religious acts of devotion during the Plague of Provence were not only organized in France but across Europe and the overseas colonies, where local ecclesiastical authorities wrote sermons and organized public fasts and processions to prevent the plague from spreading into their respective regions.

...

How did *secular* authorities respond to the crisis, however? How did the management of the Provençal plague unfold, and how was it different from that of past public health disasters? Despite the persistence of ancient understandings of disease and contagion in the eighteenth century and, as I discuss in the next section, the use of age-old measures to contain the epidemic – quarantines, sanitary lines, fumigations, and perfumings with herbs, vinegar, smoke, and other substances believed to serve as disinfectants, as well as religious acts such as prayer, processions, public fasts, and so on – the 1720 plague

[116] Jonas, *France and the Cult*, 43–4. Bérenger, *Journal du maitre d'hotel*, 19, Delta 150, ADBRM.
[117] Num. 16:48, VUL.
[118] Jonas, *France and the Cult*, 53.

marked a break from tradition in significant ways.[119] It represents a major moment in the history of centralized disaster management – a case of disaster centralism – in which efforts to suppress the spread of plague stemmed not from local, municipal governments, as was most typically the case prior to the eighteenth century, but from the capitals of the emerging nation states of Europe. In France, the government in Paris stepped in to direct local responses and mitigate the disaster after the perceived failings of municipal authorities in Marseille. Ultimately, the Plague of Provence represents both the last chapter in the book of medieval plagues and the first chapter in the book of modern disease outbreaks.

Crisis Management and "Disaster Centralism" during the Plague of Provence

The management of the 1720 epidemic was a complex and multifaceted endeavor that came from different levels of administration, touched on all aspects of everyday life, and transformed many Provençal towns into isolated police states. Traditionally in times of emergency, local authorities could wield unlimited powers to preserve order and, in times of plague, to prevent the spread of infection. We see this, for instance, in the 1668 treatise, *Ordres à observer pour empescher que la peste ne se communique hors les lieux infectez*, which granted to municipal officials the authority to do whatever necessary to prevent

---

[119] Beginning most notably with Hippocrates (460–377 BCE), and later, Galen (129–216 CE), and lasting until the late nineteenth century when miasmatic explanations of disease etiology were slowly replaced by germ theory, illness was generally understood to result from the presence of miasmas, or disease-causing foul odors or noxious vapors in the air, that threw off the balance of the four humors (or fluids) believed to determine all aspects of a person's health and personality. In humoral theory, then, the cause of disease was not understood as external to the body, like a virus or a bacterium, but as a state of humoral imbalance. For this reason, treatments or regimens would often emphasize the elimination of these corrupt vapors (e.g. by firing canons in times of plague) and the balancing of the humors through practices including bloodletting, purging (e.g. by inducing emesis or employing enemas), as well as the practice of prayer, and/or the use of stones, talismans, minerals, and brews or concoctions. Such understandings and practices persisted in Europe, largely unchanged, for centuries.

wrongdoing and to punish violators with death.[120] To some extent, this was also the case during the 1720 epidemic in southern France when municipal officials worked with representatives from the capital to manage the public health crisis. In fact, plague management during the outbreak of 1720–22 offered a nod to centuries-old standard practices in many ways. To prevent the transmission of plague to other parts of France, authorities issued strict quarantines, utilized (and, in some cases, constructed) lazarets, and employed sanitary cordons. They heavily restricted travel and regulated all movement, issuing curfews and requiring certificates of health for mobility. Smuggling practices also came under tighter scrutiny and control. Officials saw to it that food was distributed, that merchandise and other properties suspected of infection were burned, and that dogs and cats were slaughtered (in this way eliminating the rat's prominent predators, although rats, too, were to be killed if encountered).[121] Streets, homes, and merchandise likewise underwent ritual disinfections, the details of which were printed in the newspapers of cities all over Europe, including London, Amsterdam, Madrid, and others.[122] Authorities also closed or regulated markets, inns, and houses of ill repute in infected areas, and drove from the city "foreign soldiers, prostitutes, vagabonds, and

---

[120] Takeda, *Between Crown and Commerce*, 134.

[121] Jean-Jacques Manget, *Traité de la peste, et de moyens de s'en preserver*, vol. premier (Lyon: les freres Bruyset, 1722), 150.

[122] "Paris, October 1: Directions for the Precautions to be observ'd in the Provinces where there are Places infected with the Plague, and in the neighbouring Provinces, have been printed here by Royal Authority," *Evening Post* (London), September 25–28, 1721, issue 1898. "Paris, October 1: The following Directions for the Precautions to be observ'd in the Provinces where there are Places infected with the Plague ...," *Daily Courant* (London), September 27, 1721, issue 6220.
     In fact, the concept of premodern "healthscaping" highlights the fact that a desire to live in a healthy and safe urban environment was not new in the early modern period. As historian, Guy Geltner, has written, "If we define healthscaping, more broadly than modern health professionals have, as the physical, social, legal, administrative, and political process of providing urban environments with the means to promote residents' health, safety, and wellbeing, it is possible not only to demonstrate its existence as a medieval ideal ... but also to show that it was a common policy that urban governments, courts, guilds, armies, the church, and numerous other groups pursued in practice." Guy Geltner, *Roads to Health: Infrastructure and Urban Wellbeing in Later Medieval Italy* (Philadelphia: University of Pennsylvania Press, 2019), 20.

other useless people."[123] All of this took place during the 1720 plague no less than during previous outbreaks.

What makes the Plague of Provence unique is the degree to which this was all controlled and overseen from Paris, where the regent, previously at Versailles, had moved in 1715. This centralized, concentrated response to the public health crisis from 1720 to 1722 represents an example of what I term disaster centralism. From the capital, the royal government placed its men on the ground, deploying military commanders to infected areas and bestowing them with unlimited authority to manage the crisis. It intensified surveillance and police presence in infected areas; issued curfews and quarantines with directions for carrying them out in all infected towns; regulated all movement and the use of certificates of health; and prohibited movement in and out of Provence with massive military cordons (or guarded sanitary lines). Authorities in the capital also issued trade embargoes; distributed food and aid from the royal treasury; ordered towns and wealthy individuals to send funds or supplies to Provence;[124] issued all necessary *arrêts* (including a comprehensive *arrêt* that restricted all travel to and from affected areas); and, perhaps most notably, created a new *Conseil de la santé* (health council) in Paris, as well as new health bureaus in

---

[123] Manget, *Traité de la peste*, 150.

[124] This news was reported in newspapers across Europe. In October 1720, for example, the *Gazeta de Lisboa* included news of the "socorro & remedios" that the Duke Regent was sending to Marseille, including "a large number of perfumes ... which there are sorely lacking." "França, Pariz, 15 de Setembro," *Gazeta de Lisboa*, October 10, 1720, no. 41, cota F.P. 192, bobine 2, Biblioteca Nacional de Portugal (henceforth BNP). In April 1721, English newspapers, too, reported that, "The Duke Regent ha[d] given orders to Mess[ieurs] Paris [the famous Pâris brothers, financiers] to send two Millions of Livres in Specie into Provence, for the Relief of such places as are yet infected with the Plague; and Directions are likewise given to the Intendents of the neighbouring Provinces, to furnish them with all sorts of Provisions." By June, the Pâris brothers along with Samuel Bernard, who according to Saint-Simon was the richest and most famous financier in Europe, had indeed advanced two million livres "towards the Relief of the miserable Provençals (which Sum is to be repaid them in two year's time)." *London Gazette*, April 4–8, 1721, issue 5944. *Daily Courant* (London), June 1, 1721, issue 6119. The Pâris brothers were: Antoine Pâris, sometimes known as Grand Pâris (b. 1668); Claude Pâris, known as Pâris La Montagne (b. 1670); Joseph Pâris known as Pâris-Duverney (b. 1684); and Jean Pâris known as Pâris-Montmartel (b. 1690).

Provence, through which they demanded to be kept informed of any and all developments throughout the plague years.[125] The Crown was more heavily involved in the management of the 1720 outbreak than ever before, signifying a growing concentration of state oversight that would continue over the eighteenth century and ultimately survive the French Revolution.[126]

In August 1720, the State Council of the King issued one of several comprehensive *arrêts* "au sujet de la maladie contagieuse de la ville de Marseille" ("on the subject of the contagious malady of the city of Marseilles") that suspended all commerce between Marseille and the rest of Provence under pain of death until January 1723 (though it would be eased before then), much to the chagrin of local officials in the south. This decree expanded upon the earlier blockade of Marseille issued on July 31, 1720, by the *parlement* of Aix (not long before the latter was dissolved, as noted earlier, as a result of the outbreak). Through various *arrêts* in August and September, movement out of Provence beyond the natural boundaries of the rivers Rhône, Verdon, and Durance was severely restricted through the use of strict quarantines and health certificates (*certificats de santé*) and was enforced through the use of *cordons sanitaires* (guarded sanitary lines that served as barriers).[127] These military cordons involved not only city bourgeois militias and provincial levies, but also one quarter of the regular army.[128]

Although such regulations could be vulnerable to bribery and other violations, the sanitary lines were strictly regulated, and the restriction of movement severely enforced. Ordinances from the royal

---

[125] Takeda, *Between Crown and Commerce*, 127.

[126] Hildesheimer, *Le Bureau de la santé*, 156. Takeda, *Between Crown and Commerce*, 124.

[127] "Some troops are ordered towards Marseilles to hinder all communication between the infected places and the rest of the country." Mr. Pulteney to Secretary Craggs, Paris, August 27, 1720, SP 78/166, France, TNA.

[128] In his *Livre de raison*, Isnard mentions the troops sent by the king. "Livre de raison de moy, Claude Isnard, hebdomadier à Saint Agricol et prieur de Roquemartine," 24 E 11, 35–6, ADBRM.

   Eventually, the infection made it to the soldiers of the sanitary lines themselves, causing panic in nearby areas. See: Consul George Henshaw to John Carteret, secretary of state, Genoa, September 9, 1721, SP 79/13, Genoa, TNA.

government in September laid out how troops guarding the lines should behave and emphasized that no persons whatsoever were "to stir out of the said places under pain of death."[129] Even in cases where higher profile officials wished to cross the sanitary lines, the regent Philippe d'Orléans himself might step in to prevent it. Such was the case of one Sir Thomas Tipping (2nd baronet) – a young man who hoped to pass out of Provence into Languedoc with his tutor and servants in November 1720. Cardinal Dubois (the archbishop of Cambrai) and English diplomat Sir Robert Sutton petitioned the regent on Tipping's behalf, but d'Orléans refused to make an exception. As Sutton related:

I have renewed the instances which I formerly made [o]n behalf of Sir Thomas Tipping, but that gentleman being unfortunately shut up within the lines, the Regent cannot be prevailed on to make in his favour an exception to a rule hitherto very strictly observed, by granting him leave to remove into Languedoc after the performance of a quarantaine. His Royal Highness says he will not take upon himself a thing which he cannot justify, and that he is very confident the province of Languedoc would absolutely refuse to receive [him anyway].[130]

One contemporary source reported in his diary years later that whatever the "great ravages" caused by the epidemic, things would have been much worse had the royal government not put all precautions in place, "[For] the King even sent troops to surround each location that was infected and prevent any communications."[131] In fact, about half the total correspondence from 1720 to 1723 of Claude Le Blanc, the *Secrétaire d'État de la Guerre* (minister of war) during much of

---

[129] "An ordinance of the King containing 16 pages is under the press regulating the manner in which the troops that guard the passages of the infected places are to behave themselves and prohibits all persons whatsoever to stir out of the said places under pain of death." Robert Sutton to Mr. Tichell, Paris, September 10, 1721, SP 78/170, France, TNA.

[130] "The Archbishop of Cambray [Cardinal Dubois (1720–3), minister to Louis XV] cannot yet tell whether the Duke Regent will grant the favour, that Sir Thomas Tipping with his Governour and Servants may after performing a quarantaine pass out of Provence into Languedoc." Sutton to Secretary Craggs, Paris, November 29, 1720, SP 78/169, France, TNA. Also: Sutton to Secretary Craggs, Paris, November 11, 1720, SP 78/169, France, TNA.

[131] "Livre de raison de moy, Claude Isnard, hebdomadier à Saint Agricol et prieur de Roquemartine," 24 E 11, 35-6, ADBRM.

the Regency, concerned this plague barrier.[132] To this day, one can still see parts of the *mur de la peste*, or plague wall, that was erected in the Vaucluse department of Provence, where some of these military *cordons sanitaires* once stood.[133]

On September 5, 1720, the Crown appointed Charles Claude Andrault de Langeron, *maréchal* in the king's army (*Chef d'escadre des galères et maréchal des camps et armées du Roy*), as commander in chief (*commandant en chef*) of the city of Marseille and its territory.[134] While facing opposition from the local *échevins*, who resented what they perceived to be an overreach of the centralized government in violation of Marseille's local liberties, Langeron was nevertheless responsible for overseeing the massive endeavor of municipal plague management on behalf of the king.[135] Under his direction, for example, food and aid were distributed;[136] street animals were slaughtered; cannons were fired often (to dispel miasmas);[137] merchandise and other properties suspected of infection were regularly burned; and streets, merchandise, and residences regularly underwent disinfections

---

[132] Panzac, *Quarantaines et lazarets*, 60f. Brockliss and Jones, *The Medical World*, 352. Takeda, *Between Crown and Commerce*, 214.

[133] Between March and August 1721, a wall was built from Bonpas on the Durance to Sisteron. It was 100 km long, 2 m high and was preceded by a 2 m wide ditch. Monique Lucenet, "La peste, fléau majeur," Bibliothèques d'Université de Paris, www.biusante.parisdescartes.fr/histoire/medica/presentations/peste.php.

[134] Biraben, *Les hommes ...* vol. 1, 238. This appointment was officially announced to the local *échevins* on September 12, 1720.

[135] Takeda, *Between Crown and Commerce*, 153–7; Ermus, "Memory and the Representation of Public Health Crises," 780–1.

[136] A 1720 *memoire* from Saint-Rémy-de-Provence instructed the *Capitaines des Quartiers* to see to it that local bakers bake enough bread for the "one hundred homes that compose their *quartier*." Butchers, too, were to prepare enough meat ("cut it into chunks of one, two, and three pounds") for each captain's *quartier*. To receive these items, people were to appear at their windows and lower a basket on either a rope or a pole ("corde d'auffe ou de jonc d'Alicane"). The same *memoire* also ordered the slaughtering of cats and dogs, among other things. "Memoire Pour parvenir à l'execution de l'Ordonnance rendüe par M. le Premier President, le premier Novembre 1720 pour les Lieux attaqués de maladies," *Santé publique, Police sanitaire maritime, Peste de Marseille, 1720–1721*, November 2, 1720, G13, Archives historiques de la Chambre de Commerce et d'Industrie Marseille-Provence (henceforward ACCIM).

[137] *Daily Courant* (London), November 2, 1720, issue 5939.

and perfumings with vinegar or herbs including rosemary, thyme, and lavender.[138] Working with local authorities, Langeron also designated prayer days and organized religious processions; axed social events of all kinds; regulated local markets, taverns, and inns; and shuttered brothels in infected areas. The regent in Paris even sent orders to permanently banish out of Marseille all orders of monks who failed to attend the sick and offer the last rites.[139] Essentially, Langeron was charged with executing martial law, with absolute power in matters pertaining to the policing and administration of the city.[140] In September 1720, Sir Robert Sutton wrote from Paris, "They write from Marseilles that Monsieur de Langeron, commandant of that place, continues to take all possible precautions to prevent the spreading of the plague, as well by causing the dead bodies to be burned [and] by daily watering the streets which is found to be of great service."[141]

Crown control was further expressed through the creation of new *bureaux* of health in Provence, and most notably, in the spring of 1721 a new *Conseil de la santé* or Council of Health in Paris. The *Conseil* was to meet twice a week at the Louvre and consisted "of the Princes of the Blood, the Chancellour, the Marshal de Villeroy, the Comptroller General, the Secretaries of the State, and the King's First Physician, before whom all the Letters relating to the infected or suspected places are to be laid, [so] they [could] give the necessary Directions upon them."[142] Both new and previously established health bureaus in Provence were now to operate under the *Conseil* in the capital. This council was to keep careful record of, and control over, all aspects of crisis management in southern France during the plague,

---

[138] "Paris, October 1: Directions for the Precautions to be observ'd in the Provinces where there are Places infected with the Plague, and in the neighbouring Provinces, have been printed here by Royal Authority, the Substance of which is as follows," *Evening Post* (London), September 25–28, 1721, issue 1898.

[139] "The plague carries off great numbers of people at Marseilles; the Regent has sent orders to banish out of that city forever such of the orders of monks there who decline to attend the people on this occasion; the Capucins, the Jesuits, and the Recolets have not failed in their duty." Mr. Pulteney to Secretary Craggs, September 3, 1720, SP 78/166, France, TNA.

[140] Takeda, *Between Crown and Commerce*, 140.

[141] "Paris Circular," September 21, 1720, SP 78/166, France, TNA.

[142] *London Gazette*, May 20–23, 1721, issue 5957.

directing, for example, the distribution of aid from the royal treasury, the quarantining of infected towns, and the measures to be taken in cities suspected of plague.

Together, Langeron and the *Conseil* served as integral links in a tight network that connected southeastern France with the capital and allowed for centralized management and supervision.[143] Moreover, the absence of the *parlement* at Aix and the temporary closure of institutions such as the Chamber of Commerce in Marseille served to *further* augment the administrative powers of the central government. This kind of central oversight, involving regular communication between officials in the capital and those in the provinces, represents an essential element of disaster centralism. The communication of information was brought under increased royal regulation during the outbreak, as all individual *bureaux de la santé* in Provence were ordered to submit monthly registers to Paris. These consisted of information on a variety of health-related points and included such details as the number of staff employed at hospitals to dispose of bodies, updated mortality rates and number of patients, and the number and quality of beds, sheets, drugs, aromatics, provisions, and personnel – both religious and secular – available at each hospital.[144] Essentially, practices that previously rested in the hands of municipal officials were now controlled and overseen by the central government and its newly established *Conseil de la santé* in Paris.

...

Restrictions during the Plague of Provence caused significant interruptions in Mediterranean, Atlantic, and even Pacific trade networks, affecting ports from the Americas, to Europe, to the Spanish Philippines. The major port city of Marseille, like other ports in Provence and Languedoc, was bereft of the commerce and industry that represented its very lifeblood. As one account described it:

---

[143] *Because* they facilitated centralized management of the public health crisis, it is not these representatives of Paris who have been celebrated as the heroes of the 1720 plague, but local figures, such as the chevalier Nicolas Roze and Bishop Belsunce, both of whom have been memorialized in artwork, statues, literature, sermons, and even street names that commemorate the Plague of Provence. For more on this topic, see: Ermus, "Memory and the Representation of Public Health Crises."

[144] Takeda, *Between Crown and Commerce*, 143 & 127.

This commerce, which flourished such that it spread the name of the city [of Marseille] to all parts of the world and distinguished it from many other cities, was suddenly prohibited. All manufacturing ceased, as did the expedition of vessels to the port, so that all of those who worked in trade, as well as the artisans, were left without work.[145]

As the infection progressed, the situation only worsened until it seemed that all hope was lost. Any optimism that may have reigned in 1720 – when Marseillais officials wrote letters to the capital reporting that the worst was over – was temporarily lost as appearances of the plague persisted through early fall 1722. In January 1721, the *échevins* and deputies of Marseille, who only months earlier denied that plague was in Marseille, wrote: "The contagion has caused the loss of half the population of Marseille. It has proven to be the ruin of all the families, and has destroyed all industry by taking its laborers."[146] They went on to describe the partly raised buildings, homes, ships, and other structures around the port city that were abandoned mid-construction owing to a lack of funding and workers, and which now represented only sad reminders of the wealth and industry that months earlier characterized Marseille. "In such a sad situation, our neighbors have abandoned us, foreigners have distanced themselves from us, along with all the backing and support that was once ours."[147]

Without its commerce, officials argued, Marseille was lost. In July Langeron and the *échevins* of the city wrote:

Ever since this city has found itself blocked off as a result of the contagion that continues again in various places in this province, and since our foreign neighbors have refused us all commerce and have been unwilling to com-

---

[145] "Le commerce si florissant qui en a répandu le nom dans toutes les parties du monde et qui la distinguait de tant d'autres villes fut tout á coup interdit. Toutes les manufactures cessèrent de même que les expéditions des vaisseaux, de sorte que généralement tous les ouvriers occupés pour le négoce aussi bien que les artisans manquèrent de travail." "Relation de ce qui s'est passé à Marseille pendant la peste de 1720 de son principe ...," IV, 1F 80/39, ADBRM.

[146] "La contagion a fait perir presque la moitié des habitans de Marseille, elle y a ruyné toutes les familles, et detruit l'industrie, par la mortalité des ouvriers." "Les échevins et deputez du commerce de la Ville de Marseille à Monseigneur Le Duc D'Orléans," *Chambre du Commerce de Marseille, 1721–1722*, January 19, 1721, f. 3, AE BIII 42, AN.

[147] Ibid., f. 3v.

municate with us in any way, our traders have had no way of acquiring as in other times the piasters, pistoles, and other specie as well as gold or silver materials that they otherwise acquire with great ease in their trade, such that these very materials have been rendered a great rarity in this city.[148]

Letters from Marseillais officials are rife with complaints about the commercial restrictions and with appeals for them to be lifted. In a letter dated September 26, 1721, for example, the health officials (*intendants de la santé*) in Marseille maintained that the health of the realm depended on the restoration of trade relations with the Levant and Barbarie through the port of Marseille.[149] Within the city, the people suffered not only from plague and rampant crime, but from famine as well. "Il est notoriété publique que le défaut de subsistance a Marseille y a decuplé de mal de la contagion, dans les commencement," wrote one M. Niquet in 1721.[150]

Despite the plague's immediate blow to the Provençal economy and population numbers, however, the region, most notably its principal port of Marseille, was to recover its pre-plague population and surpass its former commercial eminence relatively quickly after the epidemic finally ceased. Local merchants and other officials lobbied to reopen commercial relations between Marseille and the rest of the Mediterranean. Demands to reestablish trade "as it was prior to the outbreak" began well before the end of plague in 1722, and eventually succeeded.[151] In January and February 1723, the French Crown

---

[148] "Depuis le temps que cette ville se trouve comme bloquée à cause de la contagion qui subsiste encore à quelques endroits de cette Province, et que les etrangers nos voisins ont refusé tout commerce et n'ont voulu avoir aucune communication avec nous, les negocians n'en ont pû tirer comme autres fois les piastres, pistolles [Spanish gold coin] et autres especes et matieres d'or et d'argent dont ils procuroient icy l'abondance par leur commerce, ce qui à rendu ces memes especes d'une grande rareté en cette ville." July 30, 1721, f. 191, FF 182, AMM.

[149] "M. les Intendants de la Santé de Marseille," September 26, 1721, f. 206, MAR B3 275, AN.

[150] "Sur la contagion de Provence," 1721, f. 244, MAR B3 275, AN.

[151] For example: "La chambre du commerce de Marseille demandent dans le mois d'octobre 1721 qu'il feut permis aux negocians de la dit ville d'envoyer aux ports de Ponant des marchandises non-susceptibles; elle fit voir en quoy elles concistoient qu'il ny avoit point de danger a le recevoir ... L'on se soumit des lors a telle quarantaine et a toutes les precautions que les magistrats des villes maritimes de Ponant voudroient etablir en admetant les batiments qui

marked the end of plague with *Te Deums* of deliverance.[152] Soon thereafter, Marseille reassumed its advantaged position as the capital of trade with the Levant.[153]

Yet, the Plague of Provence remains one of the most commemorated disasters in history. The epidemic has been memorialized through the construction of churches (the *Basilique du Sacré-Cœur de Marseille* was consecrated in 1947 in commemoration of the 1720 plague), the designation of street names (such as Cours Belsunce in Marseille), artworks in various mediums (paintings, statues, stained glass windows), monuments, plays, poems, and sermons. It also had a major impact on contemporary debates about the nature of contagion and would be continually referenced in the relevant literature into the twentieth century.[154] While it raged, it was among the foremost topics of concern in the contemporary record. Newspapers, government correspondence,

---

y porteroient ces marchandises. Il feut de montré combien il etoit necessaire que le Royaume feut secour et de qu'elle [ill.] c'etoit de retablir un commerce dans les etrangers s'etoient emparez au prejudice des sujets du Roy, ~~puis quil est assuré que tant que le pretexte de la contagion subsistera ces nations fairont non seulement~~ [*sic*] … Le fondement de la demande des negociants de Marseille estoit bien etabli. La peste y a cessé depuis environ une année, il ny a eu des ecoulemens de ce mal que jusques au mois de May 1721." It is worth noting the line that was struck out here, since French accusations that foreign nations were using the plague as a pretext for embargoes against France are ubiquitous in contemporary documents, especially those related to Spain. "Memoire pour etablir la necessité qu'il y a de rendre libre commerce de Marseille comme il l'etant avant la contagion," *Santé publique, Police sanitaire maritime, Peste de Marseille, 1722–1723,* January 10, 1722, G14, ACCIM. (Note: I have chosen to write out the abbreviations in this transcription.)

152   *Te Deums* in praise of God for ending the plague were sung across Europe. In Rome, for example, the Pope led a *Te Deum* on January 1, 1723. Mariano Peset, Pilar Mancebo, and José L. Peset, "Temores y defensa de España frente a la peste de Marsella de 1720," *Asclepio: Archivo Iberoamericano de Historia de la Medicina y Antropología Médica* 23 (1971): 138.

153   As one document from 1731 reads, "Le commerce du Levant êtant privatif et reüny dans la seule ville de Marseille." "Sur la question d'établir à Cadix une chambre pour diriger le Commerce que nous faisons en Espagne à l'Instar de la chambre de Marseille qui est chargée de la direction du Commerce du Levant," 1731, MAR B7 310, AN.

154   For more on this debate, see Chapter 3 on London. For an overview of the debate as it unfolded in France, see chapter 9 in Margaret DeLacy, *The Germ of an Idea: Contagionism, Religion, and Society in Britain, 1660–1730* (London: Palgrave Macmillan, 2016).

consular communications, personal letters, sermons, and diaries and memoirs across Europe and the overseas colonies all told of the hell that descended upon Marseille, Toulon, Avignon, Arles, Aix-en-Provence, and other areas of southern France, and all serve as testament to the disaster's significance. As evidenced in the chapters that follow, its influence was felt across geographic space, and its legacy stretched across decades, well beyond the plague years.

2 | *"L'état le Plus Exposé"*
The Plague of Provence in Genoa and Italy

If the efforts of the Political Government can keep the horrible evil [of plague] far from a Land and City, the significance is clear: those Leaders of the people who neglect these [measures] or who do not have them executed upon suspicion of plague will be worthy of great reproach among the people, and will have to account to God for their destructive negligence at a time of such great need for the people given to their care by divine Providence.[1]

Trade is such a universal good and of such a delicate nature, that is it absolutely necessary to nourish it with the greatest attention, and not to expose it to the slightest difficulty, [for] it thrives where it finds more freedom and flees subjection and oppression.[2]

In a letter to the secretary of state in July 1721, the British consul in Lisbon, Thomas Burnett, reported that, "All ships from Levant are obliged to perform their quarantine at Cádiz, unless it be those from Genoa, which are immediately admitted, on pretense of the great care taken by that state."[3] Some weeks earlier, John Molesworth, the British envoy in Turin wrote, "Thank God that pernicious distemper has hitherto exerted its violence at some distance from this country; tho' it has shown itself at Hyères ... the great caution and vigilance of this

---

[1] Lodovico Antonio Muratori, *Del governo della peste, e delle manière di guardarsene* (Modena: Bartolomeo Soliani Stamperia Ducale, 1714), 17. This text was later republished during the plague outbreaks of Provence and Messina (i.e. 1720, 1721, 1722, and 1743).

[2] Elizeus Burges, minister resident of Great Britain in Venice, to the Doge and Council, Venice, December 5, 1720, SP 99/62, Venice, 555, TNA.

[3] Thomas Burnett (sometimes Burnet), British consul in Lisbon, to the secretaries of state, Lisbon, July 12, 1721, SP 89/29, Portugal, f. 118, TNA.

king makes us very easy."[4] A few months later, Colonel Elizeus Burges reported of the Venetians, "[I] hope I shall be able ... to send you the account you desire, relating to the precautions [Venice] uses and the care it takes to prevent any contagion coming into its dominions. It is thought no people are more upon their guard, or understand that matter better than the Venetians do, and it is generally said the plague never came into this city from the sea."[5] Such passages by British consuls and diplomats residing in Italy are not uncommon, nor were these emissaries alone in their approval of Italian responses to the threat of plague from Provence.

For centuries, European states had looked to Italian health regulations as models for their own sanitary policies, particularly during public health crises, and the Plague of Provence was no exception.[6] Various Spanish documents, for example, suggest that officials were

---

[4] John Molesworth, British envoy extraordinary to Sardinia, to John Carteret, secretary of state, Turin, June 28, 1721, SP 92/30, Savoy and Sardinia, TNA. The king at this time was Victor Amadeus II. He was duke of Savoy from 1675 to 1730 with its capital at Turin, and king of Sicily from 1713 to 1720. When the Austrian Habsburgs obliged Victor Amadeus to exchange Sicily for Sardinia in 1720, he became king of Sardinia until his abdication in 1730. Turin remained the capital until 1798.

[5] Elizeus Burges, minister resident of Great Britain in Venice, to the secretaries of state, Venice, November 7, 1721, SP 99/62, Venice, f. 636, TNA.

[6] "The [Italian] peninsula was in fact at the forefront in Europe for the organization of preventive tools and control structures aimed at stemming the spread of the 'pestifero morbo [pestiferous disease].'" Danilo Pedemonte, "La 'pubblica salute' dello Stato genovese: il Magistrato di sanità della Repubblica come strumento di governo delle informazioni, controllo del territorio e politica economica," in *La quotidiana emergenza: I molteplici impieghi delle istituzioni sanitarie nel Mediterraneo moderno*, edited by Paolo Calcagno and Daniele Palermo (Palermo: New Digital Frontiers, 2017), 99. Also, John Henderson, *Florence Under Siege: Surviving Plague in an Early Modern City* (New Haven: Yale University Press, 2019), 3–4. It is important to note, however, that public health measures did vary across Italy. As historian John Henderson has noted, "It is ... a mistake to treat the whole of Italy as conforming to the same pattern in the development of public health measures. The models of cities such as Milan, Venice, and Genoa, with their permanent health boards and Lazaretti, have tended to dominate the historiography. Other cities often adopted more ad hoc measures or established them much later. Many created temporary Lazaretti in reaction to a particular plague epidemic, and some only gradually established permanent health boards in the later 16th century, as in the case of Turin in 1576." John Henderson, "The Invisible Enemy: Fighting the Plague in Early Modern Italy," *Centaurus* 62, no. 2 (May 2020): 266.

paying close attention to Italian reactions during the epidemic in France and were adopting many of the same practices. One from 1720 reads, "The practices, in compliance with these orders on vessel inspections, are in line with what is executed in ports of Italy."[7] Another from Barcelona offers further insight: "It is essential to proceed with the greatest precautions, because if it is deemed that these are loosened, Italy will take away their trade, as Genoa has already done with Sardinia."[8] In fact, we see this mounting interest in Italian public health measures not only during the Plague of Provence, but any time epidemic disease, especially plague, emerged in Europe. During the 1743 Plague of Messina, for example, the comte de Maurepas wrote the intendants of health in Marseille: "The Prince d'Ardore, *Ambassadeur du Roy des Deux-Siciles*, has sent me a copy of an ordinance that his court has just issued concerning the epidemic diseases that reign in Messina. I am sending it to you so that you can make use of [its] provisions ... in the deliberations you might take on occasion of these diseases."[9] These passages suggest that officials across Europe were interested in what Italian cities were doing to protect their regions. And this should come as no surprise. Italy introduced the world's first forty-day quarantine or *quarantena*,[10]

---

[7] "Lo que se practica en cumplimiento de estas ordenes en punto de visitas de embarcaciones segun lo que se executa en puertos de Italia," *Cavildos del año de 1720*, libro no. 76, f. 403v, Actas Capitulares (henceforward AC), Archivo Municipal de Cádiz (henceforward AMC). As we will see in Chapter 4 on Cádiz, vessel searches were highly controversial and roused strong opposition from foreign representatives.

[8] Don Francisco de Quesada to Marqués de Grimaldo, secretary of state, Barcelona, September 21, 1720, Estado 506, AHN. Yet another reads: "De Genova escriven amenazando a esta capital con la prohibicion del comercio, sino se guardase exactamente de tenerle con Marsella." Barcelona, September 2, 1720, Estado 506, AHN.

[9] Jean-Frédéric Phélypeaux, comte de Maurepas, to the Intendant de la Santé de Marseille, Versailles, July 10, 1743, 200 E 287, ADBRM.

[10] Dubrovnik, once known as Ragusa, may have been first to develop the concept of quarantine legislation in 1377, including a temporary plague hospital and a health office, some twenty years after its independence from the Republic of Venice. It was in Venice, however, that we saw the implementation of the *quarantena* as such (meaning forty days), and the world's first permanent lazaretto, the *lazzaretto vecchio*. See: Zlata Blažina Tomić and Vesna Blažina, *Expelling the Plague: The Health Office and the Implementation of Quarantine in Dubrovnik, 1377–1533* (Montreal: McGill-Queen's University

the first permanent lazaretto,[11] and the world's first health pass for traveling in times of disease.[12] For centuries, Italian cities were at the forefront of public health practices.

Concern for public health, however, was not the only motivation behind certain policies. During plague times, European states – including, and perhaps especially, those of Italy – sometimes imposed regulations to preserve not solely public health but their credibility, reputation, and by extension, commercial relationships. By the eighteenth century, Italian city-states prided themselves on an established public health apparatus – including an assortment of tried-and-true plague-time measures – based on a vast body of knowledge and centuries of experience with epidemic disease. A sense of competition thus existed among them as they sought to safeguard their trade while imposing appropriate safety measures. During the Great Plague Scare of 1720, this manifested itself in a sort of tit-for-tat public health diplomacy that we see also in England and Spain at this time.[13] Despite an absence of plague in Italy, as well as attempts from the mid-seventeenth century to standardize health regulations across the peninsula,[14] city-states nevertheless banned one another, at times preemptively, and at others merely in response to an existing ban. As we will see, they even dispatched representatives to observe and report on

Press, 2015), 106–7, 110; Henderson, *Florence Under Siege*, 9. For more on the forty-day quarantine, see also: Jane L. Stevens Crawshaw, *Plague Hospitals: Public Health for the City in Early Modern Venice* (New York: Routledge, 2016), 7–8. It should be noted, however, that in his book on Dubrovnik in the fourteenth and fifteenth centuries, Bariša Krekić maintained that the Venetians introduced the practice of quarantine earlier, in 1374, and that Dubrovnik then followed in 1377, but as Jane Stevens Crawshaw has observed, "the precise chronology has not been determined." Bariša Krekić, *Dubrovnik in the Fourteenth and Fifteenth Centuries: A City Between East and West* (Norman: University of Oklahoma Press, 1972), 99–101; Stevens Crawshaw, *Plague Hospitals*, 19.

[11] In 1423, the Venetians constructed Italy's first permanent lazaretto on the island of Santa Maria di Nazareth. Many other Italian cities soon followed, including Livorno, Genoa, Naples, and others. Stevens Crawshaw, *Plague Hospitals*, 20; Henderson, *Florence Under Siege*, 9.

[12] Alexandra Bamji, "Health Passes, Print and Public Health in Early Modern Europe," *Social History of Medicine* 32, no. 3 (August 2019): 441–2; Carlo M. Cipolla, *Public Health and the Medical Profession in the Renaissance* (Cambridge: Cambridge University Press, 1976), 29.

[13] See Chapters 3 and 4 of this book, respectively.

[14] Carlo M. Cipolla, *Fighting the Plague in Seventeenth-Century Italy* (Madison: University of Wisconsin Press, 1981), 46.

whether a neighboring state was taking appropriate precautions, lest all communications be cut off.

This chapter will focus on reactions to the Plague of Provence in Italy, paying special attention to the port city of Genoa. The ramifications of the threat of plague in this major seaport will begin to demonstrate the ways in which the plague in France expressed itself in European diplomacy, commerce, and crisis management beyond French boundaries. Owing to its place in the Mediterranean and its own network of information, Genoa was the primary point of entry and the main source for news about the Plague of Provence for other Italian ports.[15] For this same reason, its coasts were considered among the most exposed and, therefore, most vulnerable to infection during the epidemic both by their proximity to, and commercial relations with, Marseille. These two rival port cities maintained important connections via their maritime competition in the Mediterranean, and the Genoese consuls in Provence, especially in Marseille and Toulon, kept Genoa, and by extension much of Europe and the colonies, apprised of affairs in Marseille during the epidemic. The Republic of Genoa also maintained important relationships with some of the other port cities examined in this book, namely London and Cádiz. For example, the Genoese represented one of the largest merchant groups in Cádiz, second only to those of France, and their strong links with Spain and the Spanish Empire in the early modern period has been documented by historians such as Catia Brilli and Céline Dauverd.[16] The English, meanwhile, valued their commercial relationships with the Italians, and maintained strong interstate relations with cities including Genoa, Venice, and Livorno. Like so many other consuls and diplomats cited in this book, those of Britain in Genoa are among the most valuable sources for a transnational study on the public health crisis of 1720–22. Essentially, wherever one looks across contemporary records on the Plague of Provence – be it in the archives of Spain, France, the UK, or elsewhere in Italy – Genoa makes a regular appearance.

The chapter opens with a brief look at the history of Genoa, paying special attention to the consolidation and centralization of Italian

---

[15] Filippini, *Il Porto di Livorno e la Toscana*, 167.

[16] See: Catia Brilli, *Genoese Trade and Migration in the Spanish Atlantic, 1700–1830* (Cambridge: Cambridge University Press, 2016); Céline Dauverd, *Imperial Ambition in the Early Modern Mediterranean: Genoese Merchants and the Spanish Crown* (New York: Cambridge University Press, 2015).

and Genoese public health management throughout the early modern period. In this way, it sheds light on the origins in Italy of disaster centralism – or statist, centralized approaches to the management of disasters – which characterized reactions to the Plague of Provence across Europe. The chapter then describes the arrival of news in Genoa about the outbreak in France. Word about the plague did not begin to arrive in the capitals and port cities of Europe until late July, when a rapid spread of infections meant that the growing crisis could no longer be concealed. Denials that the disease was plague during the first crucial weeks and months of the outbreak gave way to claims over the next two years that the epidemic had ended when it in fact had not. This section, titled "Conflicting Narratives and the Invisible Commonwealth: How News of Plague Was Received in Genoa and Europe," explores implications beyond France of the campaign of misinformation that authorities in Marseille undertook to protect the commerce of the ancient port city. The chapter moves on to responses to the threat of infection from France in Genoa and Italy. One of the key underlying arguments in this book is that reactions to the Provençal plague, or any disaster, should not be considered in isolation. Officials across Europe at this time closely monitored all measures put in place in neighboring states, which served to influence how they would proceed at home. This was perhaps especially the case in parts of Italy where responses to the Great Plague Scare at times turned retaliatory. Letters from Genoa, Florence, Milan, Pisa, Venice, Rome, Lucca, Naples, Livorno, Ferrara, Urbino, Mantua, Ancona, Palermo, Messina, and others described local anxieties about the plague, as well as measures taken on the ground often modeled after, or in response to, those of other Italian cities. Central in this chapter, then, are some of the dynamics that influenced public health policy in early-eighteenth-century Italy and Europe.

Public Health Organization and the *Magistrato di sanità* in Genoa

In his book *The Voyage of Italy* (1670), Richard Lassels, Roman Catholic priest, and proponent of the Grand Tour,[17] wrote: "Genoa is one of the chief towns that stand upon the Mediterranean Sea, and one of the

---

[17] Lassels (c. 1603–68) has been credited with coining the phrase and helping to popularize the Grand Tour. Most popular in the seventeenth and eighteenth centuries, this was an educational journey, sometimes with a tutor, that

best in Italy. The common Italian proverb calls it, *Genua la Superba*: and if ever I saw a town with its Holy-day Clothes alwayes on, it was Genoa."[18] Despite a series of wars with Venice over the thirteenth and fourteenth centuries, numerous regime changes between 1300 and 1528, and sporadic encounters with plague beginning with the arrival of the Black Death in northern Italy in 1347, the Republic of Genoa, or *la Serenissima Repubblica di Genova*, was one of the foremost commercial powers and financial centers in the medieval and early modern Mediterranean world. In 1407, it even founded what would become one of Italy's "most stable and trusted public financial institutions," the *Casa di San Giorgio* (Bank of Saint George), which eventually helped administer some of Genoa's Black Sea and Mediterranean colonies in the east.[19] By the late fifteenth century, Genoese financiers were lending money to the monarchs of both France and Spain.[20] The Genoese Golden Age was not to last, however, and by the time Lassels took any of his documented voyages through Italy in the seventeenth century, the republic was in the midst of relative decline. With a dwindling fleet and a shrinking economy (compared with earlier centuries), its influence began to wane, while that of the larger European powers of Great Britain and France rapidly grew, above all after the Peace of Utrecht, which ended the War of the Spanish Succession (1701–14).[21]

aristocratic young men, and some women, took through parts of Europe, especially France and Italy, as a means of rounding out their education. Rosemary Sweet, *Cities and the Grand Tour: The British in Italy, c.1690–1820* (Cambridge: Cambridge University Press, 2012), 2, 23. See also: Jeremy Black, *The British Abroad: The Grand Tour in The Eighteenth Century* (Stroud: Sutton, 2003).

[18] Richard Lassels, *The Voyage of Italy, or a Compleat Journey Through Italy in Two Parts: With the Characters of the People, and the Description of the Chief Towns, Churches, Monasteries, Tombs, Libraries, Pallaces, Villas, Gardens, Pictures, Statues, and Antiquities: as Also of the Interest, Government, Riches, Force, &c. of All the Princes: With Instructions Concerning Travel* (Paris: Vincent du Moutier, 1670), 82–3.

[19] Thomas Allison Kirk, *Genoa and the Sea: Policy and Power in an Early Modern Maritime Republic, 1559–1684* (Baltimore: Johns Hopkins University Press, 2005), 47, 15; Christine Shaw, "Genoa," in *The Italian Renaissance State*, edited by Andrea Gamberini and Isabella Lazzarini (Cambridge: Cambridge University Press, 2012), 220.

[20] Kirk, *Genoa and the Sea*, 16.

[21] The Peace of Utrecht is discussed in more detail in Chapter 4 on Cádiz. Other Italian states that remained independent at this time include Venice, the Papal States, and the Duchy of Savoy.

Yet the Republic of Genoa was one of the very few entities in Italy
that remained independent after this war, and despite numerous challenges, it was able to adapt to changes in the political and commercial
landscapes of Europe and to maintain an influential position in Italian and European diplomacy and trade. Well into the eighteenth century, then, Genoa maintained its position as one of the most important
ports in the western Mediterranean through its relationships with
other states; its enduring commercial activity, including an extensive
merchant diaspora that extended across the western Mediterranean
and the Atlantic world;[22] its strategic geopolitical position, "essential
for controlling access to northern Italy by either land or sea;"[23] and
its prominent place in a vast network of communication that spanned
Europe and beyond. By the time the Plague of Provence emerged in
France, it also had an established health legislation and public health
structure centered around a *Magistrato di sanità* (Health Magistracy
or Health Office). For much of the late medieval to early modern
period in some Italian city-states, these institutions would serve as
tools and facilitators for the growing role of the emerging state in matters related to public health.[24] By the eighteenth century, centralized
health offices all over Europe, most notably the *Conseil de la santé* in
Paris or the *Junta de Sanidad* in Madrid – both created in response
to the Plague of Provence in 1720 – had become part and parcel of
the centralizing state.[25] As historian Frank Snowden has argued, "The
campaign against plague marked a moment in the emergence of absolutism, and more generally, it promoted an accretion of the power and
legitimation of the modern state."[26]

---

[22] For more on the eighteenth-century trade diaspora of the Genoese, see: Brilli,
Genoese Trade and Migration in the Spanish Atlantic.
[23] Brilli, *Genoese Trade and Migration in the Spanish Atlantic*, 28; Kirk, *Genoa
and the Sea*, 52, 201.
[24] Historian Ann Carmichael has written about the case of Milan by looking
at the role of its *Magistrato di sanità*, specifically its fifteenth-century
mortality registers, in the development of the state. She argues, for example,
that "Milan's mortality registers illustrate both a state interest in plague
surveillance and the recognition of individuals through registration. In their
production we see the state at work." See: Ann G. Carmichael, "Registering
Deaths and Causes of Death in Late Medieval Milan," in *Death in Medieval
Europe: Death Scripted and Death Choreographed*, edited by Joëlle Rollo-
Koster (London: Routledge, 2017), 235.
[25] See Chapters 1 and 4 of this book, respectively.
[26] Snowden, *Epidemics and Society*, 82.

The origins of Genoa's Health Office are unclear. Historian Giovanni Assereto has pointed out that a *magistrato* of health was already being referenced in documents dating to the mid-fifteenth century.[27] As in Venice and Florence, however, it is likely that officers tasked with the conservation of health had been appointed even earlier in response to the arrival of the Black Death in 1347–1351.[28] Nevertheless, it is not until the sixteenth century that we see the creation of a permanent health office in Genoa. In 1501, it was created on an ad hoc basis, and after the "very great and very horrible pestilence" of 1528, a more permanent body was developed with officials who were to be elected annually.[29] By a decree of July 1530, the health office was then given "full civil and criminal jurisdiction, with the right to sentence anyone who defied its orders to the death penalty ('etiam ad ultimum sup-plicium inclusive')."[30] It is from this point forward that we have fairly regular documentation on all matters pertaining to public health in Genoa for the first time.[31]

Over the course of the sixteenth century, all the foremost cities of northern Italy had established one of these permanent public health offices. Over time, they increasingly expanded their control, combining legislative, judicial, and executive powers in issues concerning public health, including, as historian Carlo Cipolla observed, "the recording of deaths, burials, the marketing of food, the sewage system, the disposal of byproducts of various economic activities, the hospitals, the hostelries, prostitution, and so on."[32] In this way, northern Italy – the cities of Venice, Florence, Milan, Genoa, and others – became "the most developed area in Europe in regard to health organization."[33]

---

[27] Giovanni Assereto, *"Per la comune salvezza dal morbo contagioso": I controlli di sanità nella Repubblica di Genova* (Genoa: Città del silenzio, 2011), 15.

[28] Ibid., 16.

[29] As quoted in Assereto, *"Per la comune salvezza …,"* 19. Jane Stevens Crawshaw, "The Places and Spaces of Early Modern Quarantine," in *Quarantine: Local and Global Histories*, edited by Alison Bashford (New York: Palgrave, 2016), 27; Assereto, *"Per la comune salvezza …,"* 19.

[30] Assereto, *"Per la comune salvezza …,"* 19.

[31] Ibid., 20.

[32] Cipolla, *Fighting the Plague*, 3–4. "The minor cities and the rural communities set up health boards only in time of emergency. Both the permanent boards of the major cities and the temporary boards of the minor communities were subordinate and directly answerable to the central health Magistracies of their respective capitals." Cipolla, *Fighting the Plague*, 4.

[33] Ibid., 5.

By the seventeenth century, especially after the plague epidemic of 1656–57, we see a consolidation of health legislation and a more definitive public health structure in Genoa.[34] The Great Plague of 1656 represents the last epidemic of plague in the Republic of Genoa, and one of the last in the Italian states.[35] The outbreak began in southern Italy, where it ravaged Naples and Rome, then arrived by sea in Genoa, where roughly 40–60 percent of the population perished.[36] In one burial site alone, just outside the city gates at Carbonara, as many as 1,000 bodies were buried per day.[37] In the spring of 1657, when it was clear that the plague was in fact worsening (after it had subsided in the winter), officials of the Genoese *Magistrato di sanità* set themselves to consolidating health regulations and tightening the functioning of the *Magistrato*. Strict rules, for example, were applied to prevent the flight of the very officials devising the new rules, who – by virtue of their social standing – were otherwise most likely to flee in times of plague.[38] Officials soon laid out many of the new protocols in a set of guidelines titled, "Instruzione, ed ordini per la sanità da osservarsi in tutti quei luoghi che anno giurisdizione al mare nell'una e nell'altra riviera della Serenissima Repubblica compreso il regno di Corsica, ed isola di Caprara."[39] First composed in 1661 then reprinted with some additions in

---

[34] Ibid., 40, 144. Pastore, *Crimine e giustizia in tempo di peste*, 180.

[35] The Messina Plague of 1743–4 in Sicily was the last great outbreak of plague in Western Europe.

[36] As is so often the case with disasters, especially epidemics and pandemics, the number of dead varies wildly. Some estimate that nearly half of the population perished, while others – including contemporary sources (which are sometimes inflated) – estimate that 60 percent of the population died of plague. See, for example: Henderson, *Florence Under Siege*, 23; Stevens Crawshaw, "The Places and Spaces …," 19; Kirk, *Genoa and the Sea*, 144, 176; Paul Slack, "Responses to Plague in Early Modern Europe: The Implications of Public Health," *Social Research: An International Quarterly* 87, no. 2 (Summer 2020): 410.

[37] Stevens Crawshaw, "The Places and Spaces …," 24–5.

[38] For more on some of the regulations laid out at this time, see: Assereto, "*Per la comune salvezza …*," 140–2, 48–51.

[39] "Instructions, and orders pertaining to [public] health to be observed in all those places that have jurisdiction over the sea in either riviera [or coast] of the Most Serene Republic [of Genoa] including the Kingdom of Corsica, and the island of Caprara." The full document of the *Conservatori di Sanità della Serenissima Repubblica di Genova* is published in its 1753 form in appendix 2 of Assereto, "*Per la comune salvezza …*," 167–75.

1753, the document sought to regulate issues pertaining primarily to the election and authority of health officers, and the handling of vessels that arrive at port, including, among others, the precise line of health-related questioning to be administered, the handling of animals, and the management of disinfections and bills of health.[40]

Over the next several decades, Genoa's public health legislation became increasingly centralized at the state level, and it was not alone. In the sixteenth to eighteenth centuries, public health structures were being strengthened and consolidated across Europe.[41] In some ways, northern Italy was at the forefront. In the mid-seventeenth century, we see a notable attempt to standardize health regulations across the peninsula by forming a convention, or *capitolazione*, of Italian states along the Mediterranean Sea in the name of public health, and Florence – capital of the Grand Duchy of Tuscany – led the way.[42] In 1652, amidst fears that the plague epidemic that had raged in parts of Spain since 1647 could spread to Italy, officials in Florence grappled with the challenges of obtaining accurate information and a lack of cooperation among neighboring states. They realized that in order for preventive public health measures to be effective, neighboring states would need to come together to agree upon, coordinate, and enforce them through common action.[43] Accordingly, the grand duke and his counselors devised a plan wherein Genoa and the Papal States would join Florence in adopting a set of standard health practices – pertaining to the entry of vessels, quarantining, and suspicious merchandise, and including regular communications – in the three main harbors of the Tyrrhenian Sea, namely, Genoa, Civitavecchia, and Livorno.[44]

---

[40] Assereto, "*Per la comune salvezza* …," 167–75. Among the clauses added in 1753 were instructions for the handling of corpses at port, as well as suspicious parcels, such as crates, chests, or barrels.

[41] "Despite differences in local markets and political arrangements, towns and cities across Europe strengthened their hand at plague management, met increased demands for poor relief, and fostered specialized hospital care in the sixteenth and seventeenth centuries." Sharon T. Strocchia, "Introduction: Women and Healthcare in Early Modern Europe," *Renaissance Studies* 28, no. 4 (September 2014): 507.

[42] Cipolla, *Fighting the Plague*, 34.

[43] Ibid.

[44] "To guarantee the observance and enforcement of the measures agreed upon, each state would allow the other two to station one representative of their respective health boards in its main harbor." Cipolla, *Fighting the Plague*, 34.

The plan was soon extended to include Naples, but discussions quickly fell apart, and neither Rome nor Naples ever joined the effort. Arrangements between Florence and Genoa did proceed initially, but the pact was to last only a few short years, from 1652 until 1656, when the arrival of plague in Genoa brought the partnership to an end.[45] Nevertheless, the plan marked an early and significant moment in what Cipolla called "the history of international health cooperation."[46] In his view, it represented "a revolutionary and enlightened idea which, in the interest of 'the common health,' envisaged international controls and the voluntary relinquishment of discretionary powers by fully sovereign states in the matter of public health."[47] Indeed, the proposed convention signifies a growing awareness among administrators at this time about the advantages of a standardized public health apparatus, the role of the state in crisis mitigation, the importance of cooperation between states, and what such collective health security would require. Even if the scheme was not implemented, it points to the more integrated, regulated systems that emerged in Europe by the eighteenth century and that helped pave the way for the disaster centralism of the Plague of Provence.

In the first epigraph to this chapter, written in 1714, Lodovico Antonio Muratori, scholar and librarian to the duke of Modena (at the *Biblioteca Estense*), argued that it was the responsibility of the prince, that is, of the "governo politico," to do everything in their power to defend the people, entrusted to their care by God, against the "orribil male" (horrible evil) of the plague. Failure to do so should call upon the leaders all the wrath of the people and of God for their sheer negligence at a time of such great need.[48] Moreover, he maintained, it is in the interest of both the state and its subjects to protect the populace from plague. Although a great deal of money must be spent "in Lazzeretti and maintenance of the Poor, and care of the sick, and in Guards, and Ministers," when a Plague has come, thousands of useful or necessary people for the republic would otherwise be lost:

---

[45] Ibid., 49.
[46] Ibid.
[47] Ibid., 34.
[48] Muratori, *Del governo della peste*, 17.

This great truth has to be kept in mind of Princes, Magistrates, and private individuals, that is, that there is no expense, nor inconvenience, which could equal the expenses and the terrible inconveniences of a Plague; nor could there be a better use of one's efforts and money than to preserve at once one's health and the lives of the entire Populace ... Whosoever has an understanding of economics, and much more, of Christian Charity, will readily understand the need for these preventive diligences.[49]

For Muratori, there was no question that in times of plague, it was the responsibility of the state to intervene, and failure to do so should invite the indignation of both the people and of God. Later in his book, he stressed:

The greatest good ... that can befall a People during the dangers and peril of a Contagion is to be provided with good Magistrates, who with their vigilance and prudence can arrest the Disease at the borders, or imprison it in some land or portion of the country where it has penetrated, or even to valiantly face it if it has entered the City, so that it soon suffocates and does not cause considerable slaughter. *For the Plague receives no greater strength, nor does it more readily spread, than from the disorders of the multitude when deprived of good leaders and laws* ... The vigilance of the Magistrates, by neglecting nothing ... can perform miracles on all occasions, but especially in this one, because in the end it deals with an Enemy who does not carry fiery artillery in order to forcefully cross the borders of a State, or cross the gates of a City ... Not meekness and pleasantness, but rigor is here necessary from those who govern, and this for the greater good of the Republic itself.[50]

Muratori, like others before him, likened the fight against plague to war.[51] As in warfare, the state must engage the enemy head on and spare no expense. He wrote:

---

[49] Ibid. In 1721, Muratori also published an edited translation with commentary of the *Relation de la peste de Marseille* by the physicians François Chicoyneau, François Verny, and Jean Soulier. Like his *Del governo della peste*, this one would be republished during the plague of Messina in 1743. Lodovico Antonio Muratori, *Relazione della peste di Marsiglia, pubblicata da i medici, che hanno operato in essa, con alcune osservazioni di Lodovico Antonio Muratori* (Brescia: Gian-Maria Rizzardi, 1721).

[50] Muratori, *Del governo della peste*, 34–6. Emphasis added.

[51] Samuel K. Cohn, Jr., *Cultures of Plague: Medical Thinking at the End of the Renaissance* (Oxford: Oxford University Press, 2010), 299. The language of

One must imagine that amidst the suspicion and danger of the Plague, a city is found in the same state as if it were threatened with War by a Prince or a nearby People of great power and pride who thought of occupying and devastating the territory ... The only difference is that the evils and damages of War regularly come from the Enemy and the foreigner, while those of the Plague may come from those whom we usually call friend.[52]

In likening the battle against plague to warfare – a prince's political duty par excellence[53] – Muratori was asserting that the defense against plague was a matter of state.[54] Such ideas regarding the role of the state in matters pertaining to public health and crisis helped drive the centralization of disaster management by the eighteenth century, both from the perspective of the state, which sought to expand its authority by increasing its role in more aspects of everyday life, and from the perspective of the people, who increasingly came to expect their leaders to intervene in more areas of civic life, above all in times of crisis.

As the emerging nation states of Western Europe sought to centralize their power, particularly over the seventeenth to eighteenth centuries, aspects of social welfare, including public health, were increasingly integrated into these efforts. When the first major disaster of the eighteenth century struck in 1720, European states found an opportunity to advance their centralizing ambitions. Despite the more fractured nature of the Italian city-states relative to the larger European powers of the eighteenth century, this was no less the case in parts of Italy, where centralized public health management and sophisticated networks of information had become a point of pride.[55]

---

war in the context of public health crises has become familiar to many of us during the COVID-19 pandemic. References, for example, to the "war on COVID," or to health care workers on the "front lines," have been ubiquitous in journalism, radio, television, and even in regular conversation. But the history of such military metaphors dates back at least to the sixteenth century (see Cohn, *Cultures of Plague*, 299), and possibly earlier.

[52] Muratori, *Del governo della peste*, 18.

[53] In Chapter 14 of *The Prince*, Machiavelli wrote, "A prince must have no other object or thought, nor acquire skill in anything, except war, its organization, and its discipline. The art of war is all that is expected of a ruler." Nicolo Machiavelli, *The Prince*, translated by George Bull (London: Penguin Books, 2003), 47.

[54] Cohn, *Cultures of Plague*, 299.

[55] To quote Carlo Cipolla, "how interdependent had become the health services of Northern Italy and how sensitive was their network of information." Cipolla, *Fighting the Plague*, 30.

Conflicting Narratives and the Invisible Commonwealth: How News of Plague Was Received in Genoa and Europe

As elsewhere in Europe, news of a possible plague epidemic in France arrived in Genoa nearly two months after the first cases of plague. On July 20, 1720, the Venetian consul in Genoa, Andrea Samuele Bettoni, wrote the *Provveditori e Sopraprovveditori alla Sanità* in Venice (the superintendents and supervisors of Venice's *Magistrato alla Sanità* or Health Office) to inform them of news that had arrived in Genoa from Giacomo Schinchino, the Genoese consul in Marseille. In two letters dated July 9 and 10, Schinchino briefed health officials in Genoa about some alarming deaths that had taken place in recent weeks. In one case, a porter in the lazaret of Marseille had died "in the time it takes to open a package." In another, the sailor of a vessel that had obtained a health clearance arrived at his mother's house in Marseille where, upon the unpacking of his belongings, a boy in the house (possibly his son, according to Dr. Reymond's report[56]) became ill and died soon thereafter.[57] The mother and her two small children were struck next and were at the point of death. The vessel and cargo in question, as well as the sailor's suspected belongings, were soon burned to prevent further infections. "Thus the health board [of Marseille] has declared that these accidents were caused by a *mal contaggioso* [contagious disease]."[58] Upon receipt of this news, the health office in Genoa wasted no time and moved forward with "proper orders in all the places of [their] domain to preserve it from a similar evil."[59]

The early success of Marseillais officials, physicians, health officers, and others in concealing the truth of plague in the city meant that the Italian states, along with the rest of the continent, could not initially confirm the presence of plague in France. Not until late July to August did officials beyond Provence begin learning enough information – mostly through consuls and other representatives on the ground, but also, eventually, through health magistrates in Provence – to determine

---

[56] See Chapter 1.
[57] This is the same boy described by Dr. Reymond in Chapter 1.
[58] From the *Magistrato di sanità*, Genoa, July 20, 1720, Antichi regimi, Provveditori e Sopraprovveditori alla sanità (henceforward Sanità), 644, f. 1–1v, Archivio di Stato di Venezia (henceforward ASV).
[59] Ibid.

that it was actually plague that spread in the port city.[60] As the number of new infections began to increase rapidly in July, foreign representatives from across Europe who were living in Provence began sharing with officials back home what they were learning about the growing crisis. By this time, the campaign of misinformation by those in Marseille who aimed to preserve the city's commerce was becoming well known to the rest of Europe, which moved forward with rigorous protective measures despite the protestations of officials, merchants, and others in Marseille. George Henshaw, the British consul in Genoa, for example, reported to his secretary of state in August 1720, "here is advice from the Health Office at Marseille that it is actually the plague that many die of there (tho many letters from thence pretend they are only malignant feavours)."[61] Meanwhile, Henry Davenant, British envoy to the Italian states, remarked from Genoa:

The people of Marseille have been very industrious in concealing this distemper, pretending it was only a malignant fever; but as the letters from Marseille have not been permitted to pass this week, we conclude the illness increases, and the Genovese consul writes from Toulon that the Magistracy of Marseille had at length declar'd the city was infected with the plague; it is said to be of the worst sort, people falling dead in a few hours after having taken the infection.[62]

Two months later, Davenant recommended that Britain expand its quarantine regulations to include not only vessels from Provence but all French ships and goods "more especially since 'tis reported of

---

[60] For more on this campaign of misinformation, see Chapter 1 of this book. For a published example of one of the (many) letters abroad in which the *juges conservateurs de la santé* of Marseille endeavor to minimize the seriousness of the growing crisis, see: Filippini, *Il Porto di Livorno e la Toscana*, 158n3.

[61] George Henshaw, British consul in Genoa, to Secretary Craggs, Genoa, August 20, 1720, SP 79/13, Genoa, TNA.

[62] Henry Davenant, British envoy extraordinary to the Italian states, to Secretary Craggs, Genoa, August 13, 1720, SP 79/12, Genoa, TNA. The following month, Davenant alluded to the thousands of people who fled Marseille while the plague, "concealed under the name of fever," ravaged the city for over a month: "qu'il est certain que plusieurs milliers personnes sont sortis de Marseille, et se sont introduits dans de différents endroits, après que la peste couverte sous le nom de fièvre avait fait du ravage pour plus d'un mois dans cette malheureuse ville." Henry Davenant to James Stanhope, 1st earl Stanhope, Genoa, September 8, 1720, SP 79/12, Genoa, TNA.

late that this distemper has lain disguis'd at Marseilles ever since the month of May."[63] Especially in the winter months of 1720–21, when the number of new infections in Provence temporarily subsided and claims from Provençal officials and merchants that the outbreak had ceased only intensified, it was clear to some, including Davenant, that it would be premature to accept such dangerous assertions.[64]

As the earlier passages suggest, there were several varying narratives coming out of Marseille and other parts of Provence at any given time during the epidemic. Although it was in July that cases began to multiply more rapidly, infections did not cease after the first fatalities in late May. As early as June, wealthier families were already fleeing Marseille as evidence mounted that an outbreak was unfolding. Still, the city's *échevins* and health officers played down the crisis in their correspondence. In the epidemic's earliest phase, from late May through June 1720, Marseillais health officers had joined local officials in understating the severity of the growing crisis – a decision that for a time hurt the reputation of the institution.[65] By July, however, the bureau of health came to acknowledge the presence of plague and began expanding its communications with health offices around Europe. For this reason, by the time the preceding letters were written in August 1720, the accounts of Marseillais civil administrators, the physicians they hired to misdiagnose the disease, and others began to contradict the reports of health magistrates in Marseille, who could no longer call the disease a mere fever. It was at this time that news of plague began to spread beyond Provence. It is therefore important

---

[63] Henry Davenant to Secretary Craggs, Genoa, October 9, 1720, SP 79/12, Genoa, TNA.

[64] "Comme je me suis apperçu par les lettres de France, que l'on [_] recoit extremement a Paris le mal contagieux qui afflige la Provence, jusqu'a debiter qu'il avait comme cessé, je me crois obligé d'avertir vôtre Excellence, que bien loin que les choses y aillent mieux, il semble au contraire qu'elle empirent tous les jours, puisqu'il meurent encore du monde a Marseilles, et que plusieurs endroits qui s'etoient garantis de cette maladie, en sont presentement attaquéz." Henry Davenant to Secretary Craggs, Genoa, January 14, 1721, SP 79/14, Genoa, TNA.

[65] Gilbert Buti, "L'Intendance de la Santé de Marseille au XVIIIe siècle: service sanitaire ou bureau de renseignements?," in *La quotidiana emergenza: I molteplici impieghi delle istituzioni sanitarie nel Mediterraneo moderno*, edited by Paolo Calcagno and Daniele Palermo (Palermo: New Digital Frontiers, 2017), 46.

to draw a distinction between, on the one hand, those in Provence, especially in Marseille, who continued to spread misinformation and cause confusion about the disease, and on the other hand, Provençal health officials, who, by July and August, acknowledged plague as the cause of death and began circulating information about the epidemic to health offices across Europe. These communications would ultimately find their way to the newspapers of Europe, which published letters from health bureaus, consuls, and others, throughout the crisis.[66] They not only help to demonstrate the transnational character of the Great Plague Scare of 1720 but also reveal the contradictory nature of plague-related news, especially in the earliest months of the outbreak.

The messages coming out of infected areas were mixed, and they remained as such for the duration of the epidemic. Even after it became impossible to deny that plague was in Marseille, those who wished only to preserve the economy and trade of the city merely shifted their narrative from denials that it was plague to premature claims that the crisis was over. As late as the summer of 1722, in fact, more than two years after the plague's first appearance in France, efforts by public officials to conceal the truth in Marseille persisted. The following passage is exemplary of the kind of mixed messages that came from Provence from 1720 to 1722, often forcing officials across Europe to piece together the truth for themselves:

They write from Marseilles under the 17th of last month that they still [insist] that the children of Monsieur Boeuf, together with the priest and the servant maid, which were dead there, was not occasioned by any contagious distemper, but by common sickness, notwithstanding said Monsieur Boeuf (who was conveyed to the lazaretto with several other persons for having had communication with the people that were dead) after a sicknesse of two days died also, but the Physician pretended that his death was caused by a swelling in the throat; notwithstanding ... they write from [Toulon] under the 19th of last month that they had advice from Marseilles that the death of

---

[66] In August 1720, for example, newspapers in London printed a letter from Livorno (or Leghorne) that read, "A French ship is arrived here, bound from Marseilles for Smyrna, and has brought letters from the Magistrates of Health at Marseilles advising that the Plague has been discovered in their lazaretto, where 12 persons had died of it, and 2 in the town." "Leghorne, July 27," *Daily Courant* (London), August 10, 1720, issue 5867.

Monsieur Boeuf was occasioned by a buboe under the throat, and that three more of those that were sent to the lazaretto with him were also dead, and a Priest in the cloyster of S. Vittore of Marseilles, but that nevertheless the opinions of the Physicians were various, some pretending it was pestilence, and others not.[67]

Such conflicting messages, while typical in times of crisis, posed challenges for those outside of the infected areas – not only beyond the borders of France but within them as well – who sought to understand what exactly was happening in Provence. As they contemplated how to proceed during the emerging crisis, European leaders relied more on briefings from their own representatives on the ground – above all the consuls – than on the words of Marseillais officials.[68]

Along with health magistrates, consuls and diplomats situated in France and across the Atlantic and Mediterranean worlds were major players in an extensive and significant network of information regarding the crisis. Throughout the epidemic in Provence and for many years thereafter, foreign consuls, envoys, ambassadors, merchants, and others – individuals like Davenant and Henshaw in Genoa, Burges in Venice, or the Partyets (father and son) in Cádiz[69] – found themselves petitioning the local government to stop what were seen as pernicious practices against ships bearing their nation's flag. In Venice as in Cádiz, for example, the most hated of these practices were the *fondeos* or *visites*, or searching and quarantining of foreign vessels at port, which inspired the words in defense of open trade practices in the second epigraph of this chapter. In fact, a focus on the exchange

---

[67] Consul George Henshaw to John Carteret, secretary of state, Genoa, May 5, 1722, SP 79/14, Genoa, TNA.

[68] The consulate tradition can be traced back to the twelfth and thirteenth centuries when the first ones were created in cities such as Pisa, Genoa, Messina, and Marseille. Anne Mézin, *Les consuls de France au siécle des lumières, 1715–1792* (Paris: Ministère des Affaires étrangères, 1997), 3. Consuls played a central role in this community or network of information – the "invisible commonwealth" that I discuss below. Dedicated to the interests of the states which they represented, they were integral to the transmission of information about the plague, and, importantly, about the protective measures being imposed across Europe. For this reason, consular papers from across Western Europe proved invaluable for the completion of this book.

[69] See Chapter 4 on Cádiz.

of information about the Plague of Provence – the first major disaster
to be handled from the capitals of Europe's emerging nation states,
and a dominating topic in contemporary documents across geographic
boundaries – reveals an extensive network of exchange, part of what
I term an invisible commonwealth that is traceable in communications about the public health crisis at this time. Participants in this
transnational *réseau* of correspondence looked after the interests of
the state. Unlike the concepts of the Invisible College or the Republic
of Letters of the seventeenth and eighteenth centuries, both characterized by the interchange of scientific or philosophical ideas among
groups of intellectuals, the invisible commonwealth functioned much
like an extranational community in which consuls, diplomats, and
government and public health officials exchanged information about
official matters, or incidents of common interest. From July 1720
through 1722 and beyond, the most significant topic of concern was
the Plague of Provence, and participants in this network of exchange –
which spanned Europe, the Mediterranean, and the overseas colonies –
worked to shape responses to the crisis in their respective regions
largely independent of any formal diplomatic circumstances on the
ground. While this cosmopolitan "cloud" of correspondence existed
beyond the subject of plague or public health,[70] tracing communications about this particular crisis, which so occupied contemporary
pens across the Atlantic and Mediterranean worlds, brings this

---

[70] Already by the seventeenth century, this apparatus of communication was
fully operative, with consuls, diplomats, health intendants (especially in times
of disease), and others exchanging information with one another about any
and all relevant happenings on the ground across the European continent
and across oceans. Although this transnational network was not limited to
Italy, nor to the subject of disease, it is worth noting that the health offices
of northern Italy were extremely well connected by the early modern period.
As Cipolla wrote: "In the course of the sixteenth and seventeenth centuries
the Health Magistracies of the capital cities of the republics and principalities
of northern Italy had firmly established the eminently civilized custom of
regularly informing each other of all news that they gathered on health
conditions prevailing in various parts of Italy, the rest of Europe, North
Africa, and the Middle East. Florence 'corresponded' regularly with Genoa,
Venice, Verona, Milan, Mantua, Parma, Modena, Ferrara, Bologna, Ancona,
and Lucca. The frequency of the correspondence with each one of these places
ranged from one letter every two weeks in periods of calm to several messages
a week in times of emergency." Cipolla, *Fighting the Plague*, 21.

transnational, multilingual community of male correspondents to the surface,[71] and Genoa, along with the other port cities examined in this book, played a significant part.[72]

Port cities such as Genoa, Rome, Venice, London, Madrid, Cádiz, Paris, and others held a central place in Italian and Euro-Mediterranean networks of correspondence in the seventeenth to eighteenth centuries and played a significant role in the dissemination of news about the plague in France. Mention of Genoese responses to the epidemic are commonplace in archives across the Atlantic, including those of France, Great Britain, Spain, Portugal, and other Italian states. Moreover, communications from Genoa pertaining to the plague are found in archives across Europe, most notably in the Archivio di Stato in Venice, which holds an entire *filza*, or file, on reactions in Genoa based on the letters of Genoese consuls.[73] Genoa, in fact, was the first city in Italy to learn of the outbreak in France, and news about the crisis from Genoa was printed and reprinted in newspapers all over the European continent. These dispatches and letters related a wide variety of information – from statistical information such as the number of dead in Provence, to vignettes about the victims, to episodes tied to the crisis occurring all over Europe – and they help demonstrate the interconnected and transnational nature of both eighteenth-century networks of communication and responses to the Provençal plague. In November 1720, for example, the Spanish newspaper *Gaceta de*

---

[71] The bureaucratic nature of this correspondence meant that women were largely excluded from participating in exchanges pertaining to the public health crisis. Both the absence of women and the official nature of this invisible commonwealth stand in contrast to the Republic of Letters as discussed, for example, in Dena Goodman's monumental work on the subject. See, among others: Dena Goodman, *The Republic of Letters: A Cultural History of the French Enlightenment* (Ithaca: Cornell University Press, 1994); Dena Goodman, *Becoming a Woman in the Age of Letters* (Ithaca: Cornell University Press, 2009).

[72] In an average year, the Health Bureau of Marseille, for example, sent or received 250 letters on the subject of plague, the majority of which involved Spanish and Italian health bureaus (72 percent went to or arrived from Genoa, Livorno, or Venice). In times of disease, this number surged. See: Takeda, *Between Crown and Commerce*, 115–16.

[73] See "Lettere venute dal console in Genova, n. 6, July 20, 1720–January 14, 1724," in Sanità, 644, ASV.

Madrid – one of the longest running newspapers in the world[74] – published a letter from Genoa recounting an episode that had taken place the previous month in the shores of Pisa: "From letters arriving from Pisa we have learned that in the neighboring countryside four Frenchmen were seen who had landed on the coast. A certificate of health was requested of them, but they did not have one, so they attempted to force their way inland, at which point they were shot and killed, and their corpses burned."[75] Letters like this, which came from various cities – all chief players in the dissemination of information about the Plague of Provence – helped keep Europe and the world informed about the public health crisis, above all as official information from Marseille remained contradictory at best.

Reactions to the Plague of Provence in Genoa and Italy

When news began to arrive in July 1720 that a *morbo contagioso*, or contagious disease, reigned in Provence, Genoa acted quickly. The *Cancelliere*, or chancellor, of the *Magistrato di sanità* in Genoa swiftly sent word to neighboring health offices.[76] He would later pride himself on having been the first in Italy to learn of the growing crisis in Marseille.[77] The *magistrati* then turned their attention to protecting their Genoese ports. Health officers knew they could waste no time, for the port city's proximity to Marseille meant both that it was uniquely vulnerable to infection, and that its Italian neighbors could sever commercial ties if Genoa did not impose the most rigorous measures to protect their coasts.[78] As the British envoy to Italy reported in August 1720:

There is such a constant intercourse between the river of Genoa and Marseilles, and these people have so many small ports to guard, and so many

---

[74] *La Gaceta de Madrid* ran from 1661 (under this name since 1697) until 1936, after which it continued under its new name, the *Boletín Oficial del Estado*, which remains in publication today. See: Sara Núñez de Prado, "De la Gaceta de Madrid al Boletín Oficial del Estado," *Historia y Comunicación Social* 7 (2002): 147–60.

[75] "Génova, October 22, 1720," *Gaceta de Madrid* no. 48, November 26, 1720, 190.

[76] For a published example of one of these Genoese dispatches, in this case to Livorno, see: Filippini, *Il Porto di Livorno e la Toscana*, 157n2.

[77] Assereto, "*Per la comune salvezza …*," 151.

[78] The ports of Genoa and Marseille are roughly 390 miles (630 km) apart over land, and about 200 nautical miles apart by sea. Depending on conditions, a

of their subjects in the ports of Provence and Languedoc that know all the landing places and will endeavour to fly from the Distemper, that we lye more expos'd here, than in any other part of Italy.[79]

Genoa's first orders against the "contagious disease" in Provence were published and spread across the republic on July 22, 1720, only days after the arrival of news from Schinchino, the Genoese consul in Marseille, about the nature of recent deaths in the port city.[80] In this first ordinance, Genoese health officials, or *Conservatori di sanità*, called for caution and vigilance in response to "the well-founded news that in Marseille there have been incidents of contagious disease as well as numerous deaths."[81] All trade and communications with Marseille, as well as the regions of Provence and Languedoc, were now fully suspended. This included the introduction into their "Most Serene Domain of any people, animals, cargo, vessels, and anything else, however insignificant, originating from said provinces of Provence and Languedoc, whether by direct or indirect route."[82] Genoese vessels arriving from these regions were included in the ban.[83] This ordinance was the first of many in the years that followed as Genoa confronted the threat of infection from France.

---

vessel could reach one port from the other within only two to four days. The following quote, written in 1670, recognizes the proximity of the two cities: "The ordinary wayes which an Englishman may take in going into Italy are five: to wit, either through Flanders and Germany; and so to fall in at Trent, or Treviso, and so to Venice. Or else by France, and so to Marseilles, and thence to Genoa by Sea." Lassels, *The Voyage of Italy*, 23.

[79] Henry Davenant to Secretary Craggs, Genoa, August 13, 1720, SP 79/12, Genoa, TNA. Elsewhere he wrote: "et comme cet État qui est le plus exposé, et qui prend les mesures les plus justes pour etre informé de ce qui se passe, redouble ses precautions, il sera necessaire que nous continuons a nous tenir sur nos gardes, et que nous ne reglions nos demarches que sur celles de cette Republique, qui a cause de son voisinage, ne neglige rien pour etre bien avertie de ce qui arrive en Provence." Henry Davenant to Secretary Craggs, Genoa, January 14, 1721, SP 79/14, Genoa, TNA.

[80] As described in the opening paragraph to the previous section on "Conflicting Narratives and the Invisible Commonwealth."

[81] "Conservatori di Sanità della Serenissima Repubblica di Genova, Attenzione, e vigilanza ...," Genoa, July 22, 1720, Sanità, 644, ASV.

[82] Ibid. Over the next weeks, other Italian states would quickly follow suit. Rome, for example, issued its first *editto* banning trade with Provence and Languedoc on August 3. "Editto," Roma, August 3, 1721, Bandi, collezione 1, busta 57, Archivio di Stato di Roma (henceforward ASR).

[83] "Genoa, Aug. 17," *Daily Courant* (London), September 6, 1720, issue 5890.

Throughout the plague years, Genoese responses to the crisis would evolve according to a number of factors, including the arrival of new information about the situation in Provence and shifting understandings of risk; larger diplomatic and commercial interests; and the influence of Genoa's Italian neighbors. The next few *editti*, or edicts, which came in relatively rapid succession from July through October, reflect these various considerations. Already on July 29, separate ordinances were issued that expanded upon the initial order of July 22. In one of these, Genoese health officials introduced the general use of "bollette personali della sanità" ("personal health bills") and laid out the terms for their use. The use of *bollette* and *fedi di sanità* (both are documentary proofs of health) was now made compulsory. Essentially, all judges, commissioners, officers, and deputies of health in the republic were to prohibit in their respective jurisdictions the entry of any person, "regardless of status, rank, and condition, without exception," who arrived by land or by sea from anywhere outside of the Republic of Genoa without an official bill or certificate of health from their location of origin.[84] For individuals, these bills must include the carrier's name, surname, homeland, age, and height; and for vessels, the passes must document all the relevant information pertaining to the captain, crew, passengers, cargo, and the journey (e.g. point of origin and stop-offs).[85] The order, which was to go into effect beginning on August 8, 1720, did not apply to those who traveled within the republic. As with most plague-time restrictions across Europe at this time, the new rules were to be enforced on pain of death, or loss of property and/or incarceration.[86] A separate order on the same date also prohibited communication, contact, and trade with all vessels, persons, or goods arriving in Genoa that had not yet been properly inspected, even if they had not been anywhere suspected of infection. Above all,

---

[84] "Conservatori di Sanità della Serenissima Repubblica di Genova, Desiderando noi assicurarsi ...," Genoa, July 29, 1720, Sanità, 644, ASV.

[85] Ibid. For more on the use and significance of health passes in early modern Europe, see: Bamji, "Health Passes, Print and Public Health ...," 441–64.

[86] As in other parts of Europe by the eighteenth century, the enforcement of public health measures in Italy was serious business. The following passage by English physician Samuel Sharp, writing from Venice in 1765, is revealing: "The Republick [of Venice] is extremely rigid in what regards the quarantine; and, indeed, as they border upon those countries where the plague so frequently rages, they cannot be too watchful. There is not the least connivance ever

no one was permitted to approach a vessel that at any point had been "suspended from free circulation" or spent time in quarantine; and so that no one "could claim ignorance," these vessels and areas would be marked with lines of buoys and flags.[87]

Subsequent weeks and months saw the introduction of numerous additional restrictions aimed at preventing the introduction of plague in the republic. These were tried-and-true measures that had been implemented in times of disease for centuries, and included guidelines for quarantining, disinfections (as with vinegars, herbs, sulfur, or smoke), and the cleansing of streets and homes, as well as various means of restricting public life and the gathering of crowds. In January of 1721, for example, Genoa prohibited all *Carnevale*-related gatherings or celebrations, including "all sorts of masks, *Feste di Ballo* [balls], *commedie* [*dell'arte*] performances, and any other Carnivalesque public events," with violations subject to "the gravest punishments."[88] In the fall of 1720, officials in Genoa also introduced *cordons sanitaires*, or sanitary lines, to enforce new restrictions on movement in and out of the port city. On September 11, Davenant reported: "We have 8,000 men constantly under arms to guard this coast with orders to fire on any that shall endeavor to land without bills of health to certify they don't come from places infected or under suspicion, and this rigor is used even against the subjects of the Republic. The same is practiced by the other states of Italy, and if any are caught endeavoring to get in by stealth, they are to be punished by death without trial or hopes

---

practised; all letters, to whomsoever directed, are first opened by the officers, and then smoaked [smoked] before they are delivered. Were Mr. __ to have handed over a news-paper to me, and we had been detected in the action, I must inevitably have performed quarantine in the *Lazaretto* a certain number of weeks. A few years since, a boy got on board one of these vessels performing quarantine, and stole some tobacco; he was pursued into Venice, and shot dead in the streets. There are many custom-house officers in their boats, watching the quarantine night and day, who would certainly kill the first man who should attempt to escape on shore, before the expiration of the quarantine." Samuel Sharp, *Letters from Italy, Describing the Customs and Manners of that Country in the Years 1765, and 1766* (London: R. Cave, 1767), 12–13.

[87] "Conservatori di Sanità della Serenissima Repubblica di Genova, Avendo noi fatta riflessione …," Genoa, July 29, 1720, Sanità, 644, ASV.

[88] "Duce, Govern., e Prov. della Republica di Genova," Genova, January 10, 1721, Fondo Senarega, Collegii Diversorum, 206, Archivio di Stato di Genova (henceforward ASG).

of pardon."[89] As elsewhere in Europe at this time, reports tell of various occasions on which the guards of the *cordon sanitaire* indeed fired upon unwelcome vessels. In 1721, the British consul in Genoa offered one example:

By the last advices from Provence, the Plague continues to do great mischief in severall places there, which makes this Republick as much on their guard as ever, to prevent any one landing surreptitiously all along their coast, as every now & then has been attempted by severall, & particularly last week by a boat that would have landed not far distant from this city, but they were forced to retire, the guards firing a great many shots at 'em.[90]

More than simply a response to the threat of infection, this massive deployment of forces was also a means of exhibiting Genoese efficiency to neighboring rival states.[91] The sanitary lines included both guards and vessels that were positioned at the mouth of the port to identify incoming ships and to repel those attempting to arrive from a growing list of prohibited regions.

In early August, Genoa began to cease trade relations with several areas that it declared vulnerable to infection owing to geographic location, commercial relationships with infected regions, or failure to enact proper precautions. Upon learning of the outbreak in July, the Genoese health office dispatched emissaries to various cities, including Turin and Nice, both to gather further information on the progress of the disease and to verify that the "diligences [required] by the urgency of the matter were being practiced."[92] Having learned that these states were not employing adequate protective measures in the face of the outbreak's rapid progression, trade was suspended with the states of Lyon, the Duchy of Savoy, the Principality of Piedmont with its capital of Turin, and the adjacent coastline that included Nice, Villefranche-sur-Mer, Monaco, Menton, and Oneglia (for which the Genoese had fought Savoy in the 1670s).[93] By the end of the month, Genoa would

---

[89] Henry Davenant to Secretary Craggs, Genoa, September 11, 1720, SP 79/12, Genoa, TNA.
[90] George Henshaw to Secretary Craggs, Genoa, January 7, 1721, SP 79/13, Genoa, TNA.
[91] Assereto, "*Per la comune salvezza* ...," 150–1.
[92] Translated from the original Italian as quoted in Assereto, "*Per la comune salvezza* ...," 151.
[93] "Copia di Capitolo ...," Genoa, August 3, 1720, Sanità, 644, ASV.

add the islands of Sicily and Sardinia, "with all other islands and dependencies adjacent to them, and so also the islands of Corsica and Capraia, and those of Elba, and Gorgona, Mallorca, and Menorca."[94] Once it was determined that health policies were being sufficiently observed, some of these areas, including Piedmont and Oneglia, would soon see the reopening of trade.[95] For the most part, however, the expansion of restrictions against foreign ports continued, and quickly came to include regions far removed from the outbreak in Provence. In August 1721, the Genoese Magistrate of Health began requiring that all "ships coming from the ocean, into the Mediterranean, be they English, or Dutch, or of any other nation" present "attestations of health" from the health offices of their previous destinations. Vessels that could not produce such "justifications" would not be admitted to "prattick" (or pratique, which is to say, admitted into port and granted a health clearance).[96] The new policy came in response to reports that owners of woolen goods from Provence, which "find no sales for want of trade," were designing on smuggling the cargo out on British or Dutch ships that would take the merchandise on board in Provence or Languedoc, and then take it into Genoa or Livorno "as if it came from Britain, or Holland." These ships would then give a prearranged signal offshore, and the goods would be trafficked in.[97] Such illicit activities were far from unheard of during the Plague of Provence and triggered an increased sense of urgency for officials across Europe whose concerns about smuggling in general predated the public health emergency. Like those of other regions across the Atlantic and Mediterranean worlds, administrators in Genoa – many already wary of illicit commerce – were on heightened alert against any activity that could inadvertently carry the plague into the republic. Even in July 1722, as the epidemic in Provence subsided, the Genoese Magistrate of Health warned Britain via their consul in Genoa that if they did not act to prevent British ships from journeying to Marseille,

---

[94] "Presidente, e Conservatori di Sanità della Serenissima Republica di Genova," Genoa, August 20, 1720, Sanità, 644, ASV.

[95] Assereto, "*Per la comune salvezza* …," 151.

[96] Consul George Henshaw to John Carteret, secretary of state, Genoa, August 5, 1721, SP 79/13, Genoa, TNA.

[97] Ibid.

Genoa would ban all commerce with Britain.[98] But public health measures in Genoa – as elsewhere in Italy – served other purposes, as well.
In times of disease, they helped demonstrate Genoese competency and
preparedness in matters of public health to its neighbors, and during
the Plague of Provence, they served as tools in the game of retaliatory
politics that emerged among the cities of Italy.

   Public health practices during the Provençal plague were relatively
consistent among the chief northern Italian cities, where health officers sought to hold other cities accountable, while simultaneously protecting the interests of the state in the larger balance of Italy. By the
seventeenth to eighteenth centuries, as noted earlier, the health offices
of northern Italy had created a sophisticated network of communication, keeping one another both well informed and accountable in
matters of public health, especially in times of disease. Italian states
often monitored one another, sending envoys to evaluate public health
responses in other cities. While this kind of public health oversight had
been implemented in Italy before, as during the epidemic of 1652,[99] it
was widely practiced during the Plague of Provence. Genoa, Milan,
Livorno, Venice, Rome – all sent representatives to other Italian cities.
In August 1720, the British consul in Genoa reported back home:

From Milan that Magistrate of the health have sent hither a senator on
purpose to observe whether this magistrate of the health takes the necessary
precautions against the evill they fear, that in case they did not, they might
forbid any further communication with this state, so that if the Republick
does not uniform themselves to the measures taken by their neighbours,
these would forbid all communication with them, which would soon reduce
them to a starving condition.[100]

This kind of reciprocal oversight among Italian states meant that
health and sanitation policies in times of crisis were regularly revised
in order to bring them up to the standards of neighboring states. Doing
so would prevent or reverse the imposition of sanctions – typically in

---

[98] The threat came after the Genoese Health Office learned that two British
   ships had arrived in Marseille with British goods, with more expected to
   follow. George Henshaw to John Carteret, Genoa, July 21, 1722, SP 79/13,
   Genoa, TNA.
[99] Cipolla, *Fighting the Plague*, 42.
[100] George Henshaw to Secretary Craggs, Genoa, August 20, 1720, SP 79/13,
   Genoa, TNA.

the form of trade restrictions – for failure to adopt adequate protective measures. These inter-city health evaluations also helped feed the competitive nature of Italian public health culture.

The case of Turin is an example of the kind of back-and-forth exchange of measures that was practiced among the Italian states during the Plague of Provence. In early August, the Health Office of Genoa resolved to cut all trade and communication with Turin in response to news that the region had not yet banned the introduction of French goods and had maintained communications with parts of France.[101] In response, the Health Office of Turin quickly imposed a new set of precautions that was more in line with those of other northern Italian states including Genoa. Torinese officials dispatched news of their new plague-time measures to Genoese health officials, who then reexamined their policies in an edict dated August 11, 1720:

[We] have learned from the Tribunal of Health in Turin via their letter of the 8th [of August] about the excellent and wise measures taken in the current emergency upon news of the epidemic's further progress in Marseille. [They] have deemed it for the general good to prohibit and disconnect all communication and trade not only with the said city of Marseille and the provinces of Provence and Languedoc—already banned in a previous edict—but with all the other provinces, cities, and places of France, especially the Dauphiné and Lyonnais and their countrysides, [as well as] Monaco, Menton, Barcelonne [France], and their respective dependencies ... These resolutions, and others included in their edict, have persuaded us that public salvation has been sufficiently secured in the Piedmont. For this reason, we have resolved to reopen trade with the said state, which remained suspended by our resolution of [August] 4th.[102]

In this edict, the Genoese health office not only reversed its stance on Turin but also further expanded its own list of territories deemed susceptible to infection. These included the Dauphiné, Barcelonne (France), as well as Geneva and Vaud in Switzerland. Such revisions to plague-time policies would take place regularly among the Italian states as news continued to arrive both about developments in France and responses to the plague in other parts of Italy.

---

[101] "Genova le 8 Ag° 1720," Genoa, August 8, 1720, #5, Sanità, 644, ASV.
[102] "Presidente, e Conservatori di Sanità della Serenissima Repubblica di Genova, Avendoci fatti presenti il Tribunale di Sanità di Turino ...," Genoa, August 11, 1720, Sanità, 644, ASV.

As Italian cities monitored and assessed the public health practices of their neighbors, long-standing rivalries and alliances, along with the influence of sanitary-powerhouse Venice, helped to determine how Italian states would respond to one another. In this context, the case of Livorno and Genoa is also worth noting. During the Plague of Provence, Livorno – the primary port of the Grand Duchy of Tuscany, with its capital in Florence – found itself embroiled in a "health war" against its Genoese rivals.[103] In a *terminazione* (edict) dated July 27, 1720, five days after Genoa passed its first protective measures, the Republic of Venice suspended commerce not only with Provence, but also with the states of Savoy and Piedmont, the region of Genoa ("il Genovesato"), and the islands of Sardinia, Corsica, and Sicily.[104] Other Italian cities, including Bologna and Parma, soon followed suit, and by August, the Grand Duke of Tuscany, at this time Cosimo III de' Medici, decided that Tuscany should be very cautious toward "any vessel coming from places that the Republic of Venice has banned."[105] It was Venice, then – in many ways a model republic in matters of

---

[103] Filippini, *Il Porto di Livorno e la Toscana*, 161.

[104] The ban against Genoa came as a result of its proximity and perceived exposure to Provence. Terminazione degli Illustrissimi ed Eccellentissimi Signori Sopra Provveditori e Provveditori alla Sanità, Venice, July 27, 1720, Sanità 90 (Terminazioni dei Provveditori alla sanità, 1720–1722), ASV. A note just above "il Genovesato," evidently added after the *Terminazione* was drafted, reads "per ora" ("for now"), indicating that the Venetians may not have intended to keep the suspension against Genoa in place for long. The passage reads, "In relazione à che dichiarano pure per sospesi tuti li stati della Savoia e Piemonte, come pure, [per ora] il Genovesato, l'Isole di Sardegna, Corsica, e Sicilia, in maniera tanti che le persone, merci e bastimenti da qualunque de sudetti luoghi proveniento, o sia per mare respettivamente, o sia per terra abbiano à soggiaceve à dovuti espurghi; in pena come sopra."

[105] As quoted in Filippini, *Il Porto di Livorno e la Toscana*, 160. On August 15, 1720, Rome, too, temporarily banned commercial relations with Genoa. The *editto* reads: "Et essendo giunto alla notizia della Santità Sua, che dalle Legazioni di Bologna, di Ferrara, di Romagna, e d'Urbino, dalla città d'Ancona, dal Regno di Napoli, e dalla Republica di Venezia sia stata non solamente bandita la città di Marsiglia colle due province di Provenza e di Linguadocca, ma si sia anco proceduto alla sospensione del Commercio col Genovesato, e colle isole di Sardegna, Corsica, e Sicilia, intende, e dichiara col presente editto di sospendere per ora dal commercio col rimanente de suoi stati il sopradetto genovesato e mentovate isole." "Editto," Roma, August 15, 1721, Bandi, collezione 1, busta 57, no. 50, ASR. At that time, Davenant reported to Secretary Craggs, "The Venetians use their endeavors

public health – that set the precedent and initiated a period of retaliatory public health policy during the Plague of Provence.[106] Despite the fact that on August 9 Tuscany had issued an order that expressly mimicked that of the Genoese of August 3, a new Tuscan edict on August 23 replicated that of Venice and effectively prohibited trade with Genoa ("the city of Genoa, all of the *Genovesato*, and the Riviera"), along with other regions, including those mentioned in the Venetian *terminazione* of July 27.[107]

This decision marked the beginning of a "health war" with the Republic of Genoa that came to involve nearly all of Italy and stemmed both from a genuine fear of contagion and from a long history of competition between the two rival ports. In September 1720, Genoese officials responded to the August edict by ceasing all commercial relations with Tuscany and its port of Livorno, as well as with its allies (including Massa and Lucca).[108] Other Italian cities were thus drawn into the conflict, as they exchanged not only restrictive measures but also accusations that other ports were not doing enough to defend against infection. On September 21, 1720, for example, a Genoese edict declared that Tuscany had too many unguarded coasts and that the lazarets of Livorno were not taking due diligence to protect against the plague.[109] Maintaining commercial relations with Livorno would

to persuade all the states of Italy to forbid commerce with this Republick and the Piemontese as the most expos'd. We are already shut up from the Pope's dominions, the Kingdom of Naples, and Tuscany." Henry Davenant to Secretary Craggs, Genoa, August 27, 1720, SP 79/12, Genoa, TNA. For a sample news column from Rome on the cessation of trade with Genoa, see: "Foreign Affairs, Rome, August 17," *Weekly Packet* (London), September 3–10, 1720, issue 427.

[106] "This policy, which testifies to the desire to protect Tuscany from the plague, is also due to the desire to be approved by the Venetians who inspired the entire health policy of northern and central Italy." Filippini, *Il Porto di Livorno e la Toscana*, 166.

[107] Filippini, *Il Porto di Livorno e la Toscana*, 160–1. The bando was published on August 25, 1720: "Bando per causa di Sanità," Livorno, August 25, 1720, Sanità 651, ASV.

[108] Ibid., 161.

[109] In fact, Livorno did impose measures to protect against the plague in France. In October 1720, the British consul in the port city reported thus to the secretary of state: "This Magistrate of the Health [Livorno] use all possible dilligence to preserve us in the present conjuncture of the contagion at

thus render Genoese precautions useless.[110] Accusations also flew that Livorno was to blame for the plague outbreak in the first place, since it was there that health officials and local doctors were said to have declared the *Grand Saint-Antoine* free from infection despite recent pestilential deaths on board.[111] With a certificate of health in hand, the ship's captain, Jean-Baptiste Chataud, was permitted to enter port at Marseille in May 1720. These accusations hurt the credibility, and thus the economy, of the Grand Duchy and the Livornese, who now found themselves on the defensive against Genoa (which, in turn, now enjoyed an increase in maritime traffic[112]), Venice, Rome, Naples, and others.[113] In the end, this "econo-health war," characterized by a period of retaliatory, or tit-for-tat, public health diplomacy and shifting alliances among the cities of Italy, would last beyond the end of the epidemic.[114] In February 1723, Livorno was first to ease the quarantine measures for ships and goods coming from Genoa.[115] However,

Marseilles, & spare no expense, having now made a cordon of masts of 500 yards long from the point of the Mole to the Moletta, to hinder vessels from coming into the harbour by night." Sanitary cordons were made not only of soldiers on land but of ships, as well. John Fuller, British consul in Livorno, to Secretary Craggs, Livorno, October 21, 1720, SP 98/24, Tuscany, TNA.

[110] "Presidente e Conservatori di Sanità della Serenissima Repubblica di Genova," Genoa, September 21, 1720, Sanità 644, ASV.

[111] See Chapter 1.

[112] This increase in maritime traffic ultimately resulted in the expansion of Genoa's public health apparatus via the creation of a new quarantine station at Varignano in the Gulf of La Spezia. Construction began in 1724 and was completed in 1743, the same year as the plague outbreak at Messina. Giovanni Assereto, "Polizia sanitaria e sviluppo delle istituzioni statali nella Repubblica di Genova," in *Controllare il territorio. Norme, corpi e conflitti tra medioevo e prima guerra mondiale*, edited by Livio Antonielli and Stefano Levati (Soveria Mannelli: Rubbettino, 2013), 10–11; Assereto, "*Per la comune salvezza ...*," 92–102.

[113] Filippini, *Il Porto di Livorno e la Toscana*, 178–83.

[114] "Guerra economico-sanitaria." Filippini, *Il Porto di Livorno e la Toscana*, 166.

[115] Ibid., 190. Historian Jean-Pierre Filippini provides a more detailed history of the conflict between Livorno and Genoa during the Plague of Provence, from the perspective of Tuscany, in his history of the port of Livorno. See Filippini, *Il Porto di Livorno e la Toscana*, 157–97. Giovanni Assereto and Danilo Pedemonte also touch on this. See: Assereto, "*Per la comune salvezza ...*," 92–3; Pedemonte, "La 'publicca salute,'" 113; Danilo Pedemonte, "Quando il nemico è visibile: il magistrato di sanità genovese come strumento di controllo del territorio e di politica economica," *Storia Urbana* 147 (2015): 48–9.

it took another two months – as many as eight months after the last cases of plague in France – for Genoa to reciprocate.[116]

Some of those who witnessed the conflict in Italy expressed concern about what they perceived to be the pernicious behavior of Italy's leaders. Italian officials were allowing themselves to become distracted with revenge politics rather than focusing on protecting public health. In September 1720, Davenant reported on the ordeal to James Stanhope and alleged that if the disease "slips in" ("si le mal s'y glisse"), it would be the princes' fault:

> We are very alarmed in this country about the contagious disease which reigns in Marseilles, and in my opinion, the Princes of Italy do not conduct themselves as they should in a matter of this nature: instead of directing their full attention to closing the door to the evil, they try only to suspend one another, or to refrain as it suits them to attract trade.[117]

Instead, he contended, "The states of Italy, which are not infected, should open to one another, rather than set traps, and think only of the means to guard against France, or I fear very much that the evil will spread."[118] The British envoy was not only concerned about the threat to public health, however. He also feared the detrimental effects of the closures on commerce, so much so that he worked to persuade

---

[116] Genoa eased restrictions against Livorno in April 1723. Consul George Henshaw to John Carteret, secretary of state, Genoa, April 6, 1723, SP 79/13, Genoa, TNA.

A month earlier, in March, the British consul in Genoa offered some insight: "Although the Grand Duke hath lately taken off the quarantine from vessels going to his state from hence [Genoa], yet this [Genoese] Magistrate of Health do not think fit to let vessels that come thence hither have pratick without performing a quarantine, because they have admitted [in Livorno] some vessels from France." Consul George Henshaw to John Carteret, Secretary of state, Genoa, March 29, 1723, SP 79/13, Genoa, TNA.

[117] "On est fort allarme dans ce pays au sujet du mal contagieux qui regne a Marseilles, et selon moi, les Princes d'Italy ne se conduirent pas comme il devroient dans une affaire de cette nature: au lieu de donner toute leur attention a fermer la porte au mal, ils tachent de se suspender les uns les autres, et s'interdisent a mesure qu'il leur convient pour s'attirer le commerce." Henry Davenant to James Stanhope, Genoa, September 8, 1720, SP 79/12, Genoa, TNA.

[118] The letter reads as follows: "Dans les conjectures présentes je suis bien fâché de croire que les Princes d'Italie agissant par un motif d'intérêt particulière,

the Italian states to reopen their trade. In December 1720, he wrote about the dangers of the "private pique and interest" that he believed were putting all of Europe at risk:

It is not to be conceiv'd how much trade in general suffers by the little harmony that reigns among the Princes of Italy, who have bannisht one another out of private pique and interest, insomuch that we have advice from Holland that the merchants there refused to load for these parts, being apprehensive the plague is among us. As I fear the same notion may get amongst our merchants in England, I am endeavoring, with the governor of Milan's assistance, to persuade the several states of Italy to open with one another, which might be done without any manner of danger, considering the great care that is taken upon the frontiers of France by the neighboring princes.[119]

To Davenant and many others, the exchange of embargoes among Italian cities was destructive not only because it distracted officials from the larger goal of protecting public health but also because of the threat to the economy. During the Plague of Provence, as we see throughout this book, the preservation of trade remained a major concern, and influenced European reactions to the epidemic in various ways. Even during a major public health crisis, concern for the economy never diminished but remained at the forefront.

...

Italy began to lift its plague-time regulations incrementally ("di grado in grado") beginning in early spring 1723, roughly six to eight months

---

et profitent de cette occasion de s'attirer le commerce les unes les autres, au lieu de songer aux moyens d'empêcher l'entrée à la contagion en Italie; le Pape, les Vénitiens, est le Grand Duc [of Tuscany] ont interdit ce pays, cependant je suis bien persuadé qu'ils n'ont pas les attentions qu'on a icy ... Les états d'Italie n'étant point infectez, devroient s'ouvrir entre eux, ne se point tendre des pièges, et penser seulement aux moyens de se garder de la France, ou je crains fort que le mal ne se repanda, puis qu'il est certain que plusieurs milliers de personnes sont sorties de Marseille, et se sont introduits dans de différents endroits, après que la peste couverte sous le nom de fièvre avait fait du ravage pour plus d'un mois dans cette malheureuse ville." "Extrait d'une Lettre de Monsieur D'avenant a M. le Comte Colloredo, datée le 8ᵉ Septembre 1720," Genoa, September 8, 1720, SP 79/12, Genoa, TNA. The addressee of this letter was Count Girolamo (Hieronymus) Colloredo (1674–1726), governor of the Habsburg Duchy of Milan from 1719 to 1725.

[119] Henry Davenant to M. Delafaye [possibly Charles Delafaye, Member of Parliament for Belturbet], Genoa, December 3, 1720, SP 79/12, Genoa, TNA.

after the last cases of plague in France. By April 1723, the Italian states had opened their borders to one another, but it took many more months for Genoa and Venice, for example, to lift all restrictions against France. April 1723 saw only the first steps in the normalization of trade relations. In the edict of April 29, the Health Office of Genoa declared that vessels and people from Marseille and surrounding areas would be freely admitted after a twenty-day quarantine (down from forty) and the usual disinfections. People, vessels, and merchandise "not susceptible to infection" arriving from Languedoc, however, would only need to complete a quarantine of ten days.[120] In Genoa, as in Venice and elsewhere, each subsequent edict gradually reduced the length of quarantine over the course of the year until commercial relations between Italy and France were fully reestablished.[121]

Throughout the epidemic, the Genoese spared no expense to protect their borders and to demonstrate their proficiency in matters of public health to their neighbors. By the eighteenth century, the public health structure of northern Italy was among the most developed in Europe. Particularly over the course of the early modern period, the *Magistrati di sanità*, through which this system functioned, served as instruments for the expanding role of the state. Indeed, by the end of the Plague of Provence in 1722, centralized health bureaus across

---

[120] "Presidente e Conservatori di Sanità della Serenissima Repubblica di Genova," Genoa, April 29, 1723, Sanità, 644, ASV.

[121] In late June 1723, for example, Genoa reduced the quarantine for vessels from Marseille and "other previously infected" areas from twenty days to fifteen: "Che perciò abbiamo ordinato, siccome in virtù del presente nostro Editto ordiniamo, che li Bastimenti, e Persone procedenti da oggi in avanti da Marsiglia, e altre Città, Porti, e Scali della Costa marittima di Francia altre volte infetta, invece delli giorni venti stabiliti nel nostro Editto de 29 Aprile, offernino solamente giorni quindeci di quarantena." "Presidente e Conservatori di Sanità della Serenissima Repubblica di Genova," Genoa, June 26, 1723, Sanità, 644, ASV.

Venice, too, reopened trade to France gradually, with edicts on May 22, June 30, September 2, etc. that incrementally reduced restrictions, most notably the length of quarantine, for vessels, people, and merchandise arriving from France. For example, the edict dated May 22, 1723, lessened the quarantine length for goods considered "not susceptible to infection" to twenty-eight days, and to forty days for materials considered susceptible; the next one, dated June 30, brought these numbers down to fifteen and twenty-eight days, respectively; and the edict dated September 2 lowered the number of quarantine days further to fifteen for non-susceptible goods and twenty-one for susceptible. See: "Terminatione Degl Illustrissimi, & Eccellentissimi

Europe – including the *Conseil de la santé* in Paris and *Junta de Sanidad* in Madrid that were created in response to the 1720 outbreak – had become functioning mechanisms of the emerging nation state.[122] These institutions facilitated the "disaster centralism" that characterized responses to the Provençal plague across Europe, including in Genoa and other Italian states where public health organization and networks of information had become increasingly consolidated and sophisticated over the previous centuries.

The public health structure of Genoa emerged from the Plague of Provence larger and more efficient. As a result of the outbreak in France, the Genoese magistrates of health called for the creation of a new quarantine station erected at Varignano in the Gulf of La Spezia. Under construction from 1724 until 1743 (the same year as the plague outbreak at Messina), this lazaretto further facilitated the regulation, surveillance, and patrolling of traffic into Genoa, with particular attention directed to vessels and merchandise from the Levant, from Livorno (where many goods from the Levant passed through), and from the French ports of Marseille, Toulon, Antibes, and others.[123] Through their communications with the health offices of other states, Genoese health officials also took on broader responsibilities that went beyond the preservation of public health. As historian Danilo Pedemonte has suggested, by increasing its efficiency and improving its organization in the eighteenth century, the Genoese public health apparatus became "a real structural patrimony of the Republic, often being assigned more extensive tasks than those connected to pure and simple prophylactic control."[124]

Signori Sopra Proveditori, Aggionti, e Proveditori alla Sanità," Venice, May 22, 1723, Ambasciata in Spagna, 79, segnatura precedente 87, ASV; "Terminatione Degl Illustrissimi, & Eccellentissimi Signori Sopra Proveditori, Aggionti, e Proveditori alla Sanità," Venice, June 30, 1723, Sanità, 665, ASV; "Terminatione Degl Illustrissimi, & Eccellentissimi Signori Sopra Proveditori, Aggionti, e Proveditori alla Sanità," Venice, September 2, 1723, Ambasciata in Spagna, 79, segnatura precedente 87, ASV.

[122] See Chapters 1 and 4 of this book, respectively.
[123] Assereto, "*Per la comune salvezza* ...," 94–5. For more on the new lazaretto at Varignano, see sources in footnote 112.
[124] Pedemonte, "La 'pubblica salute,'" 117. See also Assereto, "Polizia sanitaria e sviluppo delle istituzioni statali," 10–11.

After all, the need for more tightened public health surveillance did not go away with the last outbreaks of plague in Western Europe in 1720 and 1743. Plague resurfaced in Eastern Europe, Russia, and the Ottoman Empire, and newer diseases, such as yellow fever (caused by the *Aedes aegypti* mosquito), continued to threaten Europe and the overseas colonies until well into the nineteenth century. Effectively, the centuries-old, orientalist perception within Europe that plague constantly threatened from the Levant served to drive the consolidation and centralization of public health and crisis management not only in Genoa but in much of the rest of Europe, and the Plague of Provence marks a significant moment in the process.[125]

Over the course of the French epidemic, Genoese responses evolved according to various factors, including the arrival of new information about the situation in France, shifting understandings of risk, longstanding rivalries and alliances, as well as larger diplomatic and commercial interests. Thanks to its place in an extensive, transnational network of communication – an invisible commonwealth that consisted of consuls, diplomats, and others – the *Magistrato di sanità* in Genoa was the first in Italy to learn, in July 1720, that a contagious disease was spreading in Provence.[126] Its proximity to Marseille and its place in the commercial networks of the Mediterranean meant that the Republic of Genoa was considered among the most exposed to the threat of infection. Officials therefore acted quickly, sending word to other health offices in Italy, and introducing a number of protective mechanisms – quarantines, embargoes, sanitary lines both in land and at sea, mandatory certificates of health, disinfections, the cancellation

---

[125] For more on these orientalist narratives, see relevant section of Chapter 1 and the work of Nükhet Varlık, including: "Rethinking the History of Plague in the Time of COVID-19"; or "'Oriental Plague' or Epidemiological Orientalism? Revisiting the Plague Episteme of the Early Modern Mediterranean," in *Plague and Contagion in the Islamic Mediterranean: New Histories of Disease in Ottoman Society*, edited by Nükhet Varlık (Kalamazoo: ARC Humanities Press, 2017), 57–87.

[126] As discussed earlier in this chapter, news of the growing public health crisis was slow to make it out of France partly because of the campaign of misinformation in Marseille to disguise the plague as merely a malignant fever.

of public gatherings, among others – to preserve the republic from the *morbo* in France. Public health measures were employed primarily to protect Italian cities from the plague, but they also served as weapons throughout a period of retaliatory public health politics among the cities of Italy – what historian Jean-Pierre Filippini called a "health war" – during the Plague of Provence.[127] As we will see in Chapters 3 and 4, the Italian states' measures among themselves represented a microcosm of the kind of tit-for-tat, retaliatory public health diplomacy that unfolded among the larger European states during the Plague of Provence.

The case of Genoa and Italy during the Great Plague Scare serves to remind us that every act in history, every single occurrence, is the result of a multifaceted confluence of factors. The motives behind responses to the crisis in 1720 were not monolith. Beyond merely perceptions of risk and fear of contagion – significant concerns, to be sure – numerous other circumstances influenced the decisions of officials across Europe as they contemplated how to manage the threat of infection from France. The chapters that follow further illustrate that disaster and crisis management, in the eighteenth century as today, consists of a complex convergence of diverse considerations.

---

[127] We see similar dynamics among the larger states of Europe, including Great Britain and Spain. See Chapters 3 and 4, respectively.

3 | "A Scheme so Barbarous and so Destructive"

Responses to the Plague of Provence in London

[T]hese Stratagems to amuse us with Terror, thereby to let Villainy pass unregarded, and to employ us with our own Fears, that so we may not take Notice of any evil Designs against us, are not unsuccessful. The imaginary Evil spreads like the real one, and the Disease itself is not more catching than the Apprehensions of it ... This, I think, is worse than the South-Sea Scheme; we were there cajoled and wheedled into Misery, we are now frightened into it.[1]

Previous chapters have begun to examine the ways in which emergency sanitary measures – such as quarantines, *cordons sanitaires*, and commercial embargoes – could serve as convenient catalysts for control, the centralization of power, and aggressive commercial competition. This chapter adds a new dimension to the discussion by exploring the responses of a newly unified Great Britain to the Plague of Provence. It will focus on the port city of London – at this time among the largest and busiest ports in the world – and shed light on the various ramifications of the Great Plague Scare as it unfolded across the English Channel from France.

By the eighteenth century, the centralization of state power in Europe allowed for the development of disaster centralism. During the Plague of Provence, European rulers stepped in to manage the crisis, directing emergency measures and increasing communication between the capital and the provinces. Meanwhile, responses to the epidemic – or to its threat, for those outside of France – complemented the fundamental interests of the state. In Britain as elsewhere in Europe, plague-time measures reflect not only concerns over public health, but also contemporary understandings about contagion, commercial interests, and

---

[1] "To the Author of the Letters in the Weekly Journal," *The Weekly Journal or Saturday's Post* (London), October 21, 1721, issue 150.

diplomatic relationships. Taking place in the Age of Enlightenment, regarded as an era of mobility, cosmopolitanism, and intellectual dynamism (despite it also being an era in which the practice of slavery flourished), the epidemic of 1720 emerged at a time in which ideas about contagion and the usefulness of quarantine were very much in flux. This was especially true in England, where treatises from both sides of the contagionist versus anti-contagionist debate reemerged with special force as a result of the French outbreak.[2] The debate would ultimately have major implications for our understandings of disease and the history of medicine. Equally important, however, were the diplomatic realities into which news of the plague arrived in Great Britain. As we will see, the tensions that followed the Treaty of Utrecht in 1713 and the Treaty of The Hague in 1720, as well as the royal desire to curb smuggling in England, and the bursting of the South Sea Bubble just weeks prior to the arrival of plague in Marseille, all served to influence British reactions to the epidemic. Throughout the plague years, moreover, observers in London accused the government of looking to despotic France as a model for sanitary policies, but it is more likely that Britain looked instead to Spain in order to preserve British privileges in the Spanish Americas. Sanitary policies enacted in Britain from 1720 to 1722 were not unimpeded as they were in Spain, however.[3] In London, a very different political culture allowed for the emergence of a significant movement of opposition to regulations that, in the end, was effective.

The chapter begins with a brief introduction to the Quarantine Act of 1710, which served as a precursor to that of 1721. It goes on to discuss British responses to the plague in France and examines how public health regulations in Britain arose in conversation with those of other European states. It then looks at popular and intellectual reactions in London to the threat of plague, as well as the movement of opposition that arose in its wake beginning in 1720. At this time, various groups – grocers, traders, lords, and others – expressed opposition to new restrictions and sanitary regulations, and eventually succeeded

---

[2] Briefly, the anti-contagionists argued that quarantine was useless (they were miasmatists), while contagionists held that quarantining was integral for preserving against plague. More on this in the text that follows.

[3] See Chapter 4 on Cádiz and Spain.

in having many of them repealed. The final section explores the impact of the South Sea "disaster," as well as the influence of diplomatic and commercial interests, on public health measures in Britain during the Plague of Provence.

The Great European Plague Scare of 1720 in England

During the Great Northern War of the early eighteenth century, plague emerged in parts of the Polish–Lithuanian Commonwealth. According to Johann Christoph Gottwald, a physician from Danzig (Gdańsk), the outbreak first appeared in the summer of 1702 in a Swedish army hospital in Pińczów in southern Poland. From there, it is said to have spread into surrounding territories, emerging in Lviv in 1704, and gradually approaching the Prussian territories. In 1707, bubonic plague had spread into Warsaw and Kraków, after which Prussia began to enact measures against its introduction. The outbreak was at its most virulent from 1709 to 1713, in which time it spread throughout the Circum-Baltic region.[4] In response, in November 1710, Queen Anne and the English parliament passed Great Britain's first Quarantine Act.[5]

This act became necessary when earlier orders that called for a forty-day quarantine against all ships from Danzig went unheeded. Prior to its implementation, the English parliament had no say in the issuing of sanitary regulations, such as mandatory quarantines, which were issued by the king or queen in council.[6] The Quarantine Act of 1710 therefore represents the first time that a regular quarantine was issued with participation and approval from parliament. It designated Standgate Creek on the River Medway as a quarantine station, and the island of Stowfort, also along the Medway, as the designated place for the landing and airing of goods. It also set some basic terms

---

[4] Wilhelm Sahm, *Geschichte der Pest in Ostpreussen* (Leipzig: Verlag von Duncker & Humblot, 1905), 35.
[5] This was "An Act to oblige Ships Coming from Places Infected, More Effectually to Perform Their Quarentine" (1710).
[6] William Collingridge, "On Quarantine," *British Medical Journal* 1 (1897): 647. See also: Charles Mullett, "A Century of English Quarantine, 1709–1825," *Bulletin of the History of Medicine* 23, no. 6 (November–December 1949): 527–45.

for carrying out and enforcing the quarantine, and made clear that those who failed to abide by the terms of the act would be "proceeded against with the utmost severity that the law will allow of."[7] In fact, as historian Mark Harrison has observed, "The Act of 1710 placed sanitary measures in Britain on a similar footing to those in France and in theory allowed them to be used more effectively as tools of statecraft."[8] Ten years later, when a public health crisis emerged in France, Queen Anne's Quarantine Act was reissued in its original form.

On August 25, 1720, a few weeks after news arrived in London (from British diplomats abroad) that a "contagious distemper" was present in Marseille, a proclamation was issued that declared a mandatory quarantine for all ships and persons arriving from the Mediterranean according to the terms of the Quarantine Act of 1710.[9] Soon thereafter, by early September, restrictions were expanded to include all ships proceeding from the southern coasts of Spain. These were to undergo a "full quarantine, counting from the day that the ship anchors at the sites designated by customs officials."[10] Why Spain, which the British knew was untouched by the infection? In late August 1720, the Spanish Crown had effectively imposed a mandatory quarantine for vessels

---

[7] "By the Queen, A Proclamation, Requiring Quarantain to Be Performed by Ships Coming from the Baltick Sea," *London Gazette*, November 11–14, 1710, issue 4769.

[8] Mark Harrison, *Contagion: How Commerce Has Spread Disease* (New Haven: Yale University Press, 2013), 28.

[9] "By the Lords Justices ... A Proclamation, Requiring Quarentine to Be Performed by Ships Coming from the Mediterranean," *London Gazette*, August 23–27, 1720, issue 5880. Word of the pestilence in Marseille began to appear in British newspapers in the first week of August, when letters from Paris and Genoa were printed in the *London Journal*, the *London Gazette*, the *Weekly Packet*, and the *Post Man and the Historical Account*. *London Journal*, July 30–August 6, 1720, issue LIV; *Weekly Packet* (London), July 30–August 6, 1720, issue 422; *London Gazette*, August 2–6, 1720, issue 5874; *Post Man and the Historical Account* (London), August 9–11, 1720, issue 1842.

[10] "De tres dias ha, se prohibió la entrada de la embarcaciones, que viniesen de las Costas Meridionales de España, y Francia, sin que primero hagan quarentena entera, a contar desde el dia en que dieren fondo en las sitios señalados por los Oficiales de la Aduana." "Londres 13 de Septiembre de 1720," *Gaceta de Madrid*, no. 41, October 8, 1720, 162–3. "Tambien se dize, se ha da prohibir el Comercio de Levante, y precisar a que hagan quarentena las embarcaciones que salieren de las Costas Meridionales de España, y Francia." "Londres 6 de Septiembre de 1720," *Gaceta de Madrid*, no. 40, October 1, 1720, 158–9.

from all nations, including Great Britain, that approached its southern coast from Ayamonte to the Strait of Gibraltar, encompassing almost the full length of the Spanish coast along the Gulf of Cádiz.[11] The compulsory quarantines varied in length depending on a vessel's origin and its cargo. Ships were expected to brandish mandatory certificates of health, after which they would have to submit to sanitary visits and the hated *fondeos* (which involved the full unloading of a ship's cargo for inspection) on pain of having their vessel and all of its cargo burned.[12] British officials worried that Spain's stringent and unnecessary health measures would hurt Great Britain's commerce at a time when the South Sea Bubble had just burst. One English observer wrote, "The Court of Madrid has ordered the Ships of all Nations coming into any of the Ports of Spain to perform Quarantine, which will put a stop, in a great Measure, to our Trade with Spain for some Time."[13] Britain then responded with a quarantine of its own, directed specifically at Spain's southern coasts. In another major proclamation issued by the British Crown on October 14, 1720, the quarantine was extended to ships arriving from Bordeaux and "any of the ports or places on the coast of France in the Bay of Biscay," and by the end of the month, the quarantine was extended to include all ships or persons arriving from the isles of Guernsey, Jersey, Alderney, Sark, or Man.[14] It was also declared that airing grounds would henceforward be selected by customs officers, and that new quarantine ports were to be designated at London, Bristol, Portsmouth, Plymouth, and Falmouth, so that vessels could proceed to whichever was closest to the place of discharge.

The inclusion of these isles in the latest quarantine is worth a brief look. It is true that they were known to receive certain goods from Languedoc and surrounding areas that were considered "apt to retain infection," such as kid skins, silk, cotton, and human hair. But it was also recognized that the British offshore islands were major hubs for

---

[11] *Cavildos del año de 1720*, libro no. 76, ff. 399 & 485v, AC, AMC.
[12] *Cavildos del año de 1720*, libro no. 76, f. 398v, AC, AMC. See also: *Daily Post* (London), November 28, 1720, issue 362. For more on these controversial *fondeo* searches, see Chapter 4 on Cádiz.
[13] *London Journal*, October 15–22, 1720, issue LXV.
[14] Anonymous, *By the Lords Justices … A Proclamation Requiring Quarentine to Be Performed by Ships Coming from Bourdeaux, or Any of the Ports or Places on the Coast of France in the Bay of Biscay, 14 Oct. 1720* (London: John Baskett, 1720).

contraband trade, which was not only a source of anxiety insofar as the plague was concerned but also spelled trouble for the king's coffers. The final clause of the document explains it best:

And whereas a most pernicious trade is carried on by many of his Majesty's subjects by clandestinely importing goods from parts beyond the sea, to the great prejudice of his Majesty's revenue, and in defiance of his Majesty's laws, which may prove highly detrimental to the health of his Majesty's people during this time of infection abroad, we do hereby strictly charge and command all his Majesty's officers and ministers whatsoever, to take care that the laws against such illegal practices be put in execution with the utmost rigour. And we do hereby charge, forewarn, and require all his Majesty's loving subjects of what degree or condition soever, not to be aiding and assisting to, or to hold any correspondence with any persons using such practices, nor to buy, receive, or take into their custody any goods so clandestinely and unduly run and imported, but on the contrary to use their utmost endeavours to oppose and resist all persons concerned in such unlawful attempts, not only on pain of incurring his Majesty's biggest displeasure, and the severe penalties provided by law against such offenses, but as they tender their own safety, and the preservation of the welfare and safety of their country.[15]

Owing to both a heightened awareness of the dangers of smuggling during plague times and a genuine desire to help curb what had been a stubborn nuisance for years, the contagion in France served as justification for measures that could help curtail some of the illicit commerce that filtered through these islands in avoidance of port duties. Despite the protests of merchants from the isles, the terms of this proclamation would be reconfirmed on February 5, 1721, and were initially to remain in effect for three years.[16] In December 1721, however, the decision was made to end the quarantine for the islands a

---

[15] Anonymous, *By the Lords Justices, A Proclamation, Requiring Quarentine to Be Performed by Ships Coming from the Mediterranean, Bourdeaux, or Any of the Ports or Places on the Coast of France in the Bay of Biscay, or from the Isles of Guernsey, Jersey, Alderney, Sarke, or Man, 27 Octob. 1720* (London: John Baskett, 1720).

[16] "We hear that the inhabitants of the islands of Guernsey, Jersey, &c. presented their petitions last week to his Majesty, praying that the orders for ships coming from thence to England, to perform quarantine, may be revoked; but 'tis said they did not meet with their desired success." *London Journal*, December 10–17, 1720, issue LXXIII.

year earlier than planned, almost certainly because it was found to be both ineffective and counterproductive.[17] As a letter from Portsmouth printed in the *London Journal*, reported: "Smugglers are here compell'd to perform Quarantine, but some People talk as if that was advantageous to them, and gave Opportunity of running their Goods, the Customhouse Officers not daring to go on Board, tho' they see forfeited Goods there; indeed more are now run here than ever."[18] Unsurprisingly, then, smugglers found ways to dodge, and even take advantage of the new quarantine regulations.

Yet, all these initial sanitary regulations were only precursors–modeled after centuries-old guidelines and a ten-year-old document – to a more defined set of policies aimed at preventing infection and actually managing an outbreak should the plague enter British territories. By the end of 1720, King George I and his supporters decided that the terms of the first Quarantine Act were insufficient for preventing the spread of an infection the likes of which was taking place in neighboring France. As a result, in December 1720, Dr. Richard Mead (the Whig, Sir Robert Walpole's physician) was consulted and asked to compose a tract in which he would outline the best methods for the prevention of plague. It appeared soon thereafter under the title, *A Short Discourse Concerning Pestilential Contagion and the Method to Be Used to Prevent it.*[19] Armed with this treatise, the Crown issued a new act, once more with parliamentary backing.

...

[17] "And be it further Enacted, by the Authority aforesaid, That an Act ... intituled, An Act to oblige Ships coming from Places infected more effectually to perform their Quarantine; and for the better preventing the Plague being brought from Foreign Parts into Great Britain or Ireland, or the Isles of Guernsey, Jersey, Alderney, Sark, or Man; and to hinder the spreading of Infection ... shall not continue in Force any longer than until the said Twenty-fifth Day of March One Thousand Seven Hundred Twenty-three." *Journal of the House of Lords* (henceforward *JHL*), vol. 21, December 13, 1721 (London: His Majesty's Stationery Office, 1721), British History Online.

[18] "Extract of a Letter from Portsmouth, dated Sept. 16," *London Journal*, September 23, 1721, issue CXIII.

[19] Richard Mead, *A Short Discourse Concerning Pestilential Contagion and the Method to Be Used to Prevent It* (London: Printed for Sam. Buckley, 1720). It ran through seven editions within a few months. For a detailed discussion of Mead's *Discourse*, and the other plague tracts that emerged in response at this time, see: Chapter 9 in DeLacy, *The Germ of an Idea*; Arnold Zuckerman,

The new Quarantine Act of 1721 passed on January 25 and supplanted Queen Anne's Quarantine Act of 1710, which was found to be "defective and insufficient."[20] The new act built upon the previous one by outlining the steps that would be taken if the infection entered Great Britain. It took effect on February 10, 1721, and was intended to remain in force for a period of three years. Under the new provisions, quarantine would continue for vessels proceeding from infected places, and the principal officer at the British port was now to greet new arrivals with a series of questions to determine the quality of health on board. Inquiries included, among others, the name of the commander, where the cargo was picked up, where the ship had stopped, whether any ports along the way were infected, how many persons were on the vessel when it set sail, and whether there had been any deaths on board. If upon examination it appeared that someone on the vessel was infected, "then the officers of any ships of war, or forts, or garrisons … [were] to resist the entrance of such ship into any port, or to oblige such ship to depart, and to use all necessary means, by firing guns, or any kind of force and violence whatsoever." Should the master of a ship withhold information, he would suffer death as a felon, and if the master were unaware of the infection of a port he visited, of his cargo, or of any individual on his vessel, he would have to forfeit his ship along with a £200 fine. In addition, individuals were forbidden from leaving the vessel without permission during its quarantine upon pain of incurring a £200 fine and a six-month imprisonment.[21]

"Plague and Contagionism in Eighteenth-Century England: The Role of Richard Mead," *Bulletin of the History of Medicine* 78, no. 2 (Summer 2004): 273–308; Charles Mullett, *The Bubonic Plague and England: An Essay in the History of Preventive Medicine* (Lexington: University of Kentucky Press, 1956). Also: Slack, "Perceptions of Plague in Eighteenth-Century Europe": Suman Seth, *Difference and Disease Medicine, Race, and the Eighteenth-Century British Empire* (Cambridge: Cambridge University Press, 2018), 77–8, 122, 127–9; Charles Mullett, "The English Plague Scare of 1720–23," *Osiris* 2 (1936): 484–516.

[20] John Booker, *Maritime Quarantine: The British Experience, c. 1650–1900* (Surrey: Ashgate Publishing, 2007), 95. Mullett, *The Bubonic Plague and England*, 269. For a more detailed discussion of the legal process that saw the passing of this act, see Chapter 4 in Booker's *Maritime Quarantine*.

[21] Parliament of Great Britain, *A Compleat History of the Late Septennial Parliament* (London: Printed for J. Peele at Locke's-Head in Paternoster-Row, 1722), 59.

Under the terms of this new act, the king could also establish lazarets, order ships to be provided, and erect sheds and tents in designated places for use as pesthouses. Officers could compel infected persons, or those obliged to perform quarantine, "to be conveyed to some of those ships, lazarets, or tents." In other words, infected individuals and their families could be forcibly transferred to makeshift quarantine stations, and resistance was punishable by death as a felon. Refusal or escape from these designated places would likewise result in felony and death, and if anyone entered one of these areas then left without proper documentation, "[this] person shall be adjudged guilty of felony, and suffer death as a felon, without benefit of clergy."[22]

The king could also order the establishment of lines of armed guards or trenches around infected towns and could cut communication between infected places and the rest of the country, thus prohibiting any persons or goods from being carried over the lines. Justices of the peace would assign residents to keep watch day and night, with violators suffering death as felons. And if it appeared that a ship arrived, or had cargo, from an infected place, or if there were a person on board who was infected, the king could order the ship with all the goods in it to be immediately burned "for preventing the spread of infection."[23]

Quarantines in response to the Plague of Provence were also issued in the British colonies. In 1721, for example, in response to the plague in Provence, the General Court in Boston imposed a strict quarantine on all ships coming from the France and the Mediterranean, with penalties for violations including death. Measures in Boston against vessels from France were then reported in London newspapers. For example, one article read: "Those Letters add, that a Proclamation has been Published at Boston, obliging to a Quarantine all Ships that come from France, and other Countries suspected of Contagion." *Weekly Journal or British Gazetteer* (London), November 4, 1721. It is worth noting that this Bostonian quarantine against ships sailing from France took place amid a significant outbreak of smallpox in the city. It lasted from April to December 1721, and led to a major debate over inoculation, with Reverend Cotton Mather serving as passionate advocate for the practice. For more on this, see: Stephen Coss, *The Fever of 1721: The Epidemic That Revolutionized Medicine and American Politics* (New York: Simon & Schuster, 2017); John B. Blake, *Public Health in the Town of Boston, 1630–1822* (London: Oxford University Press, 1959), 74.

22 Parliament of Great Britain, *The History and Proceedings of the House of Commons from the Restoration to the Present Time*, vol. 8 (London: Printed for Richard Chandler, 1742), 195–6.

23 Parliament of Great Britain, A *Compleat History of the Late Septennial Parliament*, 57–62.

The Crown could also now prohibit ships weighing less than 20 tons burthen (tonnage of a ship in Builder's Old Measurement or BM) from leaving an English port until the master paid £500 security as a guarantee that he will not visit an infected region.[24] Essentially, for merchants, captains, officers, and all those whose work was in any way tied to English ports, the only way to avoid incurring a felony – and a rope around one's neck – was to observe all terms of the new act, beginning with a lawful quarantine confirmed in the following manner:

When a ship has perform'd quarantine, on proof made of it upon oath by the master and two persons belonging to the ship, and two credible witnesses, that the ship and persons have duly perform'd quarantine, and that they are free from infection, then the customer, &c. with two justices of the peace, are to give certificates thereof, and thereupon such ship and persons shall be liable to no further restraint.[25]

These sanitary policies were controversial both in England and abroad, and the last months of 1721 saw various changes to the new guidelines.

From the perspective of French merchants and officials, the regulations seemed unfair because they came to include *all* French ports, including those far from the epicenter of infection.[26] French officials asserted, moreover, that they had taken sufficient steps to prevent the spread of disease. It thus appeared to them that states across Europe were exploiting the epidemic to harm French commerce while advancing their own.[27] The accusation had already been directed at Spain, Genoa, and Venice, and was now being launched against Great Britain, as well. By the autumn of 1721, when Britain got word from doctors abroad that the epidemic had ceased (though it in fact had not),[28] the French government threatened them with "counter measures"

---

[24] Danby Pickering, *The Statutes at Large, from the Fifth to the Ninth Year of King George I*, vol. 14 (Cambridge: Joseph Bentham, 1765), 302.

[25] Parliament of Great Britain, A *Compleat History of the Late Septennial Parliament*, 57–62.

[26] Harrison, *Contagion*, 30.

[27] Ibid.

[28] Intendants de la Santé, Marseille, August 27, 1721, SP 78/170, France, f. 104, TNA.

if quarantine regulations were not reduced.[29] In response to French threats, reports of the plague's diminishing, and a movement of opposition to plague policies in Britain itself, the British government moved forward to suspend quarantines against French vessels on September 10, 1721.[30] By September 27, all persons arriving in Britain from French ports north of Biscay would only be subject to quarantine if they failed to carry bills or certificates of health.[31] Concerns remained, however, and on October 19, King George I gave a speech in which he expressed a need for *more* procedures to prevent the spread of infection.[32] He explicitly condemned the dangers of the clandestine running of goods, and called for fresh measures to suppress the practice.[33] Plans were also put in motion to establish a new health commission.[34] By November, commissioners of health had been appointed, but owing to a series of rumblings from the London merchant opposition that questioned the legality of such a move, the order was withdrawn less than three months later.[35]

---

[29] Robert Sutton to Lord John Carteret, Paris, September 4, 1721, SP 78/170, France, f. 108, TNA. Harrison, *Contagion*, 31.

[30] Sutton to Carteret, Paris, September 10, 1721, SP 78/170, France, f. 166, TNA. Harrison, *Contagion*, 31.

[31] Booker, *Maritime Quarantine*, 107–8. Stephen Porter, *The Great Plague* (Stroud, Sutton Publishing, 1999), 160. *Weekly Journal or Saturday's Post* (London), October 7, 1721, issue 149.

[32] *Weekly Journal or British Gazetteer* (London), October 21, 1721.

[33] "The unspeakable Misery and Desolation that has of late raged in some Parts of Europe, cannot but be a sufficient Warning to us, to use all possible Precautions to prevent the Contagion from being brought in among us; or if these Kingdoms should be visited with such a Fatal Calamity, to be in a Condition, with the Blessing of God, to stop its further Progress. And as all other Provisions will be altogether vain and fruitless, if the Abominable Practice of Running of Goods be not at once totally suppress'd, I most earnestly recommend to you, to let no other Consideration stand Competition with a due Care of Preserving so many Thousand Lives. The several Affairs which I have mentioned to you, being of the highest and most immediate Concern to the whole Kingdom, I doubt not but you will enter into the Consideration of them with that Temper, Unanimity, and Dispatch, that the Necessity and Importance of them require." *Weekly Journal or British Gazetteer* (London), October 21, 1721.

[34] Mullett, "The English Plague Scare of 1720–23," 488. Paul Slack, "Plague, Population and Political Economy in England 1550–1730," in *Le Interazioni fra economia e ambiente biologico nell'Europa preindustriale secc. XII–XVIII*, edited by Simonetta Cavaciocchi (Florence: Firenze University Press, 2010), 397.

[35] Porter, *The Great Plague*, 162.

Other measures at this time targeted local practices that directly affected the daily lives of people in London. Despite the fact that many had been implemented during previous domestic outbreaks, they nevertheless prompted their share of criticism. For example, beggars and vagrants, who were believed to "conduce to the spreading [of] any infection," were to be apprehended and carried before the justices of the peace to be dealt with according to an earlier proclamation from the time of Queen Anne's reign. Reporting a beggar or vagrant carried a reward of 2 shillings and neglecting to do so carried a penalty of 20 shillings for constables on duty.[36] Meanwhile, those in the "extreme parts of the town" who take guests in for profit, thereby crowding "15 or 20 or more to lye in a small room where it must often happen that some of them will be sick," would likewise be persecuted. Nor were meat, garbage, or offal to be permitted to stink in the markets or slaughterhouses, where offenders would be "prosecuted and punished with the utmost severity [so as to put an end to] these dangerous practices, which are most likely to produce and spread the plague in this town."[37] Public health regulations also aimed to clamp down on brandy or Geneva (gin) shops. Owners could no longer function without proper licenses, which were now made more difficult to obtain – a controversial policy at the dawn of the so-called "gin craze."[38] By keeping its clientele drunk, idle, and thus "in continued heat," these liquor shops and alehouses were believed to increase the possibility of infection, and as a result, were to be suppressed.[39] The keeping of hogs was also frowned upon, and along with the cleaning and paving of streets, walkways, and markets, was brought under tighter supervision. Regulations for the maintenance of these had previously been in force, especially "as the keeping the streets and markets paved and clean are very great preservatives against infection," but "experienced hath shewed that all those steps [had] not had

---

[36] *Daily Courant* (London), November 1, 1721, issue 6250.

[37] Ibid.

[38] For more on the eighteenth-century gin craze, see: Jessica Warner, *Craze: Gin and Debauchery in an Age of Reason* (New York: Basic Books, 2002).

[39] *Daily Courant* (London), November 1, 1721, issue 6250. In humoral theory, excessive heat (or, indeed, anything in excess) was believed to throw off one's humoral balance, which could lead to illness.

the good effect which might have been expected from them."[40] New, more rigorous controls were thus imposed. For example, high constables, petty constables, and headboroughs were to make regular visits around their assigned divisions to ensure that residents were keeping their grounds adequately clean and paved. Individuals would first be given a notice informing them of the impending date of visit in order to give them time to bring the grounds up to standards, and convictions and penalties awaited those who failed to comply.[41] Much as was done in France and Spain, orders in London also prohibited plays and feasting and demanded that alehouses close by nine o'clock in the evening.[42] And in the autumn of 1721, another controversial act was introduced allowing the king "effectually to prohibit Commerce (for the Space of One Year) with any Country that is, or shall be, infected with the Plague."[43] All of this despite the fact that the plague never spread beyond southeastern France.

From their inception, all these policies faced fierce opposition. To British traders, shopkeepers, and others, the regulations smacked of arbitrary government and an abuse of power. By February 1722, most of its clauses were repealed and nearly all provisions that touched on British disease management were reversed.[44] Only the general quarantine remained, along with the more stringent measures against smuggling that King George had requested of the House of Lords. Among these, offenders would now be judged guilty of felony, and liable to transportation, that is, transfer to a penal colony, for seven years.[45] Their ships would be burned and their tackle sold.[46] Licenses for

---

[40] Ibid.

[41] Earlier in October 1721, a notice was printed in the paper complaining about the "filth and nastiness frequently retain'd" in the markets, streets and passageways, and the animal excrement in the streets "to the great nuisance of [the] neighbours." About two weeks later, these issues were addressed in this most recent set of regulations. In many ways, they speak to the place of disease in Europe's evolving views on cleanliness and hygiene. *Daily Journal* (London), October 13, 1721, issue CCXXVII.

[42] Mullett, "English Plague Scare," 496. For Spanish reactions to the 1720 Plague of Provence, see Chapter 4.

[43] *JHL*, vol. 21, November–December 1721.

[44] Mullett, *Bubonic Plague*, 272.

[45] *Evening Post* (London), March 1–3, 1722, issue 1965.

[46] Booker, *Maritime Quarantine*, 97.

barges now also needed to be obtained from the Admiralty in order to navigate the river Thames.[47] In addition, the minimum size for ships exempt from having to pay the £500 security in order to leave the port was raised to 40 tons burthen, thus lessening the number of ships navigating the English Channel and transporting clandestine goods along the coasts of England.[48] Despite persistent protests from merchants and traders of London, it was passed on March 2, 1722, prompting a new wave of opposition.[49]

Reactions to the plague, including the movement of resistance to sanitary measures from 1720 to 1722, are many-sided and complex. The Quarantine Act of 1721 brought about a whirlwind of dissension from various sectors of society. Of particular distaste were the clauses that delineated how Great Britain would handle a domestic outbreak of plague. These included the military cordons and the forced removal of infected families to newly established pesthouses. But preventative measures, such as the burning or sinking of ships and the potential suspension of all trade with infected places, were no less controversial. Grocers and merchants joined the voices of lords and clerics both to relay their fears about the plague, and to protest what they deemed to be the destruction of their rights and liberties. Reactions, whether from fear, interest, or dissension, came from every level. It is to this medley of voices that we now turn.

"On the Repeated Outcries of the People"[50]: Popular Reactions to the Threat of Plague and Resistance to Sanitary Measures in London

The epigraph that opens this chapter is from a document featured in the *Weekly Journal or Saturday's Post* that is headed with an epigraph of its own: *Ad calamitatem quilibet rumor valet*, which is to say, "In times of calamity, every rumor is believed." This quote from Syrus' *Maxims* captures to some extent the general feeling of panic that overtook the populace during the Great Plague Scare of 1720–1722.

---

[47] *JHL*, vol. 21, March 2, 1722.
[48] Booker, *Maritime Quarantine*, 96.
[49] *JHL*, vol. 21, February 28, 1722. *JHL*, vol. 21, March 2, 1722.
[50] Parliament of Great Britain, *A Compleat History of the Late Septennial Parliament*, 63.

Despite extensive opposition to public health regulations, news of the plague outbreak in France, and thus the potential for an outbreak in England, generated rampant fear on the ground. Londoners knew, after all, about the Great Plague of London decades earlier (1665–66) that took as many as 100,000 lives – over 15 percent of the population of London and the provinces.[51] The general alarm provoked rumors that the contagion had spread into London via ships from Turkey and the Netherlands, rumors that in turn caused additional frustration. The following passage captures the aggravation:

Another great Cause of our present Terrors of the Plague is, the giving a too hasty Belief to every idle, ill-grounded Story concerning it … and after giving us about three Weeks Pain, they very modestly [tell] us again, 'twas all a Lie … Thus we are liable to the Whimsey of every petulant News-Writer, who are made the Instruments of designing men, to bring the Plague amongst us, or drive it away again, as it may serve a wicked Turn … While our Eyes are kept ready upon this great impending Ruine, we lay ourselves more open to the Injuries of wicked Men; and therefore this great Calamity is represented to us in its most horrid Colours, that thereby all other inferior Mischiefs may be lost in the Observation of it.[52]

The apprehension caused by false rumors in London stretched across the channel, as well. In October 1721, French regent Philippe d'Orléans dispatched Philippe Néricault Destouches, secretary at the French embassy in London (remembered best for his work as playwright) to the palace of George I in Kensington to give formal complaint of the false news being printed in English newspapers about the plague in France, and about the "injurious reflections against the government of France" contained therein.[53] Yet, criticism of the French government and false rumors of infection continued, despite complaints and calls for punishing those responsible. Such an appeal was published in the anonymous letter mentioned earlier: "Let the Plague itself, and not

[51] There were approximately 70,000 deaths from plague (about 15 percent of population) recorded in the *Bills of Mortality*. Allowing for those deaths that were not recorded, however, the total number could have exceeded 100,000. Porter, *The Great Plague*, 74.

[52] "To the Author of the Letters in the Weekly Journal," *The Weekly Journal or Saturday's Post* (London), October 21, 1721, issue 150.

[53] "Londres 28 de Octubre de 1721," *Gaceta de Madrid*, no. 47, November 25, 1721, 184.

the Apprehension of it, make the Alteration in us. Whoever therefore gives the Alarm, without the utmost Certainty, ought to be dealt with in as severe a manner, as our ancient Laws treated him who villainously lighted up a Beacon, when there was no approaching Danger."[54]

As rumors and the threat of plague caused widespread anxiety, so too did a fear of poverty. For many, the threat of a major disease outbreak also carried the risk of destitution, and the propagation of false rumors served to make the threat more real. During the Plague of Provence, no less than during other disease epidemics, wealthy urban residents across Europe fled the cities for the countryside, at times leaving behind a trail of starvation that resulted from want of industry and income. As one observer described it:

I need not enlarge upon the unhappy consequences of this fanciful Plague amongst us; the most insignificant Member of the Community can feel the Decay of Trade, and the Loss of public Credit, without being told of it ... we can't but justly conclude from our own Frights, that every Body will be fearful to come to a Place where the Infection is daily expected, and consequently publick Business must be laid aside, under the Pressures of an unavoidable Calamity.[55]

The "fanciful plague" was thus as damaging as the real thing, for its effects on commerce and industry were just as real. In London and surrounding areas, reports told of the decay of trade and the "miserable starving condition of their poor." Another account relates a dire situation in the town of Colchester northeast of London in Essex, where the manufacture of wool had declined such that the "once wealthy populous town" was now struggling to find money to pay the wages of "those employed in the little manufacturing that is still kept on foot there."[56]

In what was fundamentally a petition for atonement and a turning away from sin during the mandatory fasts and prayer days demanded by recent proclamations, one author, who signed their name as "The Admonisher," summarized the effects that an epidemic could have on the disadvantaged:

[54] "To the Author of the Letters in the Weekly Journal," *The Weekly Journal or Saturday's Post* (London), October 21, 1721, issue 150.
[55] Ibid.
[56] "To the Author of the London Journal," *London Journal*, December 17–24, 1720, issue LXXIV.

'Tis worthy our Notice that in contagious or publick Visitations of that Nature, the Weight of the Judgment generally falls heaviest upon the poor; not that it is more immediately sent or directed as a Plague to them, but their unhappy Circumstances, in a more especial manner, expose them to it, than others: The Rich, allarm'd by the Danger of the Infection, fly the infected Ground, and by all possible Ways shift themselves into Retreats and remote Places, that they may have the Air, and be free from the Necessity of coming into Crowds, and conversing with the Distemper'd. By this means Trade stops, Employment ceases, and the Poor wanting Work, must of consequence have their Subsistance cut off. This immediately reduces Thousands of Families to inexpressible Misery and Distress; want of Labour to them who earn their daily Bread by it, is want of Bread; and want of Bread is Perishing and Death.[57]

Then as now, for the average person, the threat of a major disease outbreak did not only mean possible illness and death, but also the possible loss of one's livelihood. And in early modern Europe, rumors of impending plague could be as harmful as the real thing.

...

As with previous disease epidemics, news of the plague in France generated rumors, fear, and calls for atonement all over Europe, but in 1720, it also bred antagonism and shook intellectual circles. The Quarantine Act of 1721 was thus controversial from the beginning. In the words of one contemporary, "As for the Quarantine Act, it [is] a Statute that has made a very great Noise, more perhaps than any other Law that has been enacted within the Memory of Man."[58] Before it even came close to running its initial course (for it would be reinstated during other public health crises into the nineteenth century), it gave rise to renewed debates about the usefulness of quarantine and the nature of contagion.

Understandings of contagion were already very much in transition in the eighteenth century. Yet the epidemic reignited discussions on the efficacy of quarantining and the nature of disease transmission, leading to an upsurge in the publication of plague tracts all over the Atlantic world; and possibly more plague tracts came out of London

[57] Ibid.
[58] Parliament of Great Britain, A *Compleat History of the Late Septennial Parliament*, 57.

at this time than anywhere else.[59] Prior to the eighteenth century, disease was generally understood as resulting primarily from the presence of miasmas, or foul odors or vapors in the air, that threw off the balance of the four humors or fluids that were believed to determine all aspects of a person's health and personality. These vapors could be released from a variety of sources, including corpses, stagnant water or swamps, and astrological events like the position of the stars or the arrival of a comet. Miasmas could also result from God's desire to punish a human population for their sins. By the later seventeenth and eighteenth centuries, however, such Galenic understandings of disease increasingly came to be perceived in opposition to those of contagionism. Ideas about the nature of contagion itself began to change, and the Plague of Provence marks a significant moment in this shift.

---

[59] Treatises that referenced the Plague of Provence would be published into the nineteenth century as debates continued. For some of the ones published *during* the epidemic, see, for example: Anonymous, *Medicina Flagellata: or, The Doctor Scarify'd* (London: Printed for J. Bateman, 1721); Richard Blackmore, *A Discourse Upon the Plague with a Preparatory Account of Malignant Fevers* (London: Printed for John Clark, 1721); Richard Bradley, *The Plague at Marseilles Consider'd: With Remarks Upon the Plague in General, Shewing its Cause and Nature of Infection, with Necessary Precautions to Prevent the Spreading of that Direful Distemper, Publish'd for the Preservation of the People of Great-Britain* (London: Printed for W. Mears, 1721); Joseph Browne, *A Practical Treatise of the Plague and All Pestilential Infections That Have Happen'd in this Island for the Last Century* (London: Printed for J. Wilcox, 1720); Daniel Defoe, *Due Preparations for the Plague, as Well as Soul and Body, Being Some Seasonable Thoughts Upon the Visible Approach of the Present Dreadful Contagion in France; the Properest Measures to Prevent It, and the Great Work of Submitting to It* (London: Bible and Dove, 1722); Explainer, *Distinct Notions of the Plague with the Rise and Fall of Pestilential Contagion* (London: Printed for J. Peele, 1722); Edmund Gibson, *The Causes of the Discontents in Relations to the Plague and the Provisions Against it, Fairly Stated and Consider'd* (London: Printed for J. Roberts, 1721); Richard Mead, *A Discourse on the Plague* (London: Printed for A. Millar, 1720); Richard Mead, *A Short Discourse Concerning Pestilential Contagion and the Methods to Be Used to Prevent il* (London: Printed for Sam. Buckley, 1720); George Pye, *A Discourse of the Plague; Wherein Dr. Mead's Notions Are Consider'd and Refuted* (London: J. Darby, 1721); Philip Rose, *A Theorico-Practical, Miscellaneous, and Succinct Treatise of the Plague, Shewing Its Nature, Signs, Causes, Prevention and Cure* (London: Printed for T. Jauncy, 1721); Charles Scarborough, *A Practical Method as Used for the Cure of the Plague in London, in 1665* (London: Printed for B. Lintot, 1722); Hans Sloane, *The First Part of the Treatise of the Late Dreadful Plague in France,*

Beginning in 1720, a major debate reemerged with particular force in Britain between the "contagionists" and "anti-contagionists." In brief, anti-contagionists argued that quarantine was useless. They were miasmatists (or miasmists), meaning that they accepted traditional,

Compared with That Terrible Plague in London, in the Year 1665, in Which Died Near a Hundred Thousand Persons (London: H. Parker, 1722); Edward Strother, *Experience'd Measures How to Manage the Smallpox; to Which Is Added, the Proper Method to Be Used in the Plague* (London: Printed for Charles Rivington, 1721).

The plague in Provence inspired medical tracts not only in Britain, but elsewhere in Europe and North America from 1720 through the nineteenth century. William Byrd II's *Discourse*, for example, was written in Virginia and reprinted in London. William Byrd II, *Discourse Concerning the Plague* (London: Printed for J. Roberts, 1721).

In German: Johann Jacob Scheuchzer, Λοιμογραφια Massiliensis: *Die in Marseille und Provence Eingerissene Pest-Seuche* (Zurich: Bodmer, 1720). In Italy, too, we see the publication (and republication, as in the case of Muratori's *Del governo della peste*) of plague tracts at this time. For example, see: Muratori, *Del governo della peste* ...; Muratori, *Relazione della peste di Marsiglia*; Domenico Gagliardi, *Consigli Preservativi, e curativi in tempo di contagio, Dati in luce in forma di Dialogo da Domenico Gagliardi, Protomedico Generale di Roma, e Stato Ecclesiastico* (Rome: Stamperia di S. Michele a Ripa Grande, 1720); Pestalozzi, the Venetian physician who settled in Lyon, also wrote a treatise at this time: Jérôme-Jean Pestalozzi, *Avis de Precaution Contre La Maladie Contagieuse de Marseille, Qui contient une idée complette de la Peste, & de ses accidens* (Turin: Chez Pierre Joseph Zappate, 1721).

Numerous plague tracts emerged in France, as well. Among them: Jean-Baptiste Bertrand, *Relation Historique de la Peste de Marseille en 1720* (Cologne: Chez Pierre Marteau, 1721); François Chicoyneau, François Verny, and Jean Soulier, *Observations et Reflexions, Touchant la Nature, les Evenemens, et le Traitment de la Peste de Marseille, Pour Confirmer ce qui est avancé dans la Relation touchant les accidens de la Peste, son Prognostic, & sa Curation, du 10 Decembre 1720* (Lyon: Chez les Freres Bruyset, 1721); Croissainte, *Journal abregé*; Antoine Deidier, *Dissertation, Où l'on établi un sentiment particulier sur la contagion de la peste, Le Latin à côté* (Paris: Chez Charles-Maurice d'Houry, 1726); Jean-Jacques Manget, *Traité de la Peste Recueilli, des meilleurs auteurs* (Geneva: Chez Philippe Planche, 1721); Helvetius, *Remèdes contre la peste* (Paris: Pierre-Auguste Lemercier, 1721). Jean d'Antrechaus, *Relation de la peste dont la ville de Toulon fut affligée en 1721, Avec des observations instructives pour la postérité* (Paris: Frères Estienne, 1726); Maurice de Tolon, *Le capucin charitable, enseignant la méthode pour remedier aux grandes miseres que la peste a coûtume de causer parmi les peuples* (Lyon: Les Freres Bruyset, 1721).

Some French plague tracts, such as that of Chicoyneau et al., were reprinted all over Europe, including Leyden, Dublin, and London. See, for example:

Galenic understandings of miasma theory as described above. For anti-contagionists, practices like trade embargoes and quarantines were useless in the face of disease-causing foul vapors, and functioned only to interrupt commerce and cause economic disaster. Contagionists, on the other hand, held that quarantines were integral for preserving against diseases like the plague. Especially by the late seventeenth to early eighteenth century, they believed that there existed some kind of infectious material. Some thought it could be a sort of chemical; others speculated that it could be a living entity, what the Dutch researcher Antoni van Leeuwenhoek had called an "animalcule" (from the Latin

François Chicoyneau, *A Succinct Account of the Plague at Marseilles, Its Symptoms, and the Methods and Medicines Used for Curing It* (Dublin: George Grierson, 1721); François Chicoyneau, François Verni, and Jean Soulier, *Beknopt verhaal, raakende de toevallen van de pest te Marseille: neevens deszelfs voorzegging en geneezing* (Leyden, 1721).

The years 1720 to 1722 also saw an explosion of traditional, full-length sermons, and many of those printed in Britain during the epidemic made their way across the Atlantic to the newspapers in the British colonies. Each is unique only in its details, choosing different biblical references to pestilence and presenting God in any of a variety of ways – God as refuge and protector in times of crisis, God as reluctant punisher, God as vengeful judge, God as merciful pardoner – for they all fundamentally shared the same message: repent, repent, repent. For some examples, see: Bishop Hugh Boulter, *A Sermon Preach'd Before the Lords Spiritual and Temporal in Parliament Assembled at the Collegiate Church of St. Peter's Westminster, on Friday, December the 16th, 1720* (London: Printed for Timothy Childe, 1720); Edward Davies, *A Sermon Preach'd on Friday Decemb. 16th 1720, Being the Day of Publick Fasting and Humiliation for the Averting God's Judgments, Particularly the Plague* (London: Printed for T. Hurt in Coventry, 1720); Thomas Newlin, *God's Gracious Design in Inflicting National Judgments: A Sermon Preach'd Before the University of Oxford at St. Mary's on Friday, Dec. 16th 1720* (Oxford: Printed at the Theatre, 1721); Bishop Joseph Wilcocks, *A Sermon Preach'd Before the Honourable House of Commons, at St. Margaret's Westminster, on Friday, Decemb. 16th 1720* (London: Printed for Timothy Childe, 1720); Obadiah Hughes, *The Good Man's Security in Times of Publick Calamity: A Sermon Preach'd in Maid-Lane, Southwark, On Occasion of the Plague in France, Published at the Request of Many That Heard It* (London: Printed for John Clark, 1722); David Jennings, *Behold the Desolations in the Earth! A Sermon Preach'd at Crosby-Square, Nov. 30, 1721, A Time of Solemn Prayer on Occasion of the Plague in France* (London: Printed for John Clark, 1721); James Paterson, *A Warning to Great-Britain in a Sermon Preach'd at Several Churches in and about London, Upon the Spreading of the Plague in France, and Now Publish'd for the Benefit of Others* (London: Printed for the Author, s.a.).

"animalculum" or "small animal") in 1676.[60] This "microscopic animal," they postulated, would be transmitted in some manner – perhaps person to person, or through the pores; perhaps by contact with a sick person, or with objects that had been in contact with a sick person.[61] For at least some contagionists, then, one major cause of disease outbreaks was commerce and the interchange of peoples and commodities that accompanied it. Measures such as trade embargoes, sanitary lines, and quarantines were thus integral for the preservation of public health. The ideas that characterized the debate between the contagionists and anti-contagionists of the eighteenth and nineteenth centuries were not new. Discussions about the nature of disease and contagion had existed in one form or another for centuries.[62] In 1720, however, the number of publications on such questions ballooned in direct response to the Plague of Provence.

The plague years also saw an upturn in dialogue and experimentation on smallpox inoculation involving some of the same figures who were writing treatises on the 1720 plague, including Dr. Edward Strother, Sir Richard Blackmore (an opponent of inoculation), and Dr. Hans Sloane (a proponent).[63] Indeed this activity flourished from the

---

[60] Along with the English polymath Robert Hooke (1635–1703), and Jesuit scholar Athanasius Kircher (1602–80) before him, Antoni Philips van Leeuwenhoek (1632–1723), at times called the "Father of Microbiology," was among the first to observe microorganisms (specifically, bacteria, which he called "animalcules") under a microscope.

[61] For more on the contagionist versus anti-contagionist debate, see, for example: Alex Chase-Levenson, *The Yellow Flag Quarantine and the British Mediterranean World, 1780–1860* (Cambridge: Cambridge University Press, 2020); DeLacy, *The Germ of an Idea*; Melvin Santer, *Confronting Contagion: Our Evolving Understanding of Disease* (Oxford: Oxford University Press, 2015); Zuckerman, "Plague and Contagionism in Eighteenth-Century England"; Paul Slack, *The Impact of Plague in Tudor and Stuart England* (London: Routledge & Kegan Paul, 1985); Mullett, *Bubonic Plague*; Mullett, "English Plague Scare."

[62] Similar ideas had been proposed much earlier, for example, by Girolamo Fracastoro in 1546, and expanded upon by Marcus von Plenciz in 1762. However, scientists and doctors did not take these seriously, widely preferring the Galenic model instead. This finally began to change in the nineteenth century when the contagionist model led to one of the biggest breakthroughs in the history of science: the development of the germ theory of disease that most famously took form with the work of Louis Pasteur in the 1850s and Robert Koch in the 1880s.

[63] Their works are listed in footnote 59.

summer of 1721 to March 1722 in particular, when Dr. Hans Sloane conducted a series of experiments on immunization. In the first of these, he successfully inoculated seven prisoners who were condemned to death.[64] In the context of the Great Plague Scare that gripped London in 1720, it was feared that smallpox, which had recently become more virulent, would represent the next great agent of death. Thus, the plague in Provence brought about in Great Britain – especially in London – a whirlwind of discussion about the nature of contagion and prevention that would continue into the nineteenth century and ultimately contribute to major advances in medicine.

...

As these great debates shook intellectual circles, criticism and protests over the new public health regulations came from individuals and groups across society. In London, anger was directed at authorities – especially King George I and the Privy Council – in response to the numerous ordinances enacted after the Quarantine Act of 1721 both to prevent infection and to manage it in the event that it entered British ports. Protests came not only from grocers, merchants, shipowners, and others who had a vested interest in policies that affected trade and commerce, but from various groups and individuals who were concerned by what appeared to be the overstepping of government authority and the implementation of ineffective policies. Responses in London at this time reveal the variety of interests that came into play in English society during the Plague of Provence.[65]

---

[64] The prisoners were promised their freedom if they submitted to the experiment. They went on to survive the trial and gain their freedom. For a more detailed discussion on the topic of smallpox inoculation in the 1720s, see: Chapter 8 in: DeLacy, *The Germ of an Idea*; Spencer J. Weinreich, "Unaccountable Subjects: Contracting Legal and Medical Authority in the Newgate Smallpox Experiment (1721)," *History Workshop Journal* 89 (Spring 2020): 22–44; Adrian Wilson, "The Politics of Medical Improvement in Early Hanoverian London," in *The Medical Enlightenment of the Eighteenth Century*, edited by A. Cunningham and R. French (Cambridge: Cambridge University Press, 1990), 4–39. See also Mullett, *Bubonic Plague*, 287–90. On the first experiment, see Wilson, "The Politics of Medical Improvement," 27.

[65] Some of the parliamentary debates that arose in response to English plague-prevention policies during the Provençal plague, including the roles of the Tories and court Whigs in these debates (which are not the focus of this chapter), are covered in Chapter 9 of: DeLacy, *The Germ of an Idea*.

Among the more controversial policies were regulations pertaining to sanitation. During the plague scare in London, new clauses in the Quarantine Act demanding stricter regulation of street cleaning at the local level prompted widespread protests. In a formal letter of complaint, the Inhabitants of the Liberty of Westminster argued that the directives and penalties set in place during the co-reign of William and Mary were sufficient for the enforcement of street cleaning and pavement maintenance in Westminster, and that the new law meant only to "take away the Jurisdiction of the Court in Westminster." In addition, they feared the prospect of corruption, namely, "the introduction of perjury, the disregard of oaths, and the incouragement of immorality and vice," on the part of the officers who would be appointed to enforce the new regulations.[66]

The Grocers of London, too, expressed their grievances over aspects of the Quarantine Act of 1721. Founded in the fourteenth century, the Worshipful Company of Grocers of the City of London, which originally included apothecaries and instrument makers, was one of London's original Livery Companies or trade associations.[67] In 1721, they drew up their formal complaint about the bill for the prevention of the clandestine running of goods. First and foremost, the grocers argued, they did not trade any goods liable to infection. Moreover, because they often had to "put several sorts of goods together, bought of different importers," it was impossible for them to acquire the necessary licenses and to provide proofs of the payment of customs dues that were necessary upon the inspection of seizure of goods.[68] The

---

[66] Anonymous, *The Case of the Inhabitants of the Liberty of Westminster, Against the Clauses, Proposed by the Justices of the Peace, to a Bill Now Passing, to Require Quarentine* (London: 1721). 816. m. 13, no. 93, British Library (henceforward BL).

[67] Deborah E. Harkness, "Maps, Spiders, and Tulips: The Cole-Ortelius-L'Obel Family and the Practice of Science in Early Modern London," in *From Strangers to Citizens: The Integration of Immigrant Communities in Britain, Ireland and Colonial America, 1550–1750*, edited by Randolph Vigne and Charles Littleton (Brighton: Sussex Academic Press, 2001), 184. John Benjamin Heath, *Some Account of the Worshipful Company of Grocers of the City of London* (London: 1829), iii, 43–4.

[68] Anonymous, *Reasons Humbly Offer'd by the Grocers of the City of London, Against Part of the Bill Now Depending in the Honourable House of Commons, Entituled, A Bill to Prevent the Bringing in the Infection, by the Clandestine Running of Goods* (London: 1721). 816. m. 13, no. 91, BL.

acquisition of such paperwork, and thus the lessening of their trade and of his Majesty's revenues, was further complicated by the fact that orders were very often received late at night for shipment the next morning, and these were usually sent off with no more than one or two hours' notice. In an appeal to reason, the grocers also questioned how it was that the dispatch of goods out of houses and shops was more conducive to infection than the seizure of said goods by the officers?

Or how can it be reconciled to Reason, that in order to prevent the bringing in the Infection, every other Person, as well as Traders, are to become Tributary and Slaves to the Will of every malicious and mercenary inferior Officer[?] ... What Publick Evil have the Traders of this City and other Parts done, that under the Pretence of preventing the Infection, their Liberties must be slided into the Hands of Officers? What good have the inferior Officers done, that they are still to be complimented with a new Power which ought not to be known in Great Britain?[69]

The grocers concluded that if the bill passed, "it would be an unsupportable Burden on every Fair Trader, not only in this City, but in every Corporation and Trading Town of Great Britain, and impracticable for them, and the Grocers in particular, to carry on their Trades ... so beneficial to the Publick."[70]

Like the Grocers of London, the shipowners, merchants, and traders of the city, many of whom sat in the House of Commons, also strongly opposed the Quarantine Act of 1721 and new anti-smuggling provisions.[71] When the bill to prevent illicit commerce was nevertheless passed on March 2, 1722, they challenged the decision on various grounds. For one, they argued that an earlier increase of 15 to 30 tons burthen for ships wishing to leave English ports without security had no proven advantages, serving only to lower customs duties, and that the new increase to 40 tons would be equally ineffectual. Punishments for violations were also a major concern for the opposition. The heavy penalties of banishment or the confiscation of one's ship were far too severe for the crimes since they did not take into account various possible circumstances. If, for example, the owner of a vessel was entirely

---

[69] Ibid.

[70] Ibid.

[71] Peggy K. Liss, *Atlantic Empires: The Network of Trade and Revolution, 1713–1826* (Baltimore: The Johns Hopkins University Press, 1983), 2–3.

innocent because the crime was committed "through the Folly or Knavery of the Sailors," then his ship would be unjustly seized. Aside from representing an injustice, such a punishment would adversely affect English trade for it would "discourage ... lending small Vessels to those who trade in them, by which a great Part of the Coast Trade is at present carried on."[72] The penalty of banishment also risked being "annexed to a very small offense" if a gentleman returned to England with "the least Trifle that has not been entered and paid Duty, though he hath not the least Design to defraud the King of His Customs, or thinks he is transgressing any Law whatsoever."[73] Of particular distaste, however, was the clause requiring licenses to be obtained from the Admiralty to navigate the Thames. The businessmen specifically opposed the fact that the law did not make exceptions for the nobility, or the lord mayor and companies, which they deemed "absurd and injurious to property." It represented "not only a great and unnecessary Indignity, but also an Invasion of Property, especially in the Case of the Barges belonging to the City of *London*, which City has an ancient Right to the Conservation of the River of *Thames*, and as high an Interest in it as is possible to be had in any Navigable River."[74]

---

[72] *JHL*, vol. 21, March 2, 1722.

[73] Ibid.

[74] Ibid. It is important to note that equally strong words were used in *support* of legislation against the clandestine running of goods. We find a good example of this in a letter by "Plowman" published in the *Weekly Journal or British Gazetteer* in 1721: "Mr. Read, By reading your Weekly Journal, I observed that you have been very active in exposing the detestable Practices of such as both wish and endeavour the Destruction of their native Country, and the subversion of the present Government; and have likewise said much of the impious Practices of the South-Sea Managers. After this, I think I may venture to tell you of another Party of Men, whose Practices are like to be of as dangerous a Consequence, and may involve the Nation in as fatal Calamities if not timely restrain'd, and that is the frequent and notorious Practice of Smugling, which is got to that head, as makes it of the highest Concern to the Publick, to put a stop to it one way or other; we have now a good and wise Parliament, which one wou'd think might easily strengthen the Laws in that Case made and provided; which makes it the stranger to all reasonable Men that nothing has been done effectually to stop this pernicious Practice; nay, tho' at this Time we run the greatest Hazard of having the Plague imported upon us, without which we are at this Time likely to become the most flourishing trading Nation in the World, since it is evident that France by that dreadful Scourge has lost all its Commerce; But I will wave this, and shew, that the Smugling Trade is of its self enough to undoe us. I am assur'd there is a Village in Sussex, about 20

Yet another group that took issue with the new health regulations were the merchants and traders of the Levant Company. Founded in 1592 as a chartered trade company, by 1720 it had roughly 200 members. A memo composed by the Company for the Privy Council in 1721 outlined their main grievances. They argued, for instance, that ships coming from Turkey that had not stopped at any infected ports should be exempt from the mandatory quarantine imposed on all ships from the Mediterranean. Instead, a certificate of health, verified by an ambassador or consul and stating that quarantine had already been satisfactorily completed elsewhere, should suffice for avoiding quarantine. They also disputed the mandatory airing of goods, claiming that it damaged merchandise such as raw silk, mohair yarn, and cotton, and rallied against the costs associated with quarantines. Because they already paid heavy customs dues on their goods, they argued, "It would be a great discouragement to Trade should the Merchant

Miles from the Sea, where there has not gone less than 5000 l. worth of Brandy at prime Cost, in about a Year; what then is run thro' the whole Kingdom, and if it be right French, as themselves say, how many Pounds of our trading Money must go to France in one Year, enough in time to bring England to extream Poverty, which will not fall on a few Men only, but on the Nation in general; But say it is not all French, as some think, but English carry'd to Sea; that is a Cheat which Justice and the Parliament out to redress and Punish ... Such men as encourage the Consumption of Foreign Commodities, are void of common Reason, and but little consult their Countries good or Interest, for if we neglect spending our own Produce, we shall in a little time bring that Land which is not rented at 100 l a Year to 60 or 70, and the Encouragers of Foreign Commodities to Ruin and Beggary. And farther I dare affirm, that these Brandy-Runners are more pernicious and hurtful to the Publick than the common Robbers on the Highway, for the one hurts only here and there a Man, but the other the whole Nation. The former spends what he gets in the Nation, but the other sends our Money into a Foreign Country; and I cannot see why one Crime shou'd be immediate Death, and not the other, I cannot see, but that it wou'd agreeably-enough suit out Excellent Constitution to make Smugling Death, especially at this time. We read in the News from France, that some Soldiers only killing a straggling Sheep or two, where there was danger of the Plague, were buried alive with the Sheep, and I cannot think out French Smuglers now, deserve much less. Besides, that the vast sums expended in this Foreign Liquor, is not only lost to the Spender, but lost to the Nation, and lost to Posterity, as much as a Man's House is, when it is burnt to Ashes ... I require you Mr. Read, to make these Lines Publick, as you are a Lover of your Country and the present Government, they being the Thoughts of a plain, honest Country Fellow, which I hope will be accepted by every one that weighs them with Reason. I am, Your loving Friend, Plowman." *Weekly Journal or British Gazetteer* (London), September 23, 1721.

be obliged to pay the Charges of Quarantine."[75] The Levant Company also called for a formal plan of compensation for those whose ships were burned because of the new regulations. If indeed ships were henceforward to be destroyed on suspicion of infection, then the proprietors should be compensated for the loss of the ship and its cargo.

Historian Mark Harrison has pointed out that this was a difficult time for the Company. For years, it had been falling behind the rival East India Company, which had lowered the price of silk. As a result, the new health regulations, which severely limited commercial exchange between British and Mediterranean ports, rendered the Levant Company vulnerable in the face of its competitors.[76] The situation was especially alarming in light of the destruction in early August 1721 of two ships that had traveled from Turkey. The *Bristol-Merchant* under the direction of Captain John Winne, and the *Turkey-Merchant* captained by John Bennet, had arrived in Britain late 1720 to early 1721. Having touched at Cyprus, where it was believed plague was recently present, the ships were confiscated, and a committee of council was formed to determine what to do with them.[77] The committee soon decided that both vessels should be destroyed along with their cargo, and that the owners should be compensated so as not to discourage trade with Turkey. On March 5, 1721, the king approved the decision, and in June 1721, a motion was made to discuss compensation for the owners once the ships were destroyed.[78] This sum was set at £23,935, and in early August, the ships and their cargoes were destroyed at Standgate Creek.[79] This, it is worth noting,

---

[75] "The Case of the Levant Company, in Relation to the Bill now depending before this Honourable House, for performing quarantine" (London: 1721?). 816. m. 13, no. 94, BL.

[76] Harrison, *Contagion*, 41–2.

[77] Booker, *Maritime Quarantine*, 103.

[78] Booker, *Maritime Quarantine*, 103. Parliament of Great Britain, *Parliamentary History of England: From the Earliest Period to the Year 1803*, vol. 7 (London: T. C. Hansard, 1811), 815.

[79] *Daily Post* (London), August 1, 1721, issue 573. *Weekly Journal or British Gazetteer*, August 5, 1721. Apparently, not all of the cargo was consumed by the fire, and we learn that in September, at least one person was caught trying to steal some of the goods: "We learn from Sheerness, that a Person was apprehended there for presuming to bring on shore half a Bale of Silk, which was part of the Goods belonging to the two Turky Ships burnt lately upon the Flats, which happened not to be consumed, and was sent Prisoner to Maidstone Goal." *London Journal*, September 23, 1721, issue CXIII.

was the only occasion on which British ships were actually destroyed in Great Britain during the Plague of Provence.

In late 1721, the City of London, described as "the Lord Mayor, Aldermen and citizens of London," also petitioned against the Quarantine Act of 1721, citing not only the dangers to the rights and privileges of the people, but also the prosperity of the kingdom.[80] In it, they tackled the clauses that allowed the king to cut communications between Great Britain and infected ports, the regulations against the clandestine running of goods, and a separate clause allowing the king additional sanitary powers. The petition, however, was rejected in a vote of forty-eight to twenty-two. It was deemed a great injustice. As one contemporary related: "it was easy to be seen that every Thing here went in favour of the Court, or the Court Favourites, [which] manifested itself further, when the Lords rejected, by a very Great Majority, the Petition of the City against the Quarentine Act."[81] Accordingly, on December 6, 1721, the City of London submitted a protest to the ratification of the act. Claiming that *"the liberty of petitioning the king* (much more than of petitioning either House of Parliament) is the birth-right of the free people of this realm ... confirmed to them soon after the revolution," the petitioners condemned the rejection of their "proper and unexceptionable" petition. They argued that because London was not only the center of credit, of trade, and of monied interest, but also the place where the plague would most likely appear, and that most suffered from the "late fatal South Sea scheme," the city was entitled "to apply for relief against some of the clauses in the Quarantine Act, and deserved to have been treated on that occasion with more indulgence and tenderness."[82] Moreover, they argued, the rejection of their petition threatened to widen the rifts that already existed and "increase the disaffection to the Government."

This formal protest was followed by another a few days later, on December 13, 1721, in which the petitioners disputed the forced removal of families suspected of infection and the drawing of lines or trenches around infected areas if the plague were to enter the

---

[80] *JHL*, vol. 21, December 6, 1721.

[81] Parliament of Great Britain, A *Compleat History of the Late Septennial Parliament*, 65.

[82] *JHL*, vol. 21, December 6, 1721. Italics as they appear in the original source.

kingdom.[83] Now, the isolation or removal of infected persons into designated places was nothing new. During previous outbreaks of plague in England, including that of 1665, the sick were expected to be shut up in their homes, away from the rest of the population, and could be removed only to established locations for the ill, such as tents, lazarets, or pesthouses. But in 1721, appeals against such acts ultimately prevailed. Petitioners argued for the repeal of this act on the grounds that the forced removal of infected persons from their homes into common lazarets or pesthouses could not be reasonably executed, and that the drawing of lines around infected towns would serve only to "disperse the rich, and by that means ... starve the poor, ruin trade, and destroy all the remains of public and private credit." Moreover, the powers expressed in these acts were unknown in the constitution, "and repugnant ... to the lenity of our mild and free Government."[84] The petitioners maintained that the measures were extraordinary enough to require military force, and would thus involve such "violent and inhuman methods" that they would "draw down the infliction of a new judgment from Heaven."[85] These strong words, with which the authors tried to put the fear of God into their adversaries, were followed by additional emphatic appeals in the newspapers of London.

One anonymous petitioner, who signed their name as Philanthropos, published their condemnatory letter in the *London Journal*.[86] The author denounced the proposed forced removal of infected persons and their families into pesthouses as a scheme "said to be contriv'd for the Suppressing of the Plague," that would "expose every one's Life and Liberty to the mercy of Officers." They invoked strong language to dispute what was deemed a great infringement of English civil liberties under the pretext of public health:

The Cruelty and Inhumanity of these Methods are so obvious, as not to need Animadversion ... A Scheme so barbarous, and so destructive of their Civil Liberties, can never be receiv'd by a Free People ... suppose our Fears were well-grounded, we ought to consider the Matter very carefully, before

---

[83] *JHL*, vol. 21, December 13, 1721. By this act, not only the infected individuals, but also those who lived with them would be removed.
[84] *JHL*, vol. 21, December 13, 1721.
[85] Ibid.
[86] *London Journal*, November 11, 1721, issue cxx.

we give up so essential a Part of our Liberty; for *Liberty once parted with, is with great Difficulty if ever afterwards regain'd.*[87]

To some, the Quarantine Act of 1721 reeked of a conspiracy to take away the freedoms that they believed made Great Britain exceptional.

In fact, among the most recurring grievances against measures of the 1721 Quarantine Act were accusations that the British monarchy was abusing its power and using the "tyrannical practices" of France as a model for England's sanitary regulations. In their letter, Philanthropos pointed out that the very scheme that was taking place in Britain had been executed in France "with utmost rigour and strictness." In broad reference to the health regulations of 1721, another critic agreed, "Some of them are so very extraordinary, that if our Protestant Parliament had not exactly copied after France, it is impossible that they could ever have been thought of ... The Barbarity and Inconsistency of these ... Clauses are so very apparent, that no Country, but an Arbitrary Government, could possibly have furnish'd us with Precedents for them."[88] This was a recurring accusation from 1720 to 1722 in particular, echoing in the chambers of parliament, and appearing in print in newspapers and pamphlets.[89] In their protest of December 13, 1721, the City of London similarly asserted:

Because, we take it, these methods were copied from France, a kingdom whose pattern, in such cases, Great Britain should not follow, the government there being conducted by arbitrary power, and supported by standing armies; and to such a country such methods do, in our opinion, seem most suitable; and yet, even in that kingdom, the powers thus exercised of late have been as unsuccessful as they were unprecedented; so that no neighbouring state hath any encouragement from thence to follow so fatal an example. In the first plague, with which we were visited *anno dom.* 1665, though none of these methods were made use of, much less authorized by Parliament, yet the infection, however great, was kept from spreading itself into the remoter parts of the Kingdom; nor did the city of London, where

---

[87] Ibid. Italics as they appear in the original source.
[88] Parliament of Great Britain, A *Compleat History of the Late Septennial Parliament*, 62.
[89] See, for instance: "December the 13th 1721," *Evening Post* (London), March 8–10, 1722, issue 1968. Parliament of Great Britain, A *Compleat Collection of the Protests of the Lords During This Last Session of Parliament* (London: Booksellers of London and Westminster, 1722).

it first appeared and chiefly raged, suffer so long or so much, in proportion to the number of its inhabitants, as other cities and towns in France have suffered, where these cruel experiments have been tried.[90]

In other words, as opponents of the act understood it, not only did the measures represent an assault on civil liberties in Great Britain but they were also completely useless in the face of infection. Essentially, theirs was an argument based on principle, namely, the principles of liberty and constitutional government that the English believed ideologically separated them from France, bolstered by one that appealed to reason and utility, which is to say, that the measures were ineffective anyway. In the end, the protests were successful. By February 12, 1722, a bill to repeal the clauses in the Quarantine Act that aimed to remove people from their homes and draw lines around infected areas received the royal assent, and by early 1723, the Quarantine Act of 1721 was no longer in force.[91]

South Sea Scheme Men, Franco-Spanish Tyranny, and Tit-for-Tat Diplomacy

Operating in the background throughout was the recent bursting in 1720 of the South Sea Bubble, in which a great number of people met financial ruin at the hands of "South-Sea Scheme-Men."[92] The financial operation was everywhere described as a disaster, a "fatal" plot, a calamity "occasion'd by the wicked Execution of the South-Sea Scheme."[93] References to it in contemporary writings quickly

---

[90] *JHL*, vol. 21, December 13, 1721.

[91] Booker, *Maritime Quarantine*, 100. As mentioned earlier, the Quarantine Act of 1721 would be reinstated in response to later disease outbreaks, including, for example, during the plague in Messina in 1743.

[92] Parliament of Great Britain, *A Compleat History of the Late Septennial Parliament*, vii. For more on the South Sea scheme, see, for example: Thomas Levenson, *Money for Nothing: The Scientists, Fraudsters, and Corrupt Politicians Who Reinvented Money, Panicked a Nation, and Made the World Rich* (New York: Random House, 2020); Richard Dale, *The First Crash: Lessons from the South Sea Bubble* (Princeton: Princeton University Press, 2004).

[93] Such references are ubiquitous in contemporary documents. Parliament of Great Britain, *The History and Proceedings of the House of Commons from the Restoration to the Present Time*, vol. 6 (London: Printed for Richard Chandler, 1742), 261.

turn into emotionally charged invectives, in which the bubble represents the evils of society, and the involvement of the intriguers are strongly condemned. Among the many voices who commented on the economic disaster was Daniel Defoe, who has been credited – or rather, blamed – for formulating the South Sea scheme.[94] In a letter entitled "All Disasters now Attributed to the South Sea," he defensively refuted the various calamities attributed to the bubble, including numerous bankruptcies and suicides. He wrote: "The South Sea Affair is now become a general Calamity, *that must be confess'd*; but as the Devil is charg'd with having a greater hand in our Crimes, than he is, or indeed can be, guilty of, so it is here."[95] Yet, the damage was real. As one contemporary described it: "I believe, it may be said with Truth, That the Executioners of this Scheme have done more Mischief to particular Persons, and to the Nation in general, in a few Months, than the most expensive War we have been at any Time ingaged in."[96] Another wrote:

What have been the Causes of these Evils is more proper for the Enquiry of this Honourable House, but there is one so notorious that we can't avoid complaining of the destructiveness and scandalous corrupt Management of the South-Sea scheme, to the Ruin of the publick, as well as private Credit, the Impoverishment of an infinite Number of Persons, and the bringing down upon us the most extensive Calamity that ever befel a Nation.[97]

[94] The man most likely to have been chief architect of the scheme was John Blunt. See Dale, 24, passim.
[95] William Lee, ed., *Daniel Defoe: His Life, and Recently Discovered Writings, Extending from 1716 to 1729*, vol. 2 (London: John Camden Hotten, 1869), 323–5. Italics are Defoe's.
[96] Archibald Hutcheson, *A Collection of Calculations and Remarks Relating to the South Sea Scheme & Stock, Which Have Been Already Published, with the Addition of Some Others, Which Have Not Been Made Publick 'Till Now* (London: 1720), 109.
[97] Parliament of Great Britain, House of Commons, "The Humble Petition of the Bailiffs, Town-Clerk, Capital Burgesses, and Other the Inhabitants of the Ancient Town of Tamworth, in the Counties of Warwick and Stafford," *A Collection of the Several Petitions of the Counties, Boroughs, &c. Presented to the House of Commons, Complaining of the Great Miseries the Nation Labours Under, by the Great Decay of Trade, Manufactuures, and Publick Credit, Occasion'd by the Mismanagements of the Late Directors of the South-Sea Company, their Aiders, Abettors, and Confederates, &c.* (London: E. Morphew, 1721), 15.

It was in this context that news of the plague – and worse, news of the Crown's responses to it – arrived in London.

Countless contemporary passages reference the South Sea scheme and its designers in relation to the "chicanery" of the Quarantine Act. As noted earlier, the City of London, for instance, cited it as one of the reasons their petitions against sanitary regulations must not be ignored. Another dissenter, the aforementioned "Admonisher," invoked the bubble when they wrote of the evils of spreading false plague rumors, which, like the conspirators of the South Sea scheme, only led to new miseries and apprehensions of another impending disaster.[98] In yet another anonymous letter, "Plowman" compares the "impious Practices of the South-Sea Managers" to the cabals of smugglers "whose Practices are like to be of as dangerous a Consequence."[99] In Britain, then, the South Sea Bubble and the Plague of Provence – or more precisely, British responses to it – represent a single moment of crisis. In some ways, the economic disaster primed Britain for the panic and waves of opposition that ensued in the wake of the Quarantine Act.

The suspicion that regulations were modeled on the "despotic principles" of France also served to drive hostility toward the Quarantine Act, yet opponents may have been pointing to the wrong Catholic kingdom. Given Anglo-Spanish relations following the treaties of Utrecht and Rastatt and that of The Hague, it seems more likely that George I and his Privy Council looked not only to France, as well as England's own history, as models for its sanitary policies, but also to Spain.[100] For one, Spain reacted quickly to the plague in France, prohibiting trade with both infected and uninfected ports, and authorizing ship burnings, death sentences, and extensive quarantines as early as the summer of 1720. The Spanish reaction may have thus served as a model for other nations, in the same way, as we saw in

---

[98] "To the Author of the Letters in the Weekly Journal," *The Weekly Journal or Saturday's Post* (London), October 21, 1721, issue 150.

[99] *Weekly Journal or British Gazetteer* (London), September 23, 1721. See footnote 74.

[100] Since the beginning of the second plague pandemic in Europe in 1347, Italian quarantine models and public health practices also influenced British and European sanitary policy. During the Provençal outbreak of 1720, Spain, for example, paid close attention to what the Italians were doing in response. For more on this, see Chapter 2 on Genoa and Italy.

Chapter 2, that some Italian reactions helped to influence Spanish ones.[101] More important, however, was Spain's treatment of Britain when plague arrived in France, and in turn, Britain's "most valuable commerce with Spain," which they hoped to preserve.[102] After the Spanish War of Succession, it was Great Britain that emerged victorious, having snatched the prized *asiento de negros* ("contract" or "agreement on the Blacks") from France – for which the South Sea Company was responsible – and gaining access to the Spanish South Sea via the annual ship allowance or *navío de permiso*, both highly coveted privileges and sources of riches for the nation that possessed them.[103] Concessions like these, after all, facilitated the lucrative business of illicit commerce.[104] For example, in June 1724, Pierre-Nicolas Partyet, the French consul in Cádiz, informed Jean-Frédéric Phélypeaux, secretary of state and the Marine in France, that José Patiño (minister of Philip V of Spain) was to meet with the Spanish monarch to apprise him of the great harm that the British right of *asiento* was causing the commerce of France and Spain, since it was being used to introduce massive amounts of merchandise, of all varieties, in the Spanish Indies.[105] Especially after the Treaty of

---

[101] Some contemporary Spanish documents on the plague made reference to Italian responses when formulating their own. For example, "Lo que se practica en cumplimiento de estas ordenes en punto de Visitas de Embarcaciones segun lo que se executa en Puertos de Italia." *Cavildos del año de 1720*, libro no. 76, f. 403v, AC, AMC.

[102] *JHL*, vol. 21, December 19, 1721.

[103] The *asiento* of 1713 contracted the South Sea Company to supply 4,800 enslaved people a year to the Spanish Indies for 30 years and granted it the right to send an annual vessel of 650 tons to trade fairs with the Spanish *flotas and galeones*. John Lynch, *Bourbon Spain, 1700–1808* (Cambridge: Basil Blackwell, 1989), 150.

[104] As historian John Lynch has pointed out, "Of course what Spain granted, it could also take away: subsequent administrations mounted fierce operations against contraband in Cádiz and America, and they did little to protect the *asiento* privileges from attack by overzealous local officials. Even so the opportunities for illicit trade were manifold ... [The South Sea] company probably controlled at least 25% of all British exports to Spain and America, immune from the formal Spanish monopoly." Lynch, *Bourbon Spain*, 150.

[105] Pierre-Nicolas Partyet to Jean-Frédéric Phélypeaux, Cádiz, June 4, 1724, AE, BI, 229, ff. 131–2, AN.

Utrecht, British trade to the Spanish Indies through Cádiz was thriving.[106] But during the recent War of the Quadruple Alliance, Britain was for a brief time "deprived of the Friendship of Spain, not easily to be retrieved."[107] The war was described as "an Interruption to one of the most valuable Branches of our Trade; and at a Time when the Nation groan'd under the Pressure of heavy Debts, occasion'd by a former long expensive War."[108] Luckily for the British, the Treaty of The Hague that followed would confirm the privileges granted to Britain in the Treaties of Utrecht and Rastatt, but these rights were by no means guaranteed given the delicate nature of Anglo-Spanish diplomacy at this time.

In the autumn of 1720, Spain imposed quarantines for all ships that approached its southern coasts from Ayamonte to Gibraltar, and violations resulted in the confiscation and burning of the ships and/or their cargoes. At this time, too, under the pretext that Britain was not doing enough to protect itself and its foreign territories against the plague, Spain began rejecting ships from Great Britain and Gibraltar, and forcing Portugal to do the same.[109] Frustrating things further, in

---

[106] Jean O. McLachlan, *Trade and Peace with Old Spain 1667–1750: A Study of the Influence of Commerce on Anglo-Spanish Diplomacy in the First Half of the Eighteenth Century* (Cambridge: Cambridge University Press, 1940), 25.

[107] *JHL*, vol. 21, December 19, 1721.

[108] Parliament of Great Britain, *The History and Proceedings VIII*, 202. Also: "the War with Spain ... does not appear to us so justifiable as we could wish; and yet it was plainly prejudicial to the Nation in sundry respects; for it occasioned an entire Interruption of our most valuable Commerce with Spain, at a Time when Great Britain needed all the Advantages of Peace, to extricate itself from that heavy National Debt it lay under: And as it deprived us of the Friendship of Spain (not easily to be retrieved), so it gave our Rivals in Trade an Opportunity to insinuate themselves into their Affections ... Nor does it appear that Great Britain has had any Fruits from this War, beyond its being restored to the same Trade we had with Spain before we began it." *JHL*, vol. 21, December 19, 1721.

[109] For example, "mas que a verdadeira causa da prohibisão [proibição] fora o exemplo de Espana em cujos portos naõ entrava algum navio Francez de ambos os mares; de sorte que em Madrid se comessava a fallar de romper o commercio com nosco por que admitiamos os do Ponente, ao que tambem se ajuntou chegar a nova de que em Inglaterra se queria usar da mesma prohibisaõ, por se dibulgar (ainda que falsamente) que a peste tinha entrado em Normandia." "Paris, 1º de Novembro de 1721," November 1, 1721,

1721, the Spanish decided to prohibit all commerce with Gibraltar and Menorca, thus targeting Britain via its other territories abroad. British ships were now also subjected to the despised sanitary visits and *fondeo* searches until well after the end of plague in Provence.[110] Rather than resulting from Britain's alleged inability to protect public health, however, Spanish regulations against the British represented both a reaction against the commercial advantages that Britain enjoyed at Spain's expense, and retaliation for their refusal to return to Spain the territory of Gibraltar, which the Spanish saw as rightfully theirs.[111] In the 1720s, tensions over Spain's loss of Gibraltar in the Treaty of Utrecht were running high.[112] It was no secret that Philip V

Ministério dos Negócios Estrangeiros (henceforward MNE), livro 790, f. 401, Arquivo Nacional Torre do Tombo (henceforward TdT). See also Harrison, *Contagion*, 32.

[110] A letter titled, "Health regulations used to oppress English trade," from Lord Cayley in Cádiz to the Duke of Newcastle, written soon after the Spanish proclamation of 1728 that formally reinforced the practice of *fondeo*, lends a voice to British frustrations with these searches: "The two or three ships that arrived here since the publication of that edict, having performed their quarantaines, are now to undergo the *Fondeo* or examination thereby directed before their cargoes can be brought ashore ... Besides the great inconveniency and loss that must accrue to the merchants from having his goods thus opened and removed backwards and forwards, he is obliged to pay these officers for doing it about six pieces of eight a day, besides their victuals; which is an excessive hardship and imposition, and the more so, as it is not only in contradiction to the very Edict itself, which said, that the several regulations therein made shall be executed with as little expense and burden to trade as possible, but no doubt will be likewise a temptation to these fellow to keep each ship under their examination as long a time as ever they can, in order to get the more by her. And what is very extraordinary, the Governour will not consent to have any more than one set of these officers to examine all the ships that arrive; so that being two, three, four or five days in clearing one ship, as they must be and sometimes longer according to their slow way of going about it, they will hardly ever be able to get through them all ... But the truth is, the Governour who is miserably covetous finds his Court very much inclined to treat us ill, and is as ready to make his Advantage of it." From archival letter transcribed in McLachlan, *Trade and Peace with Old Spain*, 192n82.

[111] For more on this, see Chapter 4 on Cádiz and Spain.

[112] In 1728, using the pretext of plague outbreaks in eastern ports, Spain would again impose quarantine for all ships coming from Gibraltar, and so the tensions continued. Indeed, Anglo-Spanish tensions over Gibraltar continue to emerge every so often to this day.

desired to have it back, nor that Great Britain refused to hand it over. As Stanhope wrote to Lord Carteret in 1723, "The king of Spain had the affair of Gibraltar as much at heart as ever."[113] Consequently, despite the protests of London merchants who opposed any retaliatory measures against Spain (since these would affect English import houses no less than Spanish exporters),[114] Britain responded to Spain's affronts, on the one hand, with a quarantine of its own (against Spanish ships), and on the other, with the Quarantine Act of 1721 and sanitary policies that were more in line with those of Spain. Officials in Britain were exasperated that the Spanish Crown appeared to be using the plague as a pretext both to slow British activity in the Spanish market and as a retaliatory tool over the Gibraltar dispute, but they could not deny the importance of their commercial relationship with Spain.

...

The Plague of Provence represents a significant event in British history, despite the infection never making it onto British shores. English reactions to the threat of plague – including public health policies, panic and rumormongering, intellectual debates, protests, and remonstrations – were influenced by a variety of factors that are revealed in the writings of those who made their voices heard during the French outbreak. A fear of "French despotism," as well as outrage about the South Sea Bubble and its scheme men, served to fuel hostility toward public health measures. Disaster centralism was employed, but it triggered waves of criticism and accusations of tyranny and oppression. This was not the case in other parts of Europe during the epidemic in France. As we will see in the next chapter, responses in Spain were quick and regulations heavy – no less heavy, in fact, than they were in France itself. Yet there exists no evidence in the archives of a major movement of opposition against the new policies. As historian Paul Cheney has written, "the comparatively underdeveloped public sphere in mainland Spain, combined with long-standing traditions of consultation in the Spanish composite monarchy, determined the way in

---

[113] James Stanhope to John Carteret, secretary of state, Madrid, January 10, 1723, SP 94/92, Spain, TNA.
[114] Harrison, *Contagion*, 41–2.

which policy debates ... unfolded."[115] In Britain, meanwhile, a more heightened suspicion of chicanery in the wake of the South Sea disaster, coupled with ideas about liberty and limited government, a growing sense of English nationalism, and a more sophisticated use of the printed word – all meant that any attempt to execute policies the likes of which were enforced in Spain and France would not go unchallenged, even though Britain's sanitary policy was, in fact, less stringent by comparison. Let us turn now to the Spanish perspective, and to reactions to the Plague of Provence in the port city of Cádiz.

---

[115] Paul Cheney, "The Political Economy of Colonization: From Composite Monarchy to Nation," in *The Economic Turn: Recasting Political Economy in Enlightenment Europe*, edited by Steven Kaplan and Sophus Reinert (London: Anthem Press, 2019), 78.

4 | *The Spanish Plague That Never Was*
*The Plague of Provence in Cádiz and Spain**

Cádiz is the hub of Europe, the Spanish Indies, and the Americas; it is the common market where all exchanges that constitute the great commerce that these two parts of the world exchange between them are carried out ... Nothing enters the Indies that does not first pass through Cádiz ... [It] therefore has, as it were, the exclusive privilege of supplying the Indies with goods; it is but a meeting point in the perpetual ebb and flow of goods, commodities, gold, silver, and fruits that come and go between the Indies and Europe.[1]

It is plain to see that [the Spanish King's] decree was devised for the purpose of inspecting our vessels, and because there has never been any form or customary way of carrying out the searches of French vessels in the coasts and ports of Spain, we stand strongly opposed to it. Furthermore, we have maintained, from time immemorial, exemptions from such visits—exemptions that are regarded as a privilege inseparable from the banner of France.[2]

---

* A version of this chapter was first published as "The Spanish Plague That Never Was: Crisis and Exploitation in Cádiz During the *Peste* of Provence," *Eighteenth-Century Studies* 49, no. 2, Special issue on Humans and the Environment in the Long Eighteenth Century (January 2016): 167–93. Copyright © 2016 American Society for Eighteenth-Century Studies. Published by Johns Hopkins University Press.

[1] The original: "Cádiz est l'Entrepôt de l'Europe et des Indes Espagnols des deux Amériques; c'est le marché commun où se font tous les échanges qui constituent le grand commerce que ces deux parties du globe font entre elles ... les Indes ne doivent rien recevoir que par l'entremise de Cádiz ... Cádiz a donc, pour ainsi dire, le privilège exclusif d'approvisionner les Indes de marchandises, mais ce n'est qu'à titre d'étape où règne un flux et reflux perpétuel de marchandises, de denrées, d'or et d'argent, et des fruits qui vont et viennent aux Indes et en Europe." "Essay sur les diverses Branches du commerce que la France fait a Cadiz, et sur le moyens généraux des les y augmenter," February 26, 1762, AE, BIII, 342, AN.

[2] "Il est aise de juger que ce Décret a été rédigé dans la veüe de parvenir a la visite de nos batimens, et car il n'y a jamais eu aucune forme n'y manière accoutumée pour visiter les vaisseaux François sur les côtes n'y dans les ports

As earlier chapters have demonstrated, the Plague of Provence influenced politics, diplomacy, public health policy, commerce, and society far beyond the reach of the infection in Provence. Different regions responded to the threat in different ways, for reasons that varied according to the territory's history and the wider diplomatic and commercial context of Europe both prior to and during the outbreak. And perhaps none emerged from the Great Plague Scare more transformed than the kingdom of Spain under King Philip V. This chapter examines some of the ramifications of the 1720 plague across the Pyrenees in neighboring Spain paying special attention to the port of Cádiz, the so-called Gateway to the Indies and one of the eighteenth-century world's most important ports.

In the 1970s, Mariano Peset, Pilar Mancebo, and José Luis Peset looked at Spanish reactions to the 1720 plague in Provence primarily in the region of Catalonia. Since then, historians such as Armando Alberola Romá, David Barnabé Gil, Alfonso Zarzoso, and others have examined Spanish experiences of (and responses to) disaster and disease during the "eighteenth century of fevers," as Peset has called it, likewise paying special attention to the eastern regions of Valencia and Catalonia.[3] One of the objectives of the present chapter is to situate

---

d'Espagne, on s'y est toujours vivement oppose, et on les a maintenu depuis un tems immémorial dans l'exception de cette visite, Exemption qui est regardée comme un privilège attache a la Bannière de France, et quien doit être inséparable." Pierre-Nicolas Partyet, "[Rapport] du commerce de France en Espagne où on Prétend visiter nos batimens sur pretexte de la santé," July 4, 1723, AE, BIII, 361, AN.

[3] See, for instance, Mariano Peset Reig and María Pilar Mancebo Alonso, "Valencia y la peste de Marsella de 1720," *Primer Congreso de Historia del País Valenciano: Celebrado en Valencia del 14 al 18 de abril de 1971* (Valencia: Universidad de Valencia, 1973): 3, 567–78; Mariano Peset and José L. Peset, *Muerte en España: Política y sociedad entre la peste y el cólera* (Madrid: Seminarios y Ediciones, 1976); Armando Alberola Romá, "Una enfermedad de carácter endémico en el Alicante del XVIII: Las fiebres tercianas," *Revista de historia moderna: Anales de la Universidad de Alicante 5* (1985): 127–40; Armando Alberola Romá and David Bernabé Gil, "Tercianas y calenturas en tierras meridionales valencianas: Una aproximación a la realidad médica y social del siglo XVIII," *Revista de historia moderna 17* (1998–99): 95–112. Alfonso Zarzoso, "¿Obligación moral o responsabilidad política?: Las autoridades Borbónicas en tiempo de epidemias en la Cataluña del siglo XVIII," *Revista de historia moderna 17* (1998–99): 73–94; Enrique Perdiguero Gil, 'Con medios humanos y divinos': La lucha contra la enfermedad y la

the 1720 Great Plague Scare within this scholarship, looking beyond the eastern territories of Spain, and stressing the significance of the Plague of Provence as a major moment in the history of disaster management and state formation – one that would in many ways set the precedent for crisis and public health management in Spain for the rest of the eighteenth century and beyond.

State formation and the centralization of disaster management go hand in hand. Spanish reactions to the French epidemic coincided with an increase in state regulation over all aspects of trade, industry, and society, including health care and crisis management, which previously rested primarily in the hands of municipal authorities. Upon receiving word of the epidemic in late July 1720, the Spanish court in Madrid quickly used the news as a pretext to impose a commercially debilitating embargo against their French competitors, along with other supervisory controls that complemented King Philip V's centralizing policies. As Antonio García-Baquero González has pointed out, Bourbon reform was concerned not merely with strengthening the absolute monarchy and aggrandizing the state, but also with bolstering commerce, especially in the ultracompetitive realm of the colonial market.[4] The development and improvement of the economy became a fundamental aspect of the Bourbon reform program in an era when the so-called Spanish monopoly over the Indies trade had been reduced to little more than an illusion.[5] In 1720, when plague threatened to penetrate the kingdom from neighboring France, the employment of disaster centralism not only supported these larger initiatives, but also

---

muerte en Alicante en el siglo XVIII," *Dynamis: Acta Hispanica ad Medicinae Scientiarumque Historiam Illustrandam* 22 (2002): 121–50; Armando Alberola Romá, "Riadas, inundaciones y desastres en el sur Valenciano a finales del siglo XVIII," *Papeles de geografía* 51–2 (2010): 23–32. On the experience of death in the borderlands of the Pyrenees, see also Raymond Sala, *Le Visage de la mort dans les Pyrénées catalanes: Sensibilités et mentalités religieuses en Haut-Vallespir, XVIIe, XVIIIe et XIXe siècles* (Paris: Economica, 1991). For a historiography of the subject of plague in Spain as of 1994, see José Luis Betrán Moya, "La peste como problema historiográfico," *Manuscrits: Revista d'història moderna*, no. 12 (1994): 283–319.

[4] Antonio García-Baquero González, "El comercio colonial en la época de Felipe V: El reformismo continuista," in *Felipe V y su tiempo: congreso internacional*, vol. 1, edited by Eliseo Serrano Martín (Zaragoza: Institución "Fernando el Católico," 2004), 75–6.

[5] Ibid., 76, 78.

helped establish working parts of a new, centralized public health structure in Spain that would far outlive the Plague of Provence.

To help contextualize Spanish responses to the Provençal plague, this chapter will first establish Spain's political backdrop and the centralizing efforts of Philip V in the years leading up to the emergence of plague (or *la peste Levantina*, as some Spaniards called it) in neighboring Provence. It will then place the epidemic within the wider framework of post-Utrecht European – especially Franco-Spanish – commerce and diplomacy before exploring the influence of this far-reaching event on commercial administration and the management of disease in Spain and the prominent Atlantic port city of Cádiz.

War and the Gallicization of the *Carrera de Indias* in the Early Eighteenth Century

When plague emerged in France in 1720, Europe was still reeling from two very busy decades of wars, treaties, financial bubbles (those of the South Sea and Mississippi), and commercial, diplomatic, and administrative restructuring. This was especially true in Spain, where a new Bourbon king, Philip V, was trying to find his place both in his new realm and in the wider balance of Europe, which over the previous decades appeared increasingly tipped toward Spain's commercial competitors.[6] Four months prior to the outbreak, in February of 1720,

---

[6] The past two decades have seen a resurgence of scholarly interest in the era of Philip V. See, for example: Antonio de Béthencourt Massieu, ed., *Felipe V y el Atlántico: III centenario del advenimiento de los Borbones* (Gran Canaria: Ediciones del Cabildo de Gran Canaria, 2002); Ricardo García Cárcel, *Felipe V y los españoles: Una vision periférica del problema de España* (Barcelona: Plaza & Janés Editores, 2002); Agustín González Encíso, *Felipe V: La renovación de España: Sociedad y economía en el reinado del primer Borbón* (Pamplona: EUNSA, 2003); Eliseo Serrano Martín, ed., *Felipe V y su tiempo: congreso internacional*, vol. 1 (Zaragoza: Institución "Fernando el Católico," 2004); Allan J. Kuethe, "La política colonial de Felipe V y el proyecto de 1720," *Orbis incognitvs: avisos y legajos del Nuevo Mundo, Homenaje al professor Luis Navarro García*, vol. 1., edited by Fernando Navarro Antolín (Huelva: Universidad de Huelva, 2007): 233–41; Catherine Désos, *Les Français de Philippe V: Un modèle nouveau pour gouverner l'Espagne, 1700–1724* (Strasbourg: Presses universitaires de Strasbourg, 2009); Pablo Vázquez Gestal, *Una nueva majestad: Felipe V, Isabel de Farnesio y la identidad de la monarquía (1700–1729)* (Madrid: Marcial Pons Historia, 2013); Trevor J. Dadson and J. H. Elliott, eds. *Britain, Spain and the Treaty of Utrecht 1713–2013* (New York:

the Treaty of The Hague ended the War of the Quadruple Alliance, which developed when Spain tried to regain by force what it had lost in the Treaties of Utrecht and Rastatt (1713 and 1714, respectively) that ended the War of the Spanish Succession. Hostilities with the Quadruple Alliance resulted in a humiliating defeat for Philip V, who was obliged to join the alliance and reconfirm in the treaty of 1720 various privileges and concessions afforded to foreign nations in 1713. In fact, disputes arising from privileges and other matters of commerce would define the limits of Anglo-Franco-Spanish cohesion and trust for the duration of Philip V's reign.[7] As a result, when news of the plague arrived in Madrid, no longer able to take back by military force what it had lost, Spain seized the opportunity to once again "correct" the balance of power in Europe the only way it could – through domestic reforms and commercial leverage. To achieve the latter, the Spanish king would have to put a check on the American contraband trade that was making his competitors rich and reduce foreign participation in the Spanish market, even if it meant violating the terms of various recent treaties.

In the years just preceding the appearance of plague in France, Philip V put forth a concentrated effort to reform Spain's imperial commerce as he tried to remedy some of Spain's perceived disadvantages in the Indies market. In April 1720, for example, only two months before the outbreak in Provence, Philip V instituted his *Real Proyecto para galeones y flotas* (Royal plan for galleons and fleets). It aimed to increase Spanish products and participation in the market while reducing that of foreigners, and to increase, too, the Crown's control over trade in the Indies. Through this project, King Philip affirmed the

---

Routledge, 2014); Christopher Storrs, *The Spanish Resurgence, 1713–1748* (New Haven: Yale University Press, 2016). Even Spanish psychiatrist Francisco Alonso-Fernández wished to examine the life of Philip V in his book: *Felipe V: El rey fantasma* (Córdoba: Editorial Almuzara, 2020).

[7] Désos, *Les Français de Philippe V*, 261. For more on post-Utrecht diplomacy and reform, see Allan J. Kuethe and Kenneth J. Andrien, *The Spanish Atlantic World in the Eighteenth Century: War and the Bourbon Reforms, 1713–1796* (New York: Cambridge University Press, 2014); Dadson and Elliott, *Britain, Spain and the Treaty of Utrecht*; Antonella Alimento and Koen Stapelbroek, eds., *The Politics of Commercial Treaties in the Eighteenth Century: Balance of Power, Balance of Trade* (Basingstoke: Palgrave Macmillan, 2017); Alfred H. A. Soons, ed., *The 1713 Peace of Utrecht and its Enduring Effects* (Leiden: Brill, 2019).

importance of establishing closer and more regular commercial relations between Spain and the Indies, which he believed to be fundamental for stimulating domestic industry, increasing royal revenue, and
thus cultivating prosperity in the kingdom.[8] The reforms that made
up the *proyecto* are significant in that they point to a renewed energy
and desire to revitalize Spanish trade and demonstrate a new Bourbon
policy of increased control over Spain's product, its commerce, and
consequently, its activity in the ports.[9]

Efforts like these, aimed at improving the situation of Spain in
the wider context of European power politics and commercial and
financial competition, become most evident in the port city of Cádiz –
eighteenth-century Spain's most important port and the official capital
for the Spanish monopoly over the Indies market. The ancient city of
Cádiz, among the oldest continually inhabited cities in Europe, has
been active as a commercial port since its founding around 1100 BCE
by the Phoenicians, who named it Gadir. For two millennia, Cádiz
remained an active seaport, linking North Africa, the Atlantic, and

---

[8] Geoffrey J. Walker, *Spanish Politics and Imperial Trade, 1700–1789*
(Bloomington: Indiana University Press, 1979), 108. According to historian
Agustín González Encíso, "the reign of Philip V saw the strengthening of
central administration, the optimization of the army and navy, and the
implementation of highly interventionist politics in various aspects of the
economy, above all that of industry." Agustín González Encíso, "La industria
en el reinado de Felipe V," in *Felipe V y su tiempo: congreso internacional*,
vol. 1, edited by Eliseo Serrano Martín (Zaragoza: Institución "Fernando
el Católico," 2004), 57. See also Jesús Pradells Nadal, *Del foralismo al
centralismo: Alicante 1700–1725* (Alicante: Universidad de Alicante, 1984),
130. Kuethe and Andrien, *Spanish Atlantic World*, 7.

[9] The best method for achieving increased contact with the Indies was the
frequent and regular dispatching of the galleons and fleets. The fleets typically
left from Seville, and after 1717, from Cádiz. When they arrived in the
Caribbean, they split up into the *flota* (smaller ships) that continued to Mexico,
while the *galeones* (larger ships) went on to Portobello or Cartagena. The *Real
proyecto* also included measures to prevent delays and prolonged stays, which
too often had detrimental effects on the ships, crews, and cargoes. Moreover,
in order to support Spanish shipyards under the terms of the *proyecto*,
only Spanish-built vessels were to be admitted in fleets (except in special
circumstances), and taxes on certain goods, such as Spanish produce, were
now 85 percent less than they had been under a previous decree of 1711. Dues
for the exporting merchant were also cut, so as to promote Spanish exports
by conducting trade with Spanish goods and produce. For more on the *Real
Proyecto*, see García-Baquero González, "El comercio colonial," 75–102.

northern Europe with the Mediterranean. In fact, no other port settlement on the Iberian Peninsula has been so often mapped.[10]

As the most active port in Spain throughout much of the eighteenth century, Cádiz serves as a valuable microcosm of Bourbon reforms, especially during the epidemic in Provence when port cities became the focal points of the Crown's preventative measures. In 1717, Cádiz officially became the dynamic epicenter for commercial activity in the Atlantic when the organs responsible for the management of the colonial convoy system called the *Carrera de Indias,* or Route to the Indies, were transferred from the inland river port of Seville.[11] From this time until the monopoly began shifting into open commerce around 1765, approximately 85 percent of all documented sailings from the Iberian Peninsula to the colonies departed from this port.[12] Foreigners were technically forbidden from trading directly with the Indies; they instead had to sell their goods to the Spanish who would then sell the foreign merchandise in the Americas. Yet by the end of the seventeenth century, despite the veil of a Spanish monopoly over commerce in the Americas, non-Spanish merchants controlled over three-quarters of all trade activity in Cádiz and the *Carrera de Indias* – all of this in a Spain that fundamentally desired to exclude foreign participation from its imperial commerce. For decades, foreigners had been making their way deeper and deeper into the market by way of concessions

---

[10] Its Phoenician founding may make it Europe's oldest Atlantic port city. Patrick O'Flanagan, *Port Cities of Atlantic Iberia, c. 1500–1900* (Aldershot: Ashgate Publishing, 2008), 82, 83.

[11] These organs were the *Casa de la Contratación* (House of Trade) and the *Consulado de cargadores a Indias* (Council of Shippers to the Indies – essentially the merchant guild). See Ana Crespo Solana, *La Casa de Contratación y la Intendencia General de la Marina en Cádiz, 1717–1730* (Cádiz: Universidad de Cádiz, 1996); Ana Crespo Solana, "El Comercio y la armada de la monarquía: La Casa de Contratación y la Intendencia General de la Marina de Cádiz, 1717-1750," *Jornadas de Historia Marítima* xxiv, no. 39 (2001): 63–78. See also, Klaus Weber and Torsten dos Santos Arnold, "Ports to 'New Worlds': Lisbon, Seville, Cádiz (15th–18th Centuries)," in *The Power of Cities: The Iberian Peninsula from Late Antiquity to the Early Modern Period,* edited by Sabine Panzram (Leiden: Brill, 2019), 321–61.

[12] O'Flanagan, *Port Cities,* 86–7. Carla Rahn Phillips, "The Growth and Composition of Trade in the Iberian Empires, 1450–1740," in *Rise of Merchant Empires: Long-Distance Trade in the Early Modern World, 1350–1750,* edited by James D. Tracy (Cambridge: Cambridge University Press, 1990), 34–101, 96. The monopoly was finally abolished in 1786.

and privileges afforded them in a variety of treaties and contracts. And among all groups of foreign merchants in Andalucía – including the Genoese, Anglo-Irish, Danish, Dutch, Portuguese, and others – it was the French who most efficiently managed to breach Spain's commercial defenses and reap the most benefits.[13] Indeed, foreign competition gradually eroded Spanish industry, while French industry saw significant gains.

The French dominated the foreign population in Cádiz, such that several historians have referred to the port from the late seventeenth to the eighteenth century as a "French colony."[14] By 1713 the French represented about 70 percent of the foreign population. French merchants also enjoyed a variety of privileges, mostly dating back to the Treaty of the Pyrenees of 1659 that reflected France's new distinction as *nación más favorecida en material commercial* (the most favored nation in commercial matters).[15] Among the terms of the treaty were the official establishment of a French consulate in Spain, protection against arbitrary imprisonment for French merchants and crewmen, the right to compose business documents in French, and, most

---

[13] Interestingly, however, the Dutch reaped the benefits of increased trade in Spanish markets after 1720 when Spain launched plague-time regulations that isolated the French and the British. For more on Dutch maritime commerce with Cádiz in particular, see the work of Ana Crespo Solana, including *El Comercio marítimo entre Amsterdam y Cádiz, 1713–1778* (Madrid: Banco de España – Servicio de Estudios, 2000); "Merchants and Observers: The Dutch Republic's Commercial Interests in Spain and the Merchant Community in Cádiz in the Eighteenth Century," *Dieciocho: Hispanic Enlightenment* 32, no. 2 (Fall 2009): 193–224; "El comercio holandés y la integración de espacios económicos entre Cádiz y el Báltico en tiempos de guerra (1699–1723)," *Investigaciones de Historia Económica* 3, no. 8 (2007): 45–76. See also: Wim Klooster and Gert Oostindie, *Realm Between Empires: The Second Dutch Atlantic, 1680–1815* (Ithaca: Cornell University Press, 2018).

[14] Among them, Henry Kamen, Albert Girard, Didier Ozanam, Manuel Bustos Rodríguez, Olivier Le Gouic, Antonio García-Baquero González and Pedro Collado Villalta, and Henri Sée.

[15] Albert Girard, *El comercio francés en Sevilla y Cádiz en tiempo de los Habsburgo* (Seville: Editorial Renacimiento, 2006), 235–6; Gaston Rambert, "La France et la politique commercial de l'Espagne au XVIIIe siècle," *Revue d'histoire modern et contemporaine* 6e, no. 4 (October–December 1959): 271; Henry Kamen, *The War of Succession in Spain, 1700–15* (Bloomington: Indiana University Press, 1969), 160. The Treaty of the Pyrenees was modeled in part after earlier treaties between Spain and England, and the Hanseatic League.

notably, the highly valued exemption from official visits or inspections of French ships and commercial vessels. This privilege was later reconfirmed on April 30, 1703, in a decree that forbade Spanish officials from boarding French ships, and again in the Treaty of Utrecht.[16] In effect, the Treaty of the Pyrenees resulted in what French consul Pierre de Catalan once called a French "liberté de commerce" (freedom of commerce) in Spain.[17] Because of it, France held the greater share of all trade that passed through Cádiz, and French goods made up the majority of foreign exports from the Gaditan port.[18] Moreover, a considerable amount of the precious metals sent to the Indies on Spanish galleons eventually made its way back to France.[19]

---

[16] Rambert, "La France et la politique commercial," 271. Kamen, *War of Succession*, 156–8.

[17] Stanley J. Stein and Barbara H. Stein, *Silver, Trade, and War* (Baltimore: Johns Hopkins University Press, 2003), 64–5. The French also enjoyed limits on commercial duties for their largest imports as a result of late seventeenth-century arrangements called the *Convenios de Eminente* (Eminente's contracts), named after the customs director in Cádiz, Francisco Báez Eminente. Imports of the cheaper and lower-quality Silesian linens, for example, remained dutied at 12 percent, while the better-quality French linens paid only 2–5 percent. The *Convenios* (agreements or contracts) worked like an unpublicized treaty system that extended to the French, Dutch, and English who traded through Cádiz beginning with the earliest of these in 1668. To the French importers in Andalucía, the privilege of the *Convenios* was considered "the foundation of their trade in Spain, without which they could not survive." Stein and Stein, *Silver, Trade, and War*, 70.

[18] Ibid., 20. Kuethe and Andrien, *Spanish Atlantic World*, 66. Already by the 1680s, French, Dutch, and English merchants supplied over 90 percent of exports from Cádiz. John Shovlin, *Trading with the Enemy: Britain, France, and the 18th-Century Quest for a Peaceful World Order* (New Haven: Yale University Press, 2021), 304. Historian Paul Cheney has estimated that France handled 39 percent of the commerce that filtered through the port city, compared with 17 percent for Genoa, 14 percent for England, and 12 percent for the United Provinces. French materials made up 75 percent of the fabric that crossed the Atlantic, stimulating industry in the regions of Brittany, Normandy, and Lyon. France also supplied the New World with profitable quantities of materials including paper, books, beaver hats, and lace. Paul Cheney, *Revolutionary Commerce: Globalization and the French Monarchy* (Cambridge, MA: Harvard University Press, 2010), 26, 27.

[19] "One estimate puts yearly averages in 1670 at twelve million l.t. [*livres tournois*] worth of gold and silver, and another, from France's diplomatic corps in 1686, puts these returns at thirteen to fourteen million." Cheney, *Revolutionary Commerce*, 27. For an exhaustive study on the flow of gold and silver from the Americas into Europe, as well as French participation in illicit trade through the port of Cádiz, see the relevant parts of chapters 3 and

When the War of the Spanish Succession began, the situation further improved for France as Philip V found himself heavily reliant on his Bourbon grandfather, Louis XIV, for weapons, funding, manpower, and guidance in the war effort. At the outbreak of the war, Jean Orry, French financier and *secrétaire du roi* for Louis XIV, and later advisor and finance minister for Philip V, was dispatched to Madrid to report on the state of finances in Spain.[20] It soon became apparent that Spain lacked the resources necessary to carry out any kind of significant military campaign.[21] Orry observed that "there is no prince more poor than the King of Spain."[22] And in 1703, in a letter to Michel Chamillart, the French minister of war the marquis de Louville wrote from Madrid, "Spain is entirely your responsibility. [It is] without troops, without money, without a navy, in a word lacking in everything that pertains to the defense of a monarchy as extensive as this."[23]

4 in Michel Morineau, *Incroyables gazettes et fabuleux métaux: Les retours des trésors américains d'après les gazettes hollandaises, XVIe–XVIIIe siècles* (Cambridge: Cambridge University Press, 1985).

[20] Orry's influence played a major role in the financial and administrative restructuring that took place under Philip V's centralizing Bourbon reforms. For more on his contributions, see Anne Dubet, *Jean Orry et la réforme du gouvernement de l'Espagne (1701–1706)* (Clermont-Ferrand: Presses Universitaires Blaise-Pascal, 2009), 15. Various studies, including those of Henry Kamen and Geoffrey J. Walker, discuss French influence on Bourbon reforms under Philip V. See also: José Miguel López García, "Sobrevivir en la corte: Las condiciones de vida del pueblo llano en el Madrid de Felipe V," in *Felipe V y su tiempo: congreso internacional*, vol. 1, edited by Eliseo Serrano Martín (Zaragoza: Institución "Fernando el Católico," 2004), 133–66.

[21] For more on financing the War of the Spanish Succession, see Concepción de Castro, "Le Conseil et les premiers ministres des Finances sous Philippe V: conflits et intégration (XVIIIe siècle)," in *Les finances royales dans la monarchie espagnole, XVIe–XIXe siècles*, edited by Anne Dubet (Rennes: Presses universitaires de Rennes, 2008), 89–102; Guillaume Hanotin, *Jean Orry: Un homme des finances royales entre France et Espagne, 1701–1705* (Cordova: Universidad de Córdoba, 2009); Dubet, *Jean Orry et la réforme*; Guy Rowlands, *The Financial Decline of a Great Power: War, Influence, and Money in Louis XIV's France* (Oxford: Oxford University Press, 2012). For more on this war in the larger Atlantic context, see Chapter 10 in Geoffrey Plank, *Atlantic Wars from the Fifteenth Century to the Age of Revolution* (New York: Oxford University Press, 2020).

[22] Quoted in Hanotin, *Jean Orry*, 65.

[23] Letter from marquis de Louville to Michel Chamillart in Madrid, August 23, 1703, as quoted and translated in Henry Kamen, *Empire: How Spain Became a World Power, 1492–1763* (New York: Harper Collins, 2003), 442. Louis de

Finding himself in an especially favorable position to exploit the commerce of the Spanish Indies, Louis XIV quickly set about breaching the monopoly further. In a letter written to Michel-Jean Amelot, the French ambassador to Spain, Louis XIV wrote, "The principal objective in the present war is the commerce of the Indies and the wealth that it produces."[24] Accordingly, one of his first aims after throwing his support behind his grandson at the start of the War of the Spanish Succession was to secure the *asiento de negros*, which he accomplished in 1701.[25] Granted to a single state or trading company at a time since the sixteenth century, this exclusive privilege permitted the French to provide Spanish America with enslaved people and much else besides. Because the *asiento* meant legal access into Spanish colonial markets, the French, like those who held it before and after, would use this privilege to smuggle merchandise of all varieties into the Spanish Americas.[26] In addition, near the start of the war in 1704, the French obtained and exploited an exclusive and very lucrative right of access to the Spanish Pacific around Cape Horn through the Straits of Magellan. This allowed for direct trade with Chile and Peru (with all their Spanish silver) from the ports of Marseille and Saint-Malo.[27]

Rouvroy, duc de Saint-Simon, *Mémoires XI*, edited by A. de Boislisle (Paris: Hachette et cie, 1895), 531. Chamillart was the minister of war for Louis XIV from 1699 until he fell out of favor in 1709. Charles-Auguste d'Allonville, marquis de Louville, was head of the king's household, or *Chef de la Maison*, for Philip V from 1700 to 1703.

[24] "Le principal objet de la guerre présente est celui du commerce des Indes et des richesses qu'elles produisent." Letter from Louis XIV to Michel-Jean Amelot, marquis de Gournay on February 18, 1708, in *Correspondance de Louis XIV avec M. Amelot, son Ambassadeur en Espagne, 1705–1709*, vol. 2, edited by M. le baron de Girardot (Nantes: Imprimerie Merson, 1864), 121.

[25] García-Baquero González, "El comercio colonial," 83.

[26] Phillips, "Growth and Composition of Trade," 95. The Portuguese and the Dutch held the *asiento* before the French in 1701. In 1713, under the terms of the Treaty of Utrecht, it was passed to the British. For more on French, Spanish, British, and Dutch interest in Spanish markets at this time, see chapter 2 in Shovlin, *Trading with the Enemy*; chapter 4 in Paul W. Mapp, *The Elusive West and the Contest for Empire, 1713–1763* (Chapel Hill: University of North Carolina Press, 2011).

[27] Wim Klooster, "Inter-Imperial Smuggling in the Americas, 1600–1800," in *Soundings in Atlantic History: Latent Structures and Intellectual Currents, 1500–1830*, edited by Bernard Bailyn and Patricia L. Denault (Cambridge, MA: Harvard University Press, 2009), 164.

This practice had already been taking place since the late seventeenth century but was now made legitimate through the war years.[28]

All these privileges proved extremely lucrative for the French. They facilitated the smuggling of French goods and allowed substantial amounts of bullion to reach France directly. This included, most notably, silver that arrived in Cádiz from the Americas and entered France through its ports, including Marseille. Indeed, geographer Patrick O'Flanagan has referred to Cádiz in the eighteenth century as the "silver city" and the silver capital of Europe, and Marseille was among the principal destinations for silver entering France.[29] In a letter to the members of the French Marine Council (*Conseil de Marine*) in 1718, Pierre-Nicolas Partyet, the consul of France in Cádiz (1716–25), reported that, while returns to France were made difficult because of a recent revocation of the right to extract gold and silver from the Indies (as a result of the escalation of the War of the Quadruple Alliance), two million piasters were still transferred from Cádiz to Marseille, "despite the vigilance of Spanish guards."[30] And the Sardinian intellectual

[28] After 1714 the French ceased their trade in these ports – a stipulation vigorously pursued by the British and Dutch after Utrecht – but the practice continued illegally, even after 1718 when Spain sent out an expedition to enforce the law and suppress French traffic in the Pacific. Madrid saw in the plague an opportunity to help control illicit French traffic in the Indies. Royal proclamations were regularly sent to the colonies that very strictly prohibited the docking of any French vessels at a Spanish port, even if the ships had not stopped in or near Provence.

[29] O'Flanagan, *Port Cities*, 86. Myriame Morel-Deledalle and Claude Badet, "Marseille aux XVIIe & XVIIIe siècles," in *Vivre en quarantaine dans les ports de Marseille aux XVIIe et XVIIIe siècles*, edited by Myriame Morel-Deladalle (Marseille: Musée d'Histoire de Marseille, 1987), 9–15, 12.

[30] Pierre-Nicolas Partyet, consul de France à Cadix, aux membres du Conseil de Marine, October 24, 1718, AE, BI, 224, ff. 392–4v, AN.

The French consulship of Cádiz was created in 1660 as a result, like other privileges, of the Treaty of the Pyrenees (Article III). This consulate represented "the most important and most productive one in Spain from the time of the treaty through the eighteenth century." Mézin, *Les consuls de France*, 672. It was the consul's responsibility to look after and protect the rights of his fellow Frenchmen abroad. The importance of this post thus grew alongside the rapid commercial growth of the seventeenth- to eighteenth-century world, when it was deemed integral that someone be assigned the role of preventing abuses in the ports, and maintaining "the good faith that must be the most solid foundation of trade," as described by one contemporary. These posts were reserved for "persons of integrity and merit," and consuls frequently appeared to take on the role of supervisors for the merchants of a nation. French

Vicente Bacallar y Sanna, marquis of San Felipe, commented on French success in Spain when he wrote, "There is no lack of money in France, and there has never been more, because for so many years they had free rein over the Indies trade, the likes of which no other nation ever managed to achieve."[31] In 1709 an official French estimate claimed a total of 180 million *livres'* worth of metal and cargo imported from the New World since 1701.[32] The arrangements that made these French privileges possible made sense during the War of the Spanish Succession, for they facilitated the import of American capital to fund the Bourbon war effort.[33] However, when Philip V began trying to shake off the yolk of French influence after the war, seeking to regain a more favorable commercial equilibrium and reduce French involvement in the Spanish Americas, such advantages represented challenges that would have to be overcome by more creative means.[34]

consuls were also expected to report to the *secrétaire d'État de la Marine*, or during the *polysynodie* (1715–18) – which included the plague years – to the *Conseil de Marine* (during the polysynody, France's secretaries of state were replaced by a number of councils). Consuls reported on anything and everything that transpired in their respective regions. As a result, the consular letters of men like Partyet serve as remarkably valuable tools for the historian. The collection of the "Correspondance des consuls de France à Cadix" in the Archives nationales in Paris runs from 1666 to 1792. It is a remarkably useful, and yet underutilized assemblage of letters covering anything and everything of social, commercial, and diplomatic interest. Pierre Ariste, *Traité des consuls de la nation française aux Pays estrangers, contenant leur origine, leurs establissemens, leurs fonctions, leurs droits, esmolumens et autres prerogatives*, 1667, manuscrit 18595, Bibliotèque nationale de France (BNF). Mézin, *Les consuls de France*, 3. Girard, *El comercio francés en Sevilla y Cádiz*, 113.

[31] "No faltaba en la Francia dinero, y nunca havia havido mas, porque tantos años tenia como libre el Comercio de las Indias, que no lograban otras Naciones." Vicente Bacallar y Sanna, marqués de San Felipe, *Comentarios de la Guerra de España, e Historia de su Rey Phelipe V El Animoso, desde el principio de su reynado, hasta la Paz General del año 1725*, tomo I (Genoa: Matheo Garvizza, 1725), 308.

[32] Rowlands, *Financial Decline*, 94.

[33] David R. Ringrose, *Spain, Europe, and the "Spanish Miracle," 1700–1900* (New York: Cambridge University Press, 1996), 99.

[34] In 1718 Spain dispatched a naval squadron to the Peruvian coast to seize several interloping French merchantmen. Ringrose notes that "direct French trade with Peru never recovered and French merchants were forced to settle for access to that market through legal channels in Cádiz." Ringrose, *Spanish Miracle*, 100.

Since the seventeenth century, despite arguments for French participation in an abating Spanish market, the Gallic encroachment on Spanish transatlantic trade had been generating a great deal of resentment toward French merchants. During the War of the Spanish Succession, for example, Ambrose Daubenton, French chief agent of commerce and marine in Spain, wrote that "the Spaniards would resolutely prefer to lose the American trade, before consenting to France's deriving the slightest benefit from it."[35] Such anti-French sentiments were expressed most explicitly in Spanish ports both on the peninsula and in the colonies. This was especially the case in Cádiz, where local Spanish merchants came together in the years just preceding the outbreak of plague in France to put an end to the practice of allowing the sons of foreigners, many of whom were of French origins, to trade in the Indies market. Originally, the right to conduct trade with the Spanish Americas belonged to the *naturales de orígen* – those born in Spain of Castilian, Navarrese, or Aragonese origin. However, a *real cédula* (royal decree) of August 14, 1620, extended this right to the sons of foreigners born in Spain (whom they called *genízaros*). Protests against this measure continued well into the eighteenth century, when Spanish merchants in Cádiz complained that extending to *genízaros* the right to conduct trade under the same conditions as the Spaniards led to prejudicial irregularities. They argued that too many foreigners used this provision as a "sinister justification" to obtain trading licenses, which they feared would eventually create a scenario in which profits remained concentrated in foreign populations and their metropolises, leaving Spaniards "dispossessed" of any lucrative involvement.[36] While tensions had been on the rise for decades, the

---

[35] Ambrose Daubenton de Villebois, French chief agent of commerce and marine in Spain, to Louis Phélypeaux, comte de Pontchartrain, August 8, 1705, in Walker, *Spanish Politics*, 23. Later, in 1754, Irishman John Boyle wrote in reference to the court at Parma, "The French hate the Spaniards, the Spaniards hate the French, and the Italians hate them both." One might say that his words resonated beyond Italy earlier in the century, as well. John Boyle, 5th earl of Cork and Orrery, "Letter VI from Bologna, Oct. 24, 1754," *Letters from Italy in the Years 1754 and 1755, by the Late Right Honourable John Earl of Corke and Orrery*, edited by John Duncombe (London: B. White, 1773), 60.

[36] Antonio García-Baquero González, *Cádiz y el Atlantico (1717–1778): El comercio colonial español bajo el monopolio gaditano* (Seville: Imprenta

frequency of protests seems to have peaked between 1717 and May 1720, when Spanish merchants in Cádiz came together to petition the king through the Council of the Indies (*Consejo de Indias*) to allow only the sons of natural-born Spaniards, and not the sons of foreigners, to conduct trade in the Spanish Indies market.[37] Upon learning of the petition, the *genízaros* of Cádiz published an appeal in which they established their legitimate right to trade out of Cádiz as natural-born Spaniards. Ultimately, they would maintain their right to trade in the *Carrera de Indias*, but grievances from both sides persisted in the ports. In 1720 Spanish officials reported to the king from the port of Barcelona that the French and their consuls were viewed with hatred ("aqui los franceses y el consul son mirados con odio").[38] Meanwhile, foreign merchants and officials complained about the various injustices committed against them in Spanish ports, more often than not in the port of Cádiz.[39]

C.S.I.C., 1976), 122. By the eighteenth century, foreign merchants were allowed to settle in Cádiz and trade with a license. See also: Margarita García-Mauriño Mundi, *La pugna entre el Consulado de Cádiz y los jenízaros por las exportaciones a Indias, 1720–1765* (Seville: Universidad de Sevilla, 1999).

[37] García-Baquero González, *Cádiz y el Atlantico*, 122–3. It was on May 25, 1720, that the ill-fated vessel, the *Grand Saint-Antoine*, arrived in Marseille allegedly carrying plague.

[38] In "Señor mio, si al Amo le llegaron quejas deste Consul de Francia ...," Barcelona, 1720, Estado 506, AHN. This same document provides one of the many accounts that emerge at this time of French merchandise being burned in the ports. It should also be mentioned that the port city of Barcelona served as the commercial capital of Catalonia, especially between 1720 and 1770, partly as a result of Bourbon centralization. Consequently, it was a major Spanish port for trade with the Levant, and thus Marseille, over the eighteenth century. See Eloy Martín Corrales, *Comercio de Cataluña con el Mediterráneo musulmán, siglos XVI–XVIII: El comercio con los "enemigos de la fe"* (Barcelona: Edicions Bellaterra, 2001), 154–63.

[39] Complaints came from the French, British, Dutch, Portuguese, and others. In August 1720, for example, Pierre-Nicolas Partyet composed his "Memoire for the gentlemen of the Marine Council, to demonstrate that the Frenchmen who come and stay in Spain to conduct trade are not treated as favorably as they would have reason to hope if the treaties concluded between the two Crowns were faithfully executed." That same month, the marquês de Tolosa, too, sent word to Lisbon "sobre las noticias que le dio el consul de la Nación Portuguesa en Cádiz de la violencia que se hacia en aquella Plaza a los Portugueses que pasaron a esta por causa de su comercio o por otras dependencias," Pierre-Nicolas Partyet to Conseil de Marine, "Mémoire

Reactions to the Plague of Provence in Spain

It was in this context that news of a deadly outbreak of disease in Marseille arrived in Madrid in late July 1720, and the administration of Philip V did everything they could both to protect Spain, and to use the epidemic to Spanish advantage. Spain acted quickly – more quickly, in fact, than did Paris.[40] As early as August 3, a *Real Provisión* (or Royal Order) from the Royal Council of Castile established the first mandatory quarantine for all ships that had passed through Marseille before arriving in Spain.[41] It also forbade all travel on land of persons who came from the vicinity of Marseille unless they could provide certificates of health (*patentes sanitarios* or *patentes de sanidad*) from their location of origin. This order was followed by various others in August and September that collectively barred commercial relations with all French ports, whether Atlantic or Mediterranean, as well as with Africa and the Levant, the islands of the Mediterranean – including Elba and Menorca (now British as a result of the Treaty of Utrecht), Nice, Monaco, Gibraltar (also now British), Portugal – various Italian ports including those of the Kingdom of Sardinia, and parts of Genoa.[42] The restrictions also included any ship bearing a French

---

à nosseigneurs du Conseil de Marine pour faire voir que les François qui viennent et demeurent en Espagne à l'occasion de leur commerce n'y sont pas traités aussy favorablement qu'ils auroient lieu de l'espérer si les traités passés entre les deux couronnes y estoient fidèlement executes," August 7, 1720, AE, 225, ff. 214–30v, AN; "Carta de Marquês de Tolosa em Madrid nos 24 de Agosto de 1720," August 24, 1720, MNE, livro 789, f. 653, TdT.

[40] As discussed in Chapter 1, the parlement of Aix issued an *arrêt* (decree) on July 31, 1720, to stop all communication with Marseille, prohibiting the movement of any more people out of the city. It was not until August 12, 1720, that the Regent sent three medical practitioners from Montpellier, doctors François Chicoyneau and François Verny and surgeon Jean Soulier, to investigate the epidemic that by then was killing as many as 400 people per day.

[41] The *Real y Supremo Consejo de Castilla* was the Spanish monarch's executive council.

[42] José Luis Fresquet Febrer, "Los medicos frente a la enfermedad en la Valencia del siglo XVIII," in *Estudios sobre la profesión médica en la sociedad valenciana, 1329–1898*, edited by José María López Piñero (Valencia: Ajuntament de València, 1998), 276. The *provisión* of August 19, for example, reads as follows: "Having just learned of the contagious disease that has befallen Marseille of France, in his desire to protect his dominions from

flag, even if it had not stopped at any port considered a threat. News of these measures was disseminated throughout all of Spain's colonies in the Atlantic and Asia, from Havana to Manila.

Vessels traveling directly from uninfected ports, including those of Great Britain and the Austrian Netherlands, could also be turned away, forced into ninety-day quarantines, or required to surrender their goods to be destroyed under the pretext of public health – reactions that may be explained in part by Spain's losses in the Treaties of Utrecht and The Hague.[43] Concessions under the terms of these treaties included the loss of various territories to the allied enemies of the Bourbons, including the island of Menorca and the ever-contentious territory of Gibraltar, which went to Great Britain; the Colônia do Sacramento (in Uruguay), which went to Portugal; and

an evil so grave, powerful and fatal, [His Majesty] has resolved not only to prohibit commerce of all persons and goods that come from Marseille, but also to prohibit absolutely the entrance of all goods and fabrics that come from any of the ports that France has in the Mediterranean, and all vessels that having traveled from Italy or other parts of the Levant have made stops in or shared commerce with Marseille; and as regards people that carry health patents from places that protect themselves from Marseille and any other French locality that this illness may have affected, may these be admitted to commerce after the ordinary visit that is customary in our ports and after observing the quarantine, having totally excluded Marseille and its territory for eight or ten leagues from its proximities; and that all ports establish vessels specifically for the guarding against contagion, or that in all customs vessels, persons of the highest caliber are assigned solely to look after and conserve the health of all that touches ground." Aviso of Don Francisco Caetano de Aragon, Barcelona, August 26, 1720, Estado 506, AHN. See also: Actas Capitulares (henceforward AC) 338, September 13, 1720, f. 135, Archivo Municipal de Murcia (henceforward AMU).

    Excluded from restrictions at this time was the main port of Genoa itself because "that port alone has secured itself" against the infection. Peset, 162. At some point, the cessation of commerce with Venice was considered, but it was decided that the other precautions would suffice. Peset and Monteano, "Valencia," 572. Like Genoa, moreover, Venice, Tuscany, and Rome had restricted commerce with much of the Mediterranean, Africa, and the Levant, which allowed Spain to point out at times that they were simply doing as these Italian states had done. See Chapter 2 on Genoa and Italy.

[43] The Peace of Utrecht comprised various documents signed over many months. The core agreements were signed on April 11, 1713, with various arrangements following soon thereafter. Its terms would be reconfirmed in later documents, including the 1721 Treaty of Madrid (or Triple Alliance of Madrid, between Great Britain, France, and Spain).

Sicily and parts of the Duchy of Milan, which were transferred to the duke of Savoy, Victor Amadeus II.[44] The rest of Milan, along with the kingdoms of Naples, Sardinia, and the Spanish Netherlands, went to Holy Roman Emperor Charles VI. Under the terms of both treaties Britain was also granted the highly coveted *asiento de negros* (to the disappointment of the French), as well as the *navío de permiso*, which authorized the English to send one annual vessel to conduct trade in the Spanish Indies. These were all extremely valuable gains for Britain because they enabled the British to participate in decades of lucrative commerce in Spanish America, both legal and illicit, much as France had already been doing for years.

Now, with the threat of plague to justify its actions, the Spanish Crown could shut Gibraltar out of Spanish commerce on the grounds that the British were not effectively enforcing protective quarantines. In doing so it could respond to Britain's refusal to return Gibraltar, the loss of which was devastating to Spanish morale given their numerous attempts to take it back.[45] At this time, too, Spain made use of its influence over Portugal by compelling it to impose restrictions against both French and British ships that wished to enter Spanish and Portuguese harbors. Portugal in turn was obliged to indulge Spain lest it, too, suffer an arbitrary quarantine.[46] By late December 1720, for example, Portugal had prohibited commerce with the whole of France, as well as all Muslim countries in the Mediterranean.[47]

---

[44] After the War of the Quadruple Alliance in 1720, Victor Amadeus II was obliged to give up Sicily in exchange for the Kingdom of Sardinia.

[45] In January 1727, for example, Spain would declare the sections on Gibraltar in the Treaty of Utrecht null and void, claiming that the British violated its terms by failing to protect Catholics by allowing Jews and Moors to live there, extending fortifications beyond allowable limits, and allowing smuggling that hurt Spanish profits. In February Spain began a siege that lasted until June, and the Utrecht terms that granted Gibraltar to the British were confirmed again in the 1729 Treaty of Seville. These disputes effectively led to the construction of the *Línea de Contravalación*, or Spanish Lines. Conflict over Gibraltar very much continues to this day. Letters, newspaper articles, and government documents dating from 1713 to today point to the unpopularity of a British Gibraltar among both the Spanish people and their government.

[46] Harrison, *Contagion*, 32, 31.

[47] "Lisboa, Jan. 9, 1721," *Gaceta de Madrid*, no. 4, January 28, 1721, 16. Portuguese regulations that prohibited all trade with France in fact began earlier, on September 20, 1720. "Lisbon," *Post Boy* (London), September 23, 1720.

The epidemic in France proved advantageous to Spain in other ways. Although the plague entered the French port at the end of May 1720, Marseillais officials did not officially acknowledge it until late July to August. As discussed in Chapters 1 and 2, they had waited as long as they could before acknowledging an epidemic of bubonic plague. Such news they knew would be detrimental to local commerce and relations with the rest of Europe.[48] Indeed, French restrictions against movements in and around Provence meant that, for a time, the region was cut off from the world. As a result, when ships could not dock in southern French ports, they would take their merchandise elsewhere, and it was often the Spaniards who benefited. In a Spanish letter, possibly from the port of Barcelona, one official reported to Madrid: "In the port of this city, many vessels from England, Scotland, Ireland, and Holland have unloaded their cargoes of codfish, salmon, eels, and herring; for since the port of Marseille is closed, everything that was destined to go there, arrives here instead."[49] The same document goes on to discuss other vessels from Dunkirk loaded with precious wheat destined for Andalucía, "as it is best that the money remain within Spain."[50]

By September 1720 the basic structure of Spain's disease-control policy had taken the shape it would hold for the rest of the eighteenth century. New restrictions required those traveling by land as well as those on vessels to carry the *patentes sanitarios* (in French, *patentes de santé*) that precisely documented all their whereabouts, whether they wished to enter Spain or move within it, and whether or not they

---

[48] Mariano Peset, Pilar Mancebo, and José L. Peset, "Temores y defensa de España frente a la peste de Marsella de 1720," *Asclepio: Archivo Iberoamericano de Historia de la Medicina y Antropología Médica* 23 (1971): 145. News made it to King Philip through communications from his authorities in Navarre, Perpignan, and Aragon. See Peset and Peset, *Muerte en España*, 30.

[49] "En el puerto desta ciudad van desembocando muchos navios Ingleses, escoceses, Irlandeses, y Olandeses, cargados de bacallaos, salmones, congríos, y arenques, que como esta cerrado el puerto de Marsella, todo lo que estava destinado para aquel, entre en este." From: "Señor mio, si al Amo le llegaron quejas deste Consul de Francia …," Barcelona, Estado 506, AHN. Though the letter is not dated or signed, it appears to be from Don Francisco de Quesada to marqués de Grimaldo. See also: Don Francisco de Quesada to marqués de Grimaldo, Barcelona, December 7, 1720, Estado 506, AHN.

[50] Ibid.

had passed through Provence. Anyone traveling without it would have their merchandise confiscated and burned. The same was done for the cargos of suspicious vessels on the coasts. In the ports and lazarets, new policies included the increased presence of a newly established health police (*policía sanitaria*); the laying out of *cordones sanitarios* (the quarantine lines); the establishment and regulation of new lazarets; and the increased regulation of coastal navigation, fisheries, taverns, inns, and markets. Measures also included the prohibition of most nonreligious public events, including the bull run. Violations of new policies were mostly enforced under pain of death, incarceration, or the confiscation of goods.[51]

The tightest controls and the most comprehensive system of surveillance were put in place in the eastern regions of Spain, in Aragon, Catalonia, and Valencia.[52] These regions not only bordered France and the Mediterranean, but during the War of the Spanish Succession had also sided with the allied enemies of the Bourbons and recognized Archduke Charles as king when he entered Barcelona in 1705.[53] Philip V saw this as an act of defiance and soon thereafter began crafting the *Nueva Planta* decrees (beginning in 1707) that aimed to consolidate the eastern territories into the Spanish kingdom, systematically replacing their leaders, courts, administration, and languages with those of Castile.[54] While this did not effectively replace all authority in the eastern territories – in fact, despite the aims of the Bourbon monarchy, there remained a great deal of continuity in some aspects of local administration – the centralizing initiatives of Philip V and his ministers did force previously independent municipalities to enter the

---

[51] Consejos 1476, October 2, 1720, f. 133v–134, AHN; Consejos 1476, August 29, 1720, f. 129v, AHN. See also Fernando Varela Peris, "El papel de la Junta Suprema de Sanidad en la política sanitaria Española del siglo XVIII," *Dynamis: Acta Hispanica ad Medicinae Scientiarumque Historiam Illustrandam* 18 (1998): 315–40, 317; Josep Barona and Josep Bernabeu-Mestre, *La salud y el Estado: El movimiento sanitario internacional y la administración española, 1851–1945* (Valencia: Universitat de Valéncia, 2008), 15.

[52] *Cavildos del año de 1720*, libro no. 76, f. 398, AC, AMC. See also Peset, Mancebo, and Peset, "Temores y Defensa de España," 149. Peset and Mancebo, "Valencia y la peste de Marsella," 567–8.

[53] Virginia León Sanz, "Felipe V y la sociedad catalana al finalizar la guerra de sucesión," *Pedralbes: Revista d'història moderna* 23 (2003): 271.

[54] Sanz, "Felipe V y la sociedad catalana," 271.

larger system of Bourbon administration to different degrees, and in many cases, to find new ways to exercise influence.[55] Indeed, it was as a result of these reforming endeavors that Philip V was later dubbed "el Animoso," or "the energetic king," a moniker meant to reflect his centralizing efforts within Spain both during and after the War of the Spanish Succession.[56] In these eastern regions, beginning as early as August 1720, soldiers and civilians were chosen to stand on twenty-four-hour watch in order to prevent clandestine vessels from disembarking in unauthorized areas and to supervise the movements and activity of the people.[57] No festivals or celebrations of any kind were allowed, and several important industries were suppressed, including the raising of pigs, bulls, and steers, as well as the fabrication of silk (owing to the foul odors, and thus possible miasmas, the raising of silkworms produced), a principal Valencian and Murcian industry in the eighteenth century that remained banned until February 1724, nearly two years after the end of the plague in France.[58]

Among the most notable of the new, kingdom-wide regulations to defend against plague, however, was the creation of Spain's first centralized Board of Health, the *Junta Suprema de Sanidad*, established on September 18, 1720, at the request of the governor of the Council

---

[55] For a look at the struggle for control in the case of Alicante after the *Nueva Planta* decrees, see Armando Alberola Romá, "La pugna por el control de la administración local en la primera mitad del siglo XVIII: El proyecto de reforma del ayuntamiento de Alicante (1747)," in *Política y hacienda el Antiguo Régimen*, edited by José Ignacio Fortea Pérez and Carmen Maria Cremades Griñán (Murcia: Universidad de Murcia, 1992): 145–54; Armando Alberola Romá, "Centralismo Borbónico y pervivencias forales: La reforma del gobierno municipal de la ciudad de Alicante (1747)," *Estudis: Revista de historia moderna*, no. 18 (1992): 147–72. For continuity in health regulations in Barcelona, see, for example: Alfonso Zarzoso, "Protomedicato y boticarios en la Barcelona del siglo XVIII," *Dynamis: Acta Hispanica ad Medicinae Scientiarumque Historiam Illustrandam* 16 (1996): 151–71.

[56] Ricardo García Cárcel, "La opinión de los españoles sobre Felipe V después de la Guerra de Sucesión," *Cuadernos de Historia Moderna Anejos* 1 (2002): 113.

[57] Peset, Mancebo, and Peset, "Temores y defensa de España," 149.

[58] Jean-Baptiste Martin Partyet to Jean-Frédéric Phélypeaux, comte de Maurepas, secrétaire d'État de la Marine, Cádiz, November 23, 1727, ff. 192–5v, AE, BI, 233, AN. This is one of the documents that mentions that commercial relations did not resume until March 1724. Also see Peset, Mancebo, and Peset, "Temores y defensa de España," 187; and Rambert, "La France et la politique commercial," 274.

of Castile, Luis de Miraval (or Mirabal) y Espínola.[59] The council was aware of the challenges involved in the implementation and execution of an empire-wide set of reforms meant to prevent the introduction of contagion in the kingdom. As a result, a centralized board was created that would direct its efforts solely to defense against biological threats, thereby freeing the royal government of this arduous task.[60] The board comprised a governor and four ministers, all members of the Royal Council (none of whom were physicians), and was to report to the king about all matters related to the plague, and later, health and disease more generally, especially as Spain battled outbreaks of yellow fever into the nineteenth century.[61] It was considered a public service, and it represents the first regular, administrative institution to record the history of Spanish health, a task it performed until it was dissolved in 1847.[62] The extension of the *Junta de Sanidad* at Cádiz

[59] Esteban Rodríguez Ocaña, "El resguardo de la salud: Organización sanitaria española en el siglo XVIII," *Dynamis: Acta Hispanica ad Medicinae Scientiarumque Historiam Illustrandam* 7–8 (1987–8): 147. Zarzoso, "¿Obligación moral o responsabilidad política?," 85. Santiago Muñoz Machado, *La sanidad pública en España: Evolución histórica y situación actual* (Madrid: Instituto de Estudios Administrativos, 1975), 82. The *Junta* was formed by Mirabal and his councillors, Jose de Castro, Pedro Jose de Grava (elsewhere spelled Lagrava), Francisco Ameller, and Luis Curriel (sometimes spelled Curiel). See also: Febrer, "Los medicos frente a la enfermedad en la Valencia," 276.

[60] Peio J. Monteano, *Ira de Dios: Los Navarros en la era de la peste, 1348–1723* (Pamplona: Gráfica Ona, 2002), 238; Varela Peris, "El papel de la Junta Suprema de Sanidad," 317–18. A *Real cédula* dated November 8, 1721, reads: "The city of Marseille of France was infected by contagious disease in the month of July of last year. From the first days of August when I had news of the calamity that France was suffering, having consulted with the governor and others of my council, I ordered the issuing of various royal provisions, and then, so as not to occupy my entire council with these orders, a junta was created, composed of said governor of my council, don Luis Curriel, and his ministers don Joseph de Castro, don Pedro Joseph de Grava y don Francisco Ameller, so that they may look after everything pertaining to the public health." "Real cédula del 8 Noviembre 1721," Libro del Acuerdo, Audiencia, 1721, f. 173, Archivo General del Reino de Valencia (henceforward ARV). Cited in Peset and Peset, *Muerte en España*, 33.

[61] Increasingly, it took over various aspects of local decision-making about matters of health. Perdiguero Gil, "Con medios humanos y divinos," 145–6. Peset and Peset, *Muerte en España*, 33.

[62] José Javier Viñes Rueda, *La Sanidad española en el siglo XIX* (Navarre: Departamento de Salud, 2006), 38–68, 44. Years after the threat of plague had subsided, the *Junta* saw an interruption in August 1742 when it was

was most active, and quickly set about the task of prohibiting maritime commerce with all French ports and much of the Mediterranean. Never before had Spain produced such a comprehensive system for the management of disease.

The new regulations caused a great deal of commotion. In Valencia, for instance, residents rushed in great numbers to obtain health certificates in case they needed to leave the city. Lines formed "from dawn until very late in the evening."[63] A letter from the Navarrese Valle del Roncal (Roncal Valley) in the Pyrenees complained that the embargo against France, which restricted the area's wool trade, would mean ruin for the people, who would suffer "the nudity, the hunger, the abandonment of their own homes and of their children."[64] And in Murcia, which essentially quarantined itself with mud walls despite lack of infection, there were reports of people scaling the newly built walls or attempting to make breaches in them to escape.[65] This led to a

---

temporarily abolished. This was not to last, however, and it was reinstated in July 1743 during outbreaks of plague in northern Africa and Messina. It was also deemed better to have a mostly inactive board of health than to dismantle it only to have to quickly recreate one when the next epidemic took place. As mentioned earlier, Spain was to become increasingly acquainted with outbreaks of yellow fever into the nineteenth century. The *Junta* was eventually replaced in part by the *Dirección General de Sanidad* under the *Ministerio de la Gobernación* that was formed with the *Cortes de Cádiz* (the *ministerio* lasted until 1977, and evolved to today's *Ministerio de Sanidad*), and by the *Real Consejo de Sanidad* in December 1855. See: Joaquín del Moral Ruiz, Juan Pro Ruiz, and Fernando Suárez Bilbao, *Estado y territorio en España, 1820–1930: La formación del paisaje nacional* (Madrid: Libros de la Catarata, 2007), 226. Muñoz Machado, *La sanidad pública en España*, 83. Ocaña, "El resguardo de la salud," 150.

[63] Peset, Mancebo, and Peset, "Temores y defensa de España," 154.

[64] "Señor, El valle de Roncal del Reyno de Navarra siempre fidelissimo a VM y siempre confiado de sus augustas," Consejos 10145, AHN. This letter is only one of many, mostly from the eastern regions of the Iberian Peninsula, requesting that exceptions to the new regulations be made, lest the people suffer from lack of industry.

[65] Officials in the city of Murcia feared that the city lay vulnerable to possible infection since it was situated near the coast and had no protective wall to speak of. Consequently, they enclosed the city with mud walls, leaving only enough doors to handle traffic, each of which would be guarded as had been done in Valencia and Aragon. Antonio Peñafiel Ramón and Concepción Peñafiel Ramón, "Repercusión de la epidemia de peste marsellesa de 1720 en la ciudad de Murcia: Realidad de un gran miedo," *Contrastes: Revista de Historia Moderna* 3–4 (1987–8): 63; September 18, 1720, ff. 139–40, AC 338, AMU.

new set of proclamations that punished such acts with 200 lashes for a nonnoble or four months of *presidio* (garrison and prison) for nobles. Meanwhile, anyone who witnessed the "crime" and failed to alert authorities would be charged a fine of 20 ducats' worth of fleece.[66] In some coastal cities, local authorities applied their own series of measures to complement those of the central government. Alicante, for example, felt markedly the effects that plague-time regulations had on the city's maritime commerce. These populations would suffer great shortages from which they would not begin to recover until after 1722.

Health Inspections and the *Fondeo* Search in the Port of Cádiz

Another regulation that emerged at this time proved to be the most controversial. The royal order of August 3, 1720, declared that all vessels arriving from the Mediterranean were subject to mandatory inspections. This might not sound like anything out of the ordinary on the surface, but the inspections of foreign vessels and warehouses – meant not only to prevent disease transfer, but also to preempt illicit commerce, confiscate goods, and extract money from victims – had been a point of contention for decades, particularly for the French, who had the closest commercial ties to Spain and were especially active in Cádiz. Prior to the 1720 plague, despite the terms of several treaties, Spanish port officials in the peninsula and the colonies conducted inspections of foreign vessels, account books, and warehouses as a measure against illicit commerce. Since the Treaty of the Pyrenees, with the exception of periods during which the terms were set aside, the searches of French cargo were prohibited. However, Franco-Spanish competition and tensions on the ground, especially in Cádiz, meant that these were nonetheless carried out, much to the dissapointment of local Frenchmen.

Searches increasingly took one of two forms. During and after the plague, they were mostly executed as *visitas de sanidad* (health visits), during which *patentes de sanidad* were submitted and Spanish port officials inspected the cargo to certify that it was free of infection or risk thereof. These continued until well into the nineteenth century, but they proved to be insufficient for Spanish port officials, who

---

[66] Ramón and Ramón, "Repercusión," 65.

desired more direct access to, and control over, foreign cargos. Consequently, during the plague in Provence, the search of foreign vessels in Spain increasingly took the form of *fondeo* or "right of access" searches. These involved the complete unloading, over a period of two or three days, of a foreign ship's cargo onto another ship (or ships) for inspection by (usually) four officials under the direction of the local governor.[67] After this rigorous, expensive, and protracted inspection, which caused delays lasting anywhere from fifteen to twenty days – a major point of contention for the French and other foreigners – the cargo was either brought ashore by the Spaniards or placed back in the foreign vessel for transport to its final destination.[68] As a measure to confirm that all cargo was accounted for and that it was free of infection, the *fondeo* sometimes represented the second step in the process of docking at a Spanish port, following twenty-four hours after the initial *visita de sanidad* and the submission to port officials of a detailed account of the ship's cargo. In addition to carrying a hefty fee, discrepancies between the account and the *fondeo* resulted in confiscations.[69]

These time-consuming inspections not only directly threatened the lucrative practice of illicit commerce, but also carried a mandatory tax that foreign merchants, consuls, and other port officials alike considered a great injustice. Throughout the seventeenth and eighteenth centuries, European nations tirelessly sought exemption from official searches of their ships, homes, account books, and warehouses in their dealings with the Spaniards. Even before 1720, Partyet, the French consul in Cádiz, often reminded French officials in his letters of the importance of protecting French privileges in Spain, above all, the exemption from these visits. Nevertheless, the inspections continued both on the peninsula and in the colonies, and the outbreak of plague in 1720 served as a solid pretext for carrying them out until long after the end of the epidemic and into the nineteenth century. Justifying trade restrictions and sanitary measures on the basis of

---

[67] Jean-Baptiste Martin Partyet, *Mémoire pour le fondeo*, November 18, 1731, MAR, B7, 310, no. 26, AN.

[68] "Mémoire sur la visite appellee fondeo," May 18, 1734, AE, BIII, 361, no. 9, AN. See Jean O. McLachlan, *Trade and Peace with Old Spain*, 192.

[69] José Canga Argüelles, *Diccionario de hacienda con aplicación a España, Tomo 2* (Madrid: Imprenta de Don Marcelino Calero y Portocarrero, 1834), 497–8.

Franco-Levantine trade relations and the possibility of a new outbreak, officials made the searches compulsory not only when Spain
received word of a disease outbreak anywhere in the Mediterranean,
but often even in times of health.

The French in Cádiz denounced *fondeo* searches as major violations
of merchant rights that served only to facilitate the arbitrary abuse of
power "under the pretext of public health," a ubiquitous phrase in
the contemporary record. Believed to exist solely as a means for the
Spanish to "little by little destroy [French] exemption from the visits
of [their] vessels," the *fondeo* searches produced endless grievances.[70]
"The *fondeo* is useless ... based on imagined pretexts," said one document.[71] The *fondeos* are expensive and cause "infinite harm," said
another; "they cause considerable delays," and "they are detrimental
to commerce," said two more.[72] In a letter dated December 23, 1720,
Partyet wrote to the French Marine Council in reference to the new
regulations, maintaining that French commerce had gone from bad to
worse because of the prohibition of French ships in Spain. He wrote,
"Many people here believe that this enormous strictness is more the
effect of political interest than of an actual fear of contagion."[73] Partyet would spend the rest of his life arguing for French merchant rights
in Cádiz, defending them against perceived injustices in the ports, and
his son, Jean-Baptiste Martin Partyet, later continued his father's
efforts when he took over the consulship.

By 1731 French concerns intensified to such a point that officials
called for the establishment of a French chamber of commerce in
Cádiz to handle Franco-Spanish commerce, "following the example
of the Chamber in Marseille for commerce with the Levant." It would

---

[70] Jean-Baptiste Martin Partyet to Jean-Frédéric Phélypeaux, November 29,
1728, AE, BI, 235, ff. 192–192v, AN.

[71] June 1749, AE, BIII, 361, AN.

[72] Jean-Baptiste Martin Partyet to Jean-Frédéric Phélypeaux, August 17, 1728,
AE, BI, 235, ff. 88–9v, AN; May 23, 1730, AE, BI, 238, ff. 185–91v, AN;
Louis de Lastre, chancelier du consulat de France à Cadix, to Jean-Frédéric
Phélypeaux, February 14, 1730, AE, BI, 238, ff. 43–5v, AN. For another
important document on French perceptions of the *fondeo*, see "Mémoire sur la
visite appelée fondeo," May 18, 1734, AE, BIII, 361, no. 9, AN.

[73] Pierre-Nicolas Partyet to Conseil de Marine, December 23, 1720, AE, BI, 225,
ff. 361v–362, AN.

be "under the command and protection of the *Ministre de la marine* [Ministry of the Navy] ... and consist of the consul and six directors or deputies that would be chosen from among the merchants."[74] It was described as "an indispensable necessity [in light of] the Spaniards' infractions against the French, and the privileges that they have given the English to the detriment of France."[75] Among these "infractions" were episodes in which British ships were allowed to bring French products into Spain with the Spanish king's permission. In 1721, for example, French traders living in Cádiz complained when James Butler, 2nd duke of Ormonde, obtained from the king of Spain a passport for two English ships to transport fabrics from Brittany to Cádiz. Reportedly, in June 1721 two English vessels (of forty and thirty cannons) transported seven to eight hundred *paquetons* of French merchandise to Cádiz and Andalucía. In a letter to the *Conseil de Marine*, Partyet angrily observed, "So it is not French goods that are prohibited here, but the French flag."[76] Yet, the French were not alone in their criticisms about the searches. Since the Treaty of Utrecht in 1713, despite an increase in French activity in the *Carrera de Indias* prior to 1720, French protests often claimed that the British and their allies were reaping all advantages at the expense of the French in the Spanish market, due in part to the privileges that were transferred from France to England in the Treaty of Utrecht (most notably, the *asiento de negros*). These objections increased exponentially after 1720, but the English, too, suffered injustices in Spanish ports. In 1722, the English statesman William Stanhope, at this time ambassador in the Spanish capital (1721–27), wrote the marquis de Grimaldo (minister of Philip V) that, according to letters he received from English merchants in Cádiz and other foreign *négociants*, the searches of vessels were not being carried out as they should, causing great inconveniences for the foreigners involved. He later wrote King Philip V to request that the governor in Cádiz only allow items genuinely suspected of infection

---

[74] "Mémoire sur la question d'establier une chambre pour diriger le commerce d'Espagne al'instar de la chambre de Marseille pour le commerce de Levant," August 1731, MAR, B7, 310, AN.
[75] Ibid.
[76] Pierre-Nicolas Partyet to Conseil de Marine, Cádiz, June 30, 1721, AE, BI, 226, ff. 147–8v, AN.

to be taken to the lazarets during the searches.[77] Countless more complaints and controversies, as well as a Franco-Spanish alliance during the War of the Polish Succession, eventually helped to end temporarily the practice of *fondeo* in 1735, but arbitrary quarantines and the *visitas de sanidad* continued, as did the grievances against them.

One of these controversies in particular was effective at bringing attention to the prejudicial practice. On June 17, 1729, Alexandre Coterel (or Cotterel), captain of the merchant ship *Le Prudent*, departed his base in Saint-Malo for Martinique and arrived at the port of Cádiz on June 20, 1730, packed with sugar. At this time, Coterel was obliged to submit to *fondeo*, at which point 160 barrels of sugar were taken from his ship. Two Spanish boats had been charged with the responsibility of holding the French ship's cargo for the *fondeo*, but these two ships were then intercepted, their men detained, and their valuable Martiniquais contents confiscated. This was done at the behest of the governor of Cádiz, Antonio Álvarez de Bohorqués, along with the director of customs, who wished to seize the cargo by carrying out what local French officials considered an obvious scheme to steal from the French.[78] The governor is said to have accused Captain Coterel of attempting to introduce the sugar as contraband in Cádiz, which the French consul in Cádiz at the time,

---

[77] Lord Stanhope to marquis de Grimaldo, Madrid, May 9, 1722, Consejos 10145, AHN. Pierre-Nicolas Partyet to Conseil de Marine, Cádiz, November 27, 1718, AE, BI, 224, ff. 454–5, AN.

Vessel searches in Venice were also a thorn in the side of representatives from Paris, London, Vienna, and other cities, who made no secret of their frustrations over the costly delays. The British dispatched numerous letters to representatives in Venice in the hopes of being exempted from the searches. One letter concludes: "E un bene si universale e d'una natura si delicata il commercio, ch'è assolutamente necessario di nutrirlo con la più grand'attentione, e non esporlo alle minime difficoltà. Riesce meglio dove trova più libertà, e fugge la soggestione e l'oppressione. È una verità questa si costante," Elizeus Burges, minister resident of Great Britain in Venice, to the Doge and Council, Venice, December 5, 1720, SP 99/62, Venice, 555, TNA. For other examples, see: Elizeus Burges, minister resident of Great Britain in Venice, to the Doge and Council, Venice, September 13, 1720, SP 99/62, Venice, 511, TNA. "Mémoire concernant le privilège d'exempt visite dont les bâtiments portants de France et d'Angleterre doivent jouir tous les ports de la Rép. de Venise," September 4, 1721, SP 78/170-1, ff. 113–37v, TNA.

[78] Jean-Baptiste Martin Partyet to Jean-Frédéric Phélypeaux, July 18, 1730, AE, BI, 239, ff. 31–6, AN.

Jean-Baptiste Martin Partyet (son of Pierre-Nicolas Partyet), argued was "as impossible as it is unheard of." Partyet described "L'affaire Coterel" (the Coterel affair) as "the greatest injustice that there has ever been."[79] Ultimately, the entire episode, including the proceedings, the loss of goods to weather damage, and the accruing interest, cost as much as 1,000 *pistolles* of gold, as well as the reputation of local Gaditan officials.

Jean-Baptiste Partyet informed Daubenton of the affair and made sure that the news made it to José Patiño, minister of Philip V, so that such abuses would cease and those responsible for them would be punished.[80] In a letter to Jean-Frédéric Phélypeaux, comte de Maurepas, he wrote, "It is hoped, for the welfare and tranquility of trade in general, that Monsieur Daubenton can see to it, together with Monseigneur, that this administrator, who is the cause of all these vexations, is dismissed."[81] Phélypeaux, secretary of state for the Marine in France, responded that as a result of this most recent offense, the Spanish king must order the suppression of the practice of *fondeo* "as soon as possible." "It is true," he wrote, "that it is important to immediately abolish the practice of *fondeo*. It stands entirely contrary to established rules, as well as to all that has been stipulated in past treaties. So long

---

[79] Jean-Baptiste Martin Partyet, *Mémoire pour le fondeo*, November 18, 1731, MAR, B7, 310, no. 2, AN.

[80] Patiño held many important positions in the first decades of the eighteenth century and is often considered Spain's first prime minister. In 1711, he became one of the first Spanish intendants, and in 1713, as superintendent of Catalonia, he oversaw the abolition of the *fueros* under the *Decretos de Nueva Planta* – a victory for Spanish absolutism (the *fueros* were ancient charters that reserved various privileges for the principalities and kingdoms that comprised the Crown of Aragon). In 1717, he was named intendant-general of Marine and president of the *Casa de la Contratación*, and in 1726, became secretary of the Office for Marine and the Indies and secretary of the Office for Finance. Later, he also held the position of secretariat of state (formally in 1733), and of war in 1730. Adrian J. Pearce, *The Origins of Bourbon Reform in Spanish South America, 1700–1763* (New York: Palgrave Macmillan, 2014), 64. For more on Patiño, see also *Chapter 3 of* Kuethe and Andrien (cited earlier), Crespo Solana on the *Casa de Contratación* (cited earlier), as well as the latter's article: "La acción de José Patiño en Cádiz y los proyectos navales de la Corona del siglo XVIII," *Trocadero: Revista de historia moderna y contemporanea*, no. 6–7 (1994–1995): 35–50.

[81] Jean-Baptiste Martin Partyet to Jean-Frédéric Phélypeaux, July 18, 1730, AE, BI, 239, f. 33v, AN.

as the practice persists, it will continue to cause various new disorders and many prejudices in our commerce with Spain."[82]

Earlier, on July 30, 1730, Daubenton received orders from Patiño ordering that Coterel's trial be transferred from local jurisdiction to the Council of Finance (*Consejo Supremo de Hacienda*). The same letter also gave orders to return to Coterel the 160 barrels of sugar that were confiscated from *Le Prudent* during the *fondeo*.[83] A few days later, Partyet reported back to Phélypeaux that his continuing efforts to end the unjust measure of *fondeo*, especially after the Coterel affair, had seen little to no progress, but that the barrels of sugar were indeed finally returned to Captain Coterel on August 8. Soon thereafter, his case proceeded to the *Consejo de Hacienda* where it was eventually settled.[84]

Although the captain won his case in September and was cleared of any false charges against him, the last we learn of *l'affaire Coterel* is that by November, the case was still pending because of the absence of the consignee of Coterel's vessel. This was possibly a witness in the case who hastily departed Cádiz to escape the outbreak of yellow fever that had arrived in the port weeks earlier.[85] Consequently, delays and excuses continually deferred the suppression of *fondeo*, much to the displeasure of the French and other foreigners in Cádiz. One French contemporary complained, "Being that there is no legitimate reason, nor basis for conducting the *fondeo*, it is of great importance to make known to his Catholic Majesty and his ministers that they must end the harassment that is as bothersome as it is costly for our trade."[86]

The short-lived Coterel affair highlighted the perceived injustices of the practice and contributed to its discontinuation for a short time

---

[82] Jean-Frédéric Phélypeaux in Compiègne to Jean-Baptiste Martin Partyet in Cádiz, August 12, 1730, AE, BI, 239, f. 75, AN.

[83] Jean-Baptiste Martin Partyet to Jean-Frédéric Phélypeaux, August 8, 1730, AE, BI, 239, ff. 70–3v, AN.

[84] Jean-Baptiste Martin Partyet to Jean-Frédéric Phélypeaux, August 15, 1730, AE, BI, 239, ff. 78–80v, AN.

[85] Jean-Baptiste Martin Partyet to Jean-Frédéric Phélypeaux, September 27, 1730, AE, BI, 239, ff. 134–7v, AN. Jean-Baptiste Martin Partyet to Jean-Frédéric Phélypeaux, November 21, 1730, AE, BI, 239, ff. 268–73v, AN. This was, in fact, the first of many outbreaks of yellow fever in the port of Cádiz.

[86] "Mémoire sur la visite appellée fondeo," May 18, 1734, AE, BIII, 361, no. 9, AN.

in August 1735. On September 12, Paul Caullet, the chancellor of the consulate of France in Cádiz, informed Phélypeaux that the royal order from the Court of Spain calling for the suppression of *fondeo* had finally arrived in Cádiz on September 5.[87] Letters from Caullet and Partyet in November and December, respectively, happily report the complete cessation of *fondeo* searches in Cádiz, but complaints against the *visitas de sanidad* persisted.[88] Alas, Spain had managed to maintain a loophole.

Some years later, however, the practice would be reinstated. It is unclear exactly when it became standard practice again, but one could speculate that it was around 1742 or 1743 – two very busy plague years in Europe. Plague outbreaks on the continent and the Mediterranean between 1742 and 1744 alarmed European authorities and may have put back into motion regulations originally imposed during the Plague of Provence. Even into the nineteenth century, when yellow fever outbreaks terrorized the Atlantic world, mention of *fondeo* searches continued in printed publications.[89] Because the 1720 plague did, after all, remain confined to Provence, Spain continually argued that their measures to prevent its spread were successful and must be reinstated time and again.

Disaster Centralism in Spain during the Plague of Provence

Progressively throughout the Plague of Provence, we see Spanish authorities' rigid intervention in trade, industry, and commercial navigation. Rather than allowing French merchants to enjoy such prearranged freedoms as the exemption from cargo searches, open access to

---

[87] Paul Caullet, chancelier du consulat de France à Cadix to Jean-Frédéric Phélypeaux, August 16, 1735, AE, BI, 246, ff. 177–81v, AN; Caullet to Jean-Frédéric Phélypeaux, August 23, 1735, AE, BI, 246, ff. 182–5v, AN; Caullet to Jean-Frédéric Phélypeaux, August 30, 1735, AE, BI, 246, ff. 186–9v, AN; Caullet to Jean-Frédéric Phélypeaux, September 12, 1735, AE, BI, 246, ff. 192–5v, AN.

[88] Caullet to Jean-Frédéric Phélypeaux, November 18, 1735, AE, BI, 246, ff. 248–51v, AN; Jean-Baptiste Martin Partyet, consul de France à Cadix to Jean-Frédéric Phélypeaux, December 6, 1735, AE, BI, 246, ff. 258–62v, AN.

[89] For example, see Comisión de Salud Pública, *Proyecto de ley orgánica de sanidad pública de la Monarquía Española* (Madrid: Imprenta de Alban y Compañía, 1822), 149–50.

Spanish ports, and lower duties, Spanish officials now used the plague as a pretext to arbitrarily inspect vessels and account books, confiscate merchandise, and demand payments. Despite protections against them in the terms of various treaties, these searches increased exponentially during and after the plague in France and became the principal cause for the grievances of foreign merchants and consuls in Spain following the 1720 plague.

There was nothing new about the suspension or restriction of trade with infected regions during plague epidemics, nor does the 1720 plague represent the first time that sanitary measures had been used to deliberately ruin another's commerce. In fact, by the eighteenth century, embargoes and quarantines were seldom imposed "solely for reasons of public health." As Mark Harrison has noted, "The question of whether to impose quarantine was a political as much as a medical one."[90] What is extraordinary about this particular case is that the severity and extent of the controls put in place, and the degree to which they were managed from the capital, had little precedent in Spanish history and were unmatched elsewhere in Europe at this time, other than in France itself. Even in parts of Italy, where trade embargoes were placed against southern France as early as July 1720, domestic measures to prevent plague did not equal those in Spain. Moreover, restrictive measures in Spain and the colonies remained in place until well after the plague had disappeared in Provence. The last significant relapse of the epidemic took place in Marseille in the autumn of 1722, after which it began to subside for good. Months later, *Te Deums* in Paris, Rome, and other cities marked the recognition that the scourge was over.[91] European cities such as Turin began lifting their trade restrictions with France as early as 1722, while others, like Genoa or Rome, waited until 1723 before allowing products from Marseille to flow into their ports.[92] Spain, however, would not lift *all* restrictions against France until March 1724 – nearly two years after the plague disappeared – and then the resumption of commerce between the two countries was slow and problematic. This was due in part to the preventative policies that persisted long after the epidemic

[90] Harrison, *Contagion*, 37, 25.
[91] "Paris, February 15, 1723," *Gaceta de Madrid*, no. 9, March 2, 1723, 34–5.
[92] "Génova, May 7, 1723," *Gaceta de Madrid*, no. 22, June 1, 1723, 86.

had vanished, including, most notably, the detested *fondeo* searches. A look at disease management in Spain prior to the Plague of Provence underscores the extent to which the policies enacted in 1720 were significantly more centralized and more extensive than those put in place during the epidemics of the seventeenth century. This is especially so if we consider that this outbreak never even made it into Spain, and that most measures remained in place long after the end of the epidemic.

At the time of the Provençal plague, Spain had not suffered a major disease epidemic since the mid-seventeenth century. In June 1647 plague entered the Iberian Peninsula through Valencia and eventually spread into Seville in Andalucía, where it became most virulent and raged until 1652.[93] Historian Antonio Domínguez Ortiz has called this "the greatest demographic catastrophe to have befallen Spain in modern times."[94] Unlike earlier plague outbreaks of the sixteenth to seventeenth centuries, the 1647 outbreak devastated Andalucía with such persistence and intensity that its socioeconomic effects would linger for many years.[95] Domínguez Ortiz puts the number of deaths within the city of Seville alone at no less than 60,000, a toll caused in large part by a lack of preventative measures.[96] Despite the virulence of this epidemic, however, and the importance of the highly populated city of Seville as the rich hub of Spain's monopoly over the Indies market at that time, the Crown's intervention remained limited. In the summer of 1649, the Crown deployed guards to the Sierra Morena mountain range to prevent movement in and out of Andalucía and created health committees that put royal judges in communication

---

[93] For more on this outbreak, see José Luis Betrán Moya, "Sociedad y peste en la Barcelona de 1651," *Manuscrits: Revista d'història moderna* 8 (January 1990): 255–82. And for a study on the measures taken in Madrid to protect itself (not the rest of the realm) from the plague while it raged in Valencia, see: Elvira Arquiola, Jose Luis Peset, Mariano Peset, and Santiago La Parra, "Madrid, villa y corte, ante la peste de Valencia de 1647–1648," *Estudis: Revista de historia moderna* 5 (1976): 29–46.

[94] Antonio Domínguez Ortiz, *La Sociedad Española en el Siglo XVII: El Estamento nobiliario*, vol. 1 (Granada: Universidad de Granada, 1992), 71.

[95] Ibid.

[96] Antonio Domínguez Ortiz, *Historia de Sevilla: La Sevilla del siglo XVII* (Seville: Universidad de Sevilla Secretariado de Publicaciones, 1986), 74. Other estimates claim that a quarter of the city's population perished. In any case, a sizable percentage of the population died during the epidemic.

with municipal magistrates for the first time.[97] Yet the establishment in the capital of a permanent, centralized *Junta de Sanidad* – a notable product of Spain's disaster centralism – that could manage, collect information about, and report on public health in the realm did not come to fruition until 1720 when Spain learned of the epidemic in Provence. By the seventeenth century there did exist local *Juntas de Salud* or boards of health put in place at a municipal level in some of the most important ports on the peninsula, but because of their local and often provisional nature, these were powerless in the face of major outbreaks like that of Seville.[98] They lacked, for instance, the efficient system of communication that the centralized *Junta* of 1720 established – a defect that some considered to be one of the principal difficulties that authorities faced in 1647.[99] In Barcelona, too, where the elements that would represent the city's public health legislation were implemented between 1460 and 1530, the epidemic of 1647 presented a challenge for the *Consell de Cent* (Council of One Hundred), the local governing body that was later abolished by Philip V under the *Decretos de Nueva Planta*.[100] Unable to prevent the infection from entering Barcelona, the *Consell de Cent* was primarily responsible for managing the crisis and preventing its spread, which proved an impossible task. As a result, many were compelled to flee the city, including members of the local government, which in turn lessened support for public authority and thus aggravated an already critical situation.[101]

Along with the practice of prayers and processions meant to ward off divine ire, disease control by the mid-seventeenth century in Spain consisted of defensive measures that aimed to restrict the movements of peoples or products. Local authorities could regulate people's movements by requiring that they obtain permits, or *cédulas*, from the municipal *Cabildo* (local government) in order to pass city walls, or by

---

[97] James Casey, *Early Modern Spain: A Social History* (London: Routledge, 1999), 39.

[98] Juan Ignacio Carmona García, *La Peste en Sevilla* (Seville: Ayuntamiento de Sevilla, 2005), 224.

[99] James Casey, *España en la Edad Moderna: Una historia social* (Madrid: Editorial Biblioteca Nueva, 2001), 76–7; Casey, *Early Modern Spain*, 39.

[100] José Luis Betrán Moya, *La peste en la Barcelona de los Austrias* (Lleida: Editorial Milenio, 1996), 259.

[101] Betrán Moya, "Sociedad y peste," 270–3.

employing quarantine lines, essentially cordoning off infected areas to prevent the spread of disease. In plague times local festivals were often suspended, and local and central authorities commonly issued trade restrictions that limited and monitored the entrance into Spain of any persons or materials coming from an infected port. This happened, for example, when news arrived in Spain that there was plague in Holland in 1663 and then in London from 1665 to 1666. Madrid prohibited any commercial dealings with ports of either country, though prohibitions were lifted soon thereafter.[102] Still, communication networks and plague prevention measures throughout the seventeenth century were much more fragmented than they were by 1720, when Spain was both trying to maintain a position of influence in the commercial and diplomatic milieu of Europe and working to reform and consolidate Spain from within. In essence, for most of the early modern era, municipal and regional governments, rather than a more centralized state, were primarily responsible for preventing and managing public health – particularly in times of disease.[103]

...

The Plague of Provence and the Great Plague Scare that ensued allowed the Spanish Crown the opportunity to impose a variety of measures meant to complement administrative centralization and control, and to attempt to regain the commercial footing that it had lost over the previous several decades, all under the veil of plague prevention. These efforts ultimately failed, since the Spanish Crown could not effectively subdue foreign dominance over the Indies trade; indeed, France's involvement in the Indies market both through Cádiz and through its own increasing presence in the Atlantic only intensified during the eighteenth century. Nevertheless, working parts of the new centralized system for plague prevention in Spain were born of

---

[102] The Great Plague of London raged through September 1666 and took an estimated 100,000 lives. Still, by October 1667, commercial restrictions had been lifted. Monteano, *Ira de Dios*, 226–7.

[103] Kristy Wilson Bowers, *Plague and Public Health in Early Modern Seville* (Rochester: University of Rochester Press, 2013), 90. This slowly began to change beginning with Philip II (r. 1580–98). However, "Definitive change in Spain came in the eighteenth century, after the rise of the Bourbon dynasty to the throne" in the person of Philip V. Bowers, 99.

the plague in Provence and continued well into at least the nineteenth century, resulting in major changes in the management of both public health and customs inspections. Among these changes were the *Junta de Sanidad*, the increased use of lazarets, the health patent policy, the highly contested *visitas de sanidad* and *fondeo* searches, and the use of arbitrary extended quarantines. At this time, too, all of Spain saw a significant increase in communication between the Crown and administrators in the provinces, especially along the borders and in the ports. Beginning with one José Fornés, for example, a Spanish physician sent to Marseille to confirm the presence of plague, "inspectors" were designated at the beginning of each major outbreak of disease, assigned with the task of investigating the epidemic and reporting back to Madrid – a tradition that also continued into the nineteenth century. Customs inspections and the public health system emerged more centralized and bureaucratized. The rise of state power increasingly offered countries like Spain the ability to respond to the threat or impact of epidemics and other disasters in ways that complemented the fundamental interests of the state. The administration of Philip V was capable of launching a centralized system of laws, royal decrees, and provisions during the French plague, the likes of which had never been known in Spain, all as a result of the Spanish plague epidemic that never was. Efforts to extend this disaster centralism to the colonies, however, would prove more of a challenge.

5 | Entangled Empires
The Great Plague Scare in the Colonies

Thank God the plague is in Marseille, and that for a long time you will not have ships from this city. Prevail over the sale of your merchandise and be certain to get the best deal possible on the goods of your island.[1]

It is appropriate [for the Spanish] to cut off communications [with the French], because their sole guiding principle and policy is, under any pretext, to introduce their trade and take the silver.[2]

On April 6, 1721, François de Pas de Mazencourt, marquis de Feuquières (c. 1660–1731) and Charles Bénard (1622–1728), the *gouverneur général* and *intendant*, respectively, of the French colony of Martinique, wrote the Marine Council (*Conseil de Marine*) in Paris to confirm that they had taken the necessary precautions to protect against the contagion that reigned in Provence.[3] "These have so far proved unnecessary," they wrote, "because the island has not seen a vessel from the Mediterranean in over a year, which does inexpressible harm to the islands by the lack of provisions which these vessels have accustomed to bring. [And] the prices for oil, soap, and other merchandise from Provence and Languedoc are exorbitant."[4] Writing from the administrative capital of Fort Royal (now known as Fort-de-France), the officials also requested that the physician Sieur LeDran, who was

---

[1] François de Pas de Mazencourt, marquis de Feuquières, *gouverneur general* of Martinique (henceforward, Feuquières) to *Son altesse sérénissime, Monseigneur l'amiral* (Louis-Alexandre de Bourbon, head of the *Conseil de Marine*), Fort Royal, May 9, 1721, Col. F3 26, f. 472, ANOM.

[2] Alexandro Wauchop to the marqués de Casafuerte, composed aboard a *paquebot*, February 21, 1723, Audiencia de México 380, f. 17, Archivo General de Indias (henceforward AGI).

[3] Feuquières served as *gouverneur général* of Martinique from 1717 to 1727. Bénard served as *intendant* from 1719 to 1723.

[4] Feuquières and Bénard to the *Conseil de Marine*, Fort Royal, April 6, 1721, Col. C8B 7, f. 42, ANOM.

back in Paris, return to the island. He was much needed there as a result of "the imminent inclement weather which has already started to be felt since the heat and drought began two months earlier than usual." Indeed, they insisted that if LeDran could not make residence in Fort Royal, a different doctor should be sent in his stead, since the island's sole surgeon, Sieur Heudes, was in too great a demand by the inhabitants. They related that the former commander of Saint Lucia had died of yellow fever ("mal de Siam" or malady of Siam) on the island within three days and without any help, because Heudes had been lodged with Mr. and Mrs. de la Touche who had been at the point of death for a month. "The profession of doctor and surgeon," they added, "is excellent in Martinique, because there are always so many diseases, and we pay handsomely so that in a short time, [these physicians] make an honest fortune."[5]

As this letter suggests, the European colonies were in a unique position during the public health crisis in France. They existed in a sort of middle ground, torn in some ways between the demands of the metropole and the needs of the colony; reliant on, and under the command of the metropole in theory, but quite often acting independently in practice. After all, no one understood the needs of the colonies better than those on the ground, in lands unknown to most of the Europeans who ruled over them. For this reason, officials in the metropole sometimes granted administrators in the colonies some independence by advising them to act as they saw fit in various situations. Meanwhile, in other cases, colonial autonomy functioned behind a façade of strict allegiance to the wishes of the Crown. In both instances, however, colonial governors, intendants, viceroys, and others often did whatever was necessary to get by, including, as we will see, in times of crisis and upheaval. And this was not only the case in the French colonies but in the wider eighteenth-century colonial world in both the Americas and Asia. Both France and Spain, for example, sought to restrict foreign and illicit commerce throughout the eighteenth century, and both wished for their respective colonies to be solely dependent on the metropole for goods. Neither, however, was ever able to clamp down completely on contraband trade, even during public health crises like the Plague of Provence, despite the constant barrage of letters from officials in

[5] Ibid.

Europe demanding as much. Instead, commerce and trade, both legal and illicit, continued throughout the plague years, even with attempts by the crowns of Europe to restrict it. Consequently, while disaster centralism seemed ostensibly to extend from Europe to the colonies during the Plague of Provence – as the metropoles dispatched orders to protect against the spread of plague and monitored activities on the ground – local economic concerns, as well as the need for foods, fabrics, supplies, and personnel, often outweighed concerns about public health.

But the situation in the colonies was unique in other ways as well. Nowhere is the interconnectedness of the eighteenth-century world and the invisible commonwealth (as discussed in Chapter 2) more manifest than in the European colonies, where colonial governors, intendants, merchants, and others networked, interacted, and struggled to balance the demands and expectations of the metropole with broader colonial realities. And in the colonial world of 1720, perhaps no relationship was more intertwined, or more contentious, than that between France and Spain. To protect against the spread of infection during the Plague of Provence, European states, including France, dispatched restrictions against French ships and merchants across the colonies, from Quebec to Boston to Buenos Aires; from New Spain to Havana to Manila; but some of the most noteworthy and most revealing accounts that emerge in the historical archives deal with Spanish and French reactions to the plague, and the ways in which these intersected. Even so, few works in the English language have focused on Franco-Spanish colonial relations in the eighteenth century and have instead concentrated on the Spanish and British or the British and French in the Atlantic.[6] This chapter reveals how the Great Plague

---

[6] On British and French or Spanish relations in the Atlantic, see, for example: J. H. Elliott, *Empires of the Atlantic World: Britain and Spain in America 1492–1830* (New Haven: Yale University Press, 2006); Trevor Burnard and John Garrigus, *The Plantation Machine: Atlantic Capitalism in French Saint-Domingue and British Jamaica* (Philadelphia: University of Pennsylvania Press, 2016); Jorge Cañizares-Esguerra, ed., *Entangled Empires: The Anglo-Iberian Atlantic, 1500–1830* (Philadelphia: University of Pennsylvania Press, 2018). On Franco-Spanish colonial relations in the eighteenth century, see: Henri Sée, "Esquisse de l'histoire du commerce français à Cadix et dans l'amérique espagnole au XVIIIe siècle," *Revue d'histoire modern* 3e, no. 13 (January–February 1928): 13–31; Ronald Hilton, "Spaniards in Marseilles in the XVIIIth

Scare unfolded in the colonies, paying special attention to the port city of Fort Royal, Martinique – at this time, the richest French colony, and a hugely important administrative center for the French Antilles[7] – and to interactions between the French and Spanish in the Americas. The chapter then examines anti-French and anti-foreign reactions to the Great Plague Scare in the Spanish colonies. As we will see, relationships between the major European powers during the Plague of Provence expressed themselves in unique ways in the colonies, where the demands of the metropole were not always in line with the needs or wants of these far-flung outposts.

Century," *Bulletin Hispanique* 40, no. 2 (1938): 176–85; Allan Christelow, "French Interest in the Spanish Empire During the Ministry of the Duc de Choiseul, 1759–1771," *The Hispanic American Review* 21, no. 4 (November 1941): 515–37; Rambert, "La France et la politique commercial de l'Espagne au XVIIIe siècle," 269–88; Didier Ozanam, "La colonie française de Cadix au XVIIIe siècle, d'après un document inédit (1777)," in *Melanges de la Casa de Velazquez*, tome 4, edited by Centre National de la recherche scientifique (Paris: Éditions E. de Boccard, 1968), 259–347; Charles Frostin, "Les Pontchartrain et la pénétration commerciale française en Amérique espagnole (1690–1715)," *Revue Historique* 245, no. 498 (April–June 1971): 307–36; John Robert McNeill, *Atlantic Empires of France and Spain: Louisbourg and Havana, 1700–1763* (Chapel Hill: University of North Carolina Press, 1985); Antonio García-Baquero González and Pedro Collado Villalta, "Les Français à Cadix au XVIIIe siècle: La colonie marchande," in *Les Français en Espagne à l'époque modern, XVIe–XVIIIe siècles, ouvrage collectif*, edited by Centre national de la recherche scientifique (Paris: Éditions du Centre national de la recherche scientifique, 1990), 173–96; Girard, *El comercio francés en Sevilla y Cádiz*; Manuel Bustos Rodríguez, "Les associations de commerce autour de la 'Carrera de Indias' au XVIIIe siècle," in *Le commerce atlantique franco-espagnol: acteurs, négoces et ports, XVe–XVIIIe siècle*, edited by Jean-Philippe Priotti and Guy Saupin (Rennes: Presses universitaires de Rennes, 2008), 275–84; Olivier Le Gouic, "Des négociants français aux portes des Indes: Les Lyonnais à Cadix au XVIIIe siècle," in *Le commerce atlantique franco-espagnol: acteurs, négoces et ports, XVe–XVIIIe siècle*, edited by Jean-Philippe Priotti and Guy Saupin (Rennes: Presses universitaires de Rennes, 2008), 285–317; François Crouzet, "La rivalité commerciale franco-anglaise dans l'empire espagnol, 1713–1789," *Histoire: Economie et Société* 31 (2012/13): 19–29.
7 Bernard Moitt, *Women and Slavery in the French Antilles, 1635–1848* (Bloomington: Indiana University Press, 2001), 39. For French Royal administrators, Martinique was the most important Caribbean colony and one of its most important overseas possessions until as late as the 1760s. Saint-Domingue typically gets most of the attention in this context, but from a strategic, royal perspective, Martinique was *cléf des îles* and more valuable: "The island of Martinique is the most advantageous, and therefore la cléf des

Responses to the Plague of Provence in the French Colonies

Before air travel and the trans-Atlantic telegraph cable, word traveled slowly across oceans. For much of 1720 authorities in the European colonies had no idea that plague was in France. Moreover, the confusion in the early days of the outbreak discussed in Chapters 1 and 2 meant that even Paris could not confirm plague in Provence until weeks after the epidemic began. As a result, official news of the plague, and the accompanying orders to implement appropriate precautions, did not begin going out to the French colonies until as late as the fall of 1720 when the *Conseil de Marine*[8] wrote colonial officials of the French *Îles du Vent et Sous-le-Vent de l'Amérique,* or French Antilles, with the information.[9] In a letter dated October 2, the *Conseil* wrote the governor-general and intendant of Martinique – the aforementioned Feuquières and Bénard – as well as the heads of Saint-Domingue and Cayenne, with directions on how to proceed in light of the epidemic in Marseille. Relating that the contagion had already

îles [the key to all the others], which makes it essential to conserve, and of the greatest importance." "Mémoire de fortification et de guerre défensive avec des observations sur la non valleur des terres incultes de la Martinique pour mettre cette colonie à une perfection d'agriculture à sa juste valleur en augmentant les habitations et le Dommaine du Roy," Rochemore, March 8, 1765, 13 DFC, f. 244, ANOM. Cited in: Arad Gigi, "The Materiality of Empire: Forts, Labor, and the Colonial State in the French Lesser Antilles, 1661–1776" (PhD diss., Florida State University, 2018), 51; see also 10, 215–16.

[8] Established during the regency's polysynody on November 3, 1715, to replace the *secrétaire d'État à la Marine,* the *Conseil de Marine* was abolished only eight years later, in 1723, and the *secrétaire* reestablished. Among its responsibilities was the administration of the colonies.

[9] By the early eighteenth century, the French had founded and occupied numerous colonies in the Americas. Among *les Îles Sous-le-Vent* or French Leeward Islands of the French Antilles (French West Indies) was the French colony of Saint-Domingue, now Haiti, which occupied the western third of the island of Hispaniola. Most French colonies at this time, however, were in *les Îles du Vent,* or Windward Islands, which included Martinique (founded in 1635), Marie Galante, Saint-Christophe, Saint-Barthélémy, Saint-Martin, Grenada, Saint-Croix, and Guadeloupe (the latter of which was considered part of the Leeward Islands in some documents). Other possessions included those of Canada, as well as French Louisiana, and French Guiana. See: James Pritchard, *In Search of Empire: The French in the Americas* (Cambridge: Cambridge University Press, 2004), xvii.

caused several nations, including France, to take necessary precautions, the Marine Council now insisted that the island colonies do the same. First, the colonial officials were ordered to designate new, more isolated locations where vessels arriving from the coasts of the Mediterranean could anchor until the doctor or surgeon charged with ship inspections had produced his report confirming a ship's health. While the vessel awaited the all-clear, no one on board was to disembark, no merchandise could be unloaded, and all unauthorized communication between those on board and those on land was strictly forbidden. The Council also instructed these officials to take any additional precautions they deemed necessary, and to communicate those orders to the colonies of Guadeloupe and Grenada.[10]

Feuquières and Bénard acted accordingly, and in April 1721, they issued an *Ordonnance sur la peste*, or plague ordinance, that added to the October 1720 orders. It prohibited, on pain of death, the captain or shipmaster (*maître de navire*) of any vessel from Marseille, Languedoc, or any port of the Mediterranean from anchoring in the harbors of the French Antilles without having first received authorization from the local *commandant du quartier*, or district commander; nor could anyone on these vessels come on land, bring anyone on board from the shore, or even communicate with those on the other ships anchored in the harbor, likewise on pain of death. The ordinance also required that the captains and commanders in the harbors of the island colonies notify all captains coming from the ports of the Mediterranean about the restrictions, or they would need to answer for any violations. These stipulations, moreover, applied to "all inhabitants, merchants, and other persons of whatever quality and condition they may be."[11]

Similar ordinances were issued across the French Atlantic colonies, from Cayenne in the south to Quebec in the north.[12] On paper, if not always in practice, all prohibited the entry of vessels from the

---

[10] *Conseil de Marine* to Feuquières and Bénard, Paris, October 2, 1720, Col. B 42, f. 298v, ANOM.

[11] M. Durand-Molard, "Ordonnance sur la peste," *Code de la Martinique, nouvelle edition*, tome 1 (Saint-Pierre, Martinique: Imprimerie de Jean-Baptiste Thounens, 1807), 164–5.

[12] On October 20, 1721, the governor-general of New France, Philippe de Rigaud, marquis de Vaudreuil, and the intendant, Michel Bégon de la Picardière, introduced similar quarantine regulations, designating the

Mediterranean that were not first granted authorization prior to their arrival. For those ships that *were* granted access to French colonial harbors, ordinances included strict guidelines for anchoring and for the inspection of merchandise and crew by the designated surgeon or physician; quarantines of varying lengths; and the prohibition of movement for the captain, crew, and cargo, as well as restrictions on their ability to communicate with nearby ships and those on land. And for vessels that nevertheless arrived from anywhere near the infected areas of France without prior authorization, all the colonies had at their disposal the option of burning the ship and cargo.

It is unclear how often these unwelcome vessels were actually destroyed in the French colonies, however. Some of the episodes that emerge in contemporary documents indicate that the practice could be very controversial, despite the fact that it would have been done, at least in theory, in the name of public health. The Sète affair, as I call it, which unfolded primarily on the island of Martinique from 1721 to 1722, is telling of the kind of controversy the arrival of a ship from the Mediterranean coast of France could cause during the Plague of Provence. It also sheds light on some of the rivalries that existed between merchants from different French ports in the early eighteenth-century Atlantic world.

...

On the evening of April 25, 1721, a merchant ship called *Les États de Languedoc* from the port city of Sète in the province of Languedoc, France, ran aground as it arrived off the coast of Le Prêcheur near Saint-Pierre in Martinique. The vessel was carrying merchandise destined for the island including flour, oil, cheeses, wines, eau-de-vie (a brandy), anchovies, and other goods. The captain, Jean-Baptiste

Isle-aux-Coudres in Quebec for any ships arriving from the Mediterranean. Upon arrival, vessels were to fly their distress signal, and fire three cannon or swivel-guns shots – or three musket shots if they had nothing else – every fifteen minutes for an hour, and repeat the same signal every two hours, until "those whose duty it is to board the vessels will be cognizant of their arrival." Moreover, any cargo that was removed prior being declared free of infection would be burned on the spot "without further formality or judicial procedure." These regulations remained in until 1724. John J. Heagerty, *Four Centuries of Medical History in Canada*, vol. 2 (Toronto: Macmillan Company of Canada Limited, 1928), 25–6.

Bordes (also, Bordés or Borde), communicated to the local who was on watch that he would need two boats to lighten his load so that he could set his vessel afloat.[13] Upon learning of the ship's arrival, a Saint-Pierre merchant named Rieussec, to whom the vessel was addressed, immediately contacted Feuquières and Bénard to see to it that the captain's request was granted. Now, if this vessel had come from the *Ponant* (the Atlantic coast of France), the request for assistance would not have been of much concern, especially since the ship was carrying numerous kinds of goods of which the island was in need. During the Plague of Provence, however, when much of the world was on high alert against any vessels from southern France or anywhere in the Mediterranean, the arrival in Martinique of this ship from Languedoc launched a weeks-long scandal that at least temporarily pitted the island's topmost officials against local merchants and residents.

As word quickly spread throughout Martinique that a ship from Languedoc was anchored near Le Prêcheur, the entire population of the island was gripped by fear of infection from the French vessel, and on April 30, five days after its arrival, the governor and intendant reported that a large mob had gathered at Fort Royal in protest. The people demanded that Captain Bordes and his vessel be forced to depart the coasts of the island at once, or else the people would burn the entire vessel along with its cargo. Further, they would force the crew to disembark and strip naked, shave their heads, and have them bathe repeatedly in the ocean. After all, they argued, the owners of the vessel, "who know that the port of Sète is very close to Marseille where the plague has reigned for a long time," should have known that it would not be received in the islands. And if the plague passed to the islands, they feared, the colonies would be quickly depopulated and "lost without resource."[14]

---

[13] Feuquières and Bénard to the *Conseil de Marine*, no. 3, Fort Royal, April 25, 1721, Col. F3 252, 43, ANOM.

[14] "Memoire pour le Sieur Bordes capitaine commandant le vaisseau de Cete …," no. 7, Fort Royal, April 30, 1721, Col. F3 252, 50–2, ANOM. See also: The deputies of the inhabitants and merchants of Saint-Pierre to Feuquières and Bénard, no. 8, Saint-Pierre, May 2, 1721, Col. F3 252, 54–7, ANOM; The deputies of the inhabitants and merchants of Saint-Pierre to Feuquières and Bénard, no. 8, Saint-Pierre, May 12, 1721, Col. F3 252, 85–7, ANOM.

[15] "Veu le requette cy dessus a nous presantée par divers habitans et negocians …," no. 8, Fort Royal, May 2, 1721, Col. F3 252, 58, ANOM.

Yet, Feuquières and Bénard maintained that since the vessel in question was not in seaworthy condition according to the declaration made to them by Captain Bordes and his crew, they were "unable to send it back whence it came in accordance with the petitioners' request."[15] Although the governor and intendant were more than willing to take reasonable precautions for the preservation of public health, upon review of the letters of health (*lettres de santé*) from the duc de Roquelaure[16] and from the intendant of Languedoc, Louis de Bernage, they did not, in fact, suspect that the vessel from Sète was infected with plague. Consequently, the proposal from the merchants to burn the vessel and its cargo with no compensation whatsoever seemed nothing short of "violent" to the officials. They also feared that the king and his council would disapprove of the ship's burning, especially given the complaints that the shipowners (*armateurs*) would almost certainly take to the king against the colonial officials.[17]

But there were further reasons for Feuquières and Bénard's wariness. From their perspective, the entire ordeal was being driven not by a genuine fear of infection but by the avarice of a group of merchants who had much to gain from the prohibition of ships from Languedoc and Marseille. On May 8, 1721, they reported to the Marine Council in Paris:

The greater part of this terror which is so widely spread among our inhabitants and traders comes only from the insinuation of the merchants of Nantes and Bordeaux established in this island which have always preserved an implacable hatred for the merchants of Marseille and Languedoc, because they wish to have sole rights of commerce in these islands. The Council will easily remember that the trade syndicate of Nantes and Bordeaux did all they could to obtain from his majesty that the Compagnie de Cette [Sète Company[18]] be forbidden to trade in these islands in view of the fact that they had permission to go to the Levant, and the just refusal of their request has only served to foment their hatred for this Company. Some have even gone as far as ... Sieur Goujon, a merchant of Nantes, who wrote some time

---

[16] Roquelaure was *Lieutenant Général des Armées du Roi* (lieutenant general of the King's Armies) and *commandant en chef* (commander in chief) of the province of Languedoc.

[17] "Veu le requette cy dessus a nous presantée par divers habitans et negocians ...," no. 8, Fort Royal, May 2, 1721, Col. F3 252, 58, ANOM.

[18] Sète was developed by financiers from Montpellier in the 1660s in order to provide the province of Languedoc with an adequate port. Some of these

ago to his son in St. Pierre, using terms that even the most Jewish of Jews would not use: "Thank God that we are freed from Marseillais commerce as a result of the plague. You should not have to worry about seeing a ship from this area for a long time. Take advantage for the sale of your merchandise, [for] it appears that sugar will drop considerably."[19]

Feuquières and Bénard argued that these merchants of Bordeaux and Nantes, "who fomented this uproar by the desire to sell their goods at higher prices," should be responsible for the value of any burned property, above all, the younger Goujon, who "has been at the head of this whole affair and has been most insistent, having drawn up and presented all the requests that have been addressed to us."[20] To the officials, then, the movement on the island to destroy the ship from Sète was not driven by a legitimate concern for public health but by long-standing rivalries between France's Atlantic and Mediterranean ports. These disputes had grown over the previous decades primarily in reaction to Marseille's privilege as a free port and its monopoly over Levantine trade. Now, they were being blamed for the discord that unfolded when ships from these Mediterranean ports arrived in Martinique during the Plague of Provence.

Nevertheless, after much deliberation, and in consultation with other officials of the island, Feuquières and Bénard ultimately bowed to the demands of the merchants and their supporters, resolving to burn the vessel and much of its cargo "only to appease the noise of the people."[21] But they could not act quickly enough. By now, two weeks after the

---

financiers went on to form two Sète trading companies in 1669 and 1676. The latter, which succeeded the former, is the one mentioned in this passage. Initially formed to supply wine and eau-de-vie throughout the Mediterranean, it soon expanded to include trade in the Levant. J. K. J. Thomson, *Clermont-de-Lodève, 1633–1789: Fluctuations in the Prosperity of a Languedocian Cloth-Making Town* (Cambridge: Cambridge University Press, 1982), 149–50.

[19] Feuquières and Bénard to the *Conseil de Marine*, Fort Royal, May 8, 1721, Col. C8A 28, ff. 51v–52, ANOM. The epigraph to this chapter quotes a different instance in which Feuquières cites this same passage from a letter allegedly written six months earlier, around November 1720, by the elder Goujon for his merchant son in Saint-Pierre. Note, the offhand antisemitic remark.

[20] Feuquières and Bénard to the *Conseil de Marine*, Fort Royal, May 8, 1721, Col. C8A 28, f. 57, ANOM; Feuquières to head of the Marine Council, Fort Royal, May 9, 1721, Col. F3 26, f. 472, ANOM.

[21] Feuquières and Bénard to the *Conseil de Marine*, Fort Royal, May 8, 1721, Col. C8A 28, f. 57, ANOM.

ship's arrival, the situation in Martinique had escalated to the point that the governor and intendant feared a revolt and even feared for their lives. On May 9, 1721, Feuquières wrote Louis-Alexandre de Bourbon, head of the Marine Council, of the "ill will, disobedience, and rebellion" that the inhabitants and traders of the island had demonstrated since the arrival of the ship from Sète.[22] "The residents always harbor the idea of revolt," he related, "[and] I have every reason to believe that the current *esprit de sédition* [spirit of sedition] has been suggested to them by the emissaries of merchants from Nantes who cannot suffer that any others trade in these islands, and who (you know, *Monseigneur*) do everything in their power to prevent the ships from Sète from coming here."[23] On May 13, 1721, Feuquières and Bénard even learned of a possible plot in St. Pierre to assassinate them if they did not burn the ship.[24]

Feuquières' fear that the people might rise in revolt was not unfounded. He remembered all too well the events, only three years earlier, that led to his assuming the position as *gouverneur général* of Martinique in the first place. As evident from the story with which this chapter opens, the metropole could not always ensure that the colonies were adequately stocked with food and supplies. Too often left to fend for themselves, colonists engaged in illicit trade with their Spanish, English, and Dutch neighbors, outside of the closed system of commerce that France desired to maintain with its colonies.[25] Consequent efforts to clamp down on the unregulated trade, while never fully successful, nevertheless triggered opposition in the colonies, sometimes to the point of revolt.[26] This is what occurred in May

---

[22] S.A.S. (*Son altesse sérénissime*) Louis-Alexandre de Bourbon, comte de Toulouse (1678–1737) was one of the sons of Louis XIV and his mistress Françoise-Athénaïs, marquise de Montespan. In these letters, he is referred to as "l'amiral" because of his role as *grand amiral de France* (grand admiral of France).

[23] Feuquières to head of the Marine Council, Fort Royal, May 9, 1721, Col. F3 26, f. 472 & 472v, ANOM.

[24] Feuquières and Bénard to the *Conseil de Marine*, Fort Royal, May 13, 1721, Col. C8A 28, f. 60v, ANOM.

[25] Pritchard, *In Search of Empire*, 256; Laurie Marie Wood, "Îles de France: Law and Empire in the French Atlantic and Indian Oceans, 1680–1780" (PhD diss., University of Texas at Austin, 2013), 212.

[26] As Bertie Mandelblatt has maintained, "[W]hile famine and starvation were real problems in French Caribbean colonies throughout this period, they

1717 when metropolitan administrators were sent to Martinique to help bring an end to smuggling on the islands.[27] Soon after the arrival of a new governor-general and intendant, La Varenne and Ricouart, respectively, colonial residents began to gather. They protested both the attempts to clamp down on illicit commerce, and a four-year-old levy on enslaved people, the *octroi*, that had already incited protests in Guadeloupe two years earlier.[28] The uprising at this time even included calls for independence and the formation of a republic on the island.[29] Siding with the protesters, a group of militia officers and soldiers resolved to arrest La Varenne and Ricouart while they dined in the town of Le Diamant.[30] With the support of the *Conseil supérieur* (Superior Council), the island's highest court, the demonstrators promptly placed the two officials on a ship headed back to France

often served to mask the real subject at stake in these commercial debates – colonists' insistence on their right to trade with foreigners and metropolitan merchants' entrenched opposition to this perceived violation of their commercial privileges." Bertie Mandelblatt, "How Feeding Slaves Shaped the French Atlantic: Mercantilism and the Crisis of Food Provisioning in the Franco-Caribbean During the Seventeenth and Eighteenth Centuries," in *The Political Economy of Empire in the Early Modern World*, edited by Sophus A. Reinert and Pernille Røge (Basingstoke: Palgrave Macmillan, 2013), 194.

[27] The revolt that ensued, called Le Gaoulé, unfolded only weeks after the French Crown issued the *Lettres patentes*, or royal charters, of April 1717, intended to help curtail illicit commerce with foreign merchants. Mandelblatt, "How Feeding Slaves Shaped the French Atlantic," 202–3; "Lettres patentes du roi portant reglement du commerce dans les colonies françaises …," April 1717, Col. A 25, ANOM.

[28] In 1715, between 400 and 500 colonists took up arms to protest the new *octroi* tax on slaveowners. See Pritchard, *In Search of Empire*, 256. The officials' full names are Antoine, marquis d'Arcy de La Varenne, and Louis-Balthazar de Ricouart, comte de Herouville. In Saint-Domingue, too, a revolt broke out beginning in late 1722. In fact, as historian Malick Ghachem has observed, "anti-corporate revolt was already something of an established tradition in the French Caribbean going back to the later 17th century." Malick W. Ghachem, "'No Body to Be Kicked?' Monopoly, Financial Crisis, and Popular Revolt in 18th-Century Haiti and America," *Law & Literature* 28, no. 3 (2016): 416.

[29] See, for example, the letter of Pierre Le Bègue, lieutenant of the king at Martinique, September 16, 1717, Col. C8B 4, ANOM. See also chapter 13 of: Jacques Petitjean Roget, *Le Gaoulé: La révolte de la Martinique en 1717* (Fort-de-France: Société d'histoire de la Martinique, 1966).

[30] Wood, "Îles de France," 218–19.

with a number of documents explaining their actions.[31] France, meanwhile, barely batted an eye at the insubordination.[32]

This revolt, known as the *Gaoulé* from a Creole term for "uprising," signified a unity between colonial residents and elites of the island against metropolitan officials. As historian Laurie Wood has argued, "It also demonstrated that local elites were not tied to the decisions of the governor and intendant as the sole leaders of the colony."[33] Feuquières, himself a Creole notable[34] who had served as governor of Grenada and Guadeloupe before succeeding the ousted La Varenne, knew this history all too well, and often revealed his distrust of the people in letters to Paris. In 1720, a year before the Sète affair, he related to the Marine Council that the loyalty of the people was "very unsteady." Having just completed a general tour of the island, he reported that "he received no cooperation during his inspection; many militia officers failed to present themselves for review, and few local officials could be trusted."[35] And in May 1721, he wrote: "It is quite sad and even more painful for officers like Mr. Bénard and I, entrusted as we are with the power of his Majesty, to find ourselves exposed to the whims of a wicked people … lacking the forces to oppose them or to make them return to their duties."[36]

Accordingly, the primary concern for colonial authorities during the Plague of Provence not only consisted of "protecting [the] colonies from a disease that would lose them entirely to the king," but of preserving them, too, from being lost to *rebellion*.[37] Indeed, conflicts between the French Crown and the Superior Council of Martinique – and its colonies across the eighteenth-century Americas – would arise every so often throughout the island's colonial history, prompting its

---

[31] Pritchard, *In Search of Empire*, 257; Wood, "Îles de France," 219. For more on Le Gaoulé, see also: Roget, *Le Gaoulé*.

[32] Pritchard, *In Search of Empire*, 257. "Conseils in the colonies were created with many of the same personnel and functions as well-respected metropolitan courts like the parlements, like the role of *conseiller*, or magistrate." Wood, "Îles de France," 7.

[33] Wood, "Îles de France," 215.

[34] Wood, "Îles de France," 222.

[35] Pritchard, *In Search of Empire*, 258.

[36] Feuquières to head of the Marine Council, Fort Royal, May 9, 1721, Col. F3 26, f. 473, ANOM.

[37] Ibid.

leaders to periodically request help from Paris. In 1726, for example, Du Rieux, the king's lieutenant at Fort Royal, urged the comte
de Maurepas, then the French minister of the Marine, "to remedy
against [the] independence, and against *the republican and tyrannical
spirit* that [the island's Superior Council] wishes to exercise."[38] And in
1721, wishing to prevent "a second rebellion" amidst the 1721 Sète
crisis, Feuquières, too, called for support from Paris:

> I have many times related the absolute necessity that there be stronger garri-
> sons here, and at least two good, well-armed frigates to maintain the author-
> ity of the king and contain the inhabitants; since the Council has informed
> me that this is impossible ... I had resolved not to speak of it anymore; but
> the case today is very serious ... [the king's] interest, the preservation of
> his colonies, and his authority depend so much on the assistance necessary
> for the maintenance of both, that as long as we do not continuously have
> at least one strong and well-armed vessel, and if a reinforcement of four
> companies ... are not sent ... we will never be able to restrain these people,
> who are so strongly inclined to disobedience; and supposing that we can
> avoid with precautions and our temperaments all the insults of which they
> are more than capable, we can only very weakly assert the authority of the
> king.[39]

Yet it would take weeks for the Marine Council to even see this
renewed request for reinforcements to help reestablish the authority
of the king. In fact, we do not begin to see responses to the Sète affair
from the *Conseil* until July 12, 1721, two months after the letters
requesting backup.[40] By the time Paris dispatched two armed vessels
to Martinique, the entire affair had been over for months. Officials on
the island were thus forced to handle the crisis alone, without guidance or assistance from Paris.

The Sète affair, then, which unfolded in part because of plague-time
regulations that restricted the entry of ships from anywhere near the

---

[38] Emphasis added. Pierre Henri Miraillet Du Rieux, lieutenant of the king at
   Martinique, to Jean-Frédéric Phélypeaux, comte de Maurepas, *secrétaire
   d'État à la Marine* at this time, Martinique, April 15, 1726, Col. C8B 9,
   no. 36, ANOM; Pritchard, *In Search of Empire*, 257.

[39] Feuquières to head of the Marine Council, Fort Royal, May 9, 1721, Col. F3
   26, f. 473v, ANOM.

[40] Feuquières to Louis-Alexandre de Bourbon, Fort Royal, September 22, 1721,
   Col. C8A 28, f. 276, ANOM.

infected coasts of France, reveals a great deal about how difficult it was to control the colonies in times of crisis, and relatedly, the extent to which the colonies were often left to act on their own in the early eighteenth century. In the French Antilles at least, where the possibility of rebellion seemed ever-present, the real threat exposed by the Plague of Provence was not the loss of the colonies to disease but to revolt. The Sète affair – like the Gaoulé and so many other early eighteenth-century uprisings in the islands – reveals the "spirit of sedition" and the "republican and tyrannical spirit" of the colonial islands many decades before the Age of Revolutions.[41] And yet, colonial officials like Feuquières and Bénard were often forced to deal with very real problems on the ground with little help or direction from the metropole. On the surface, France's inability to promptly assist colonial officials during upheavals like the Gaoulé or the Sète affair partly resulted from the fact that it could take anywhere from five to eight weeks on average, but sometimes quite a bit more,[42] for correspondence to cross the Atlantic. The Marine Council did, after all, dispatch the two armed vessels that Feuquières had requested during the Sète affair a few months after it was all over. The larger issue was the inability of France's absolutism to function effectively in the colonies. As historian James Pritchard has observed, absolutism was simply not

---

[41] Feuquières to head of the Marine Council, Fort Royal, May 9, 1721, Col. F3 26, f. 472 & 472v, ANOM; Du Rieux to Maurepas, Martinique, April 15, 1726, Col. C8B 9, no. 36, ANOM.

[42] On average, it took anywhere from five to eight weeks for mail between the metropole and the Atlantic colonies to arrive in either direction. At times, however, it could take much longer – as long as five or six months. When a letter was mailed from Paris to Martinique, for example, it had to travel to the coast where it might have to wait for favorable conditions to depart (e.g. from La Rochelle and Rochefort this could take at least a month; it would then travel the five to eight weeks across the Atlantic, sometimes more, because travel west to the Americas was slower than travel east to Europe from the Atlantic colonies). So by the time responses to the Sète affair from the Marine Council began to arrive in Martinique, the ordeal was long over. For more on travel times across the Atlantic in the eighteenth century, see chapter 3 of Kenneth J. Banks, *Chasing Empire Across the Sea: Communications and the State in the French Atlantic, 1713–1763* (Montreal: McGill-Queen's, 2006). For his estimate of five to seven weeks westbound from Europe and six to eight weeks eastbound from the Antilles, see 77–8. See also: Kenneth Banks, "Communications and 'Imperial Overstretch': Lessons from the Eighteenth-Century French Atlantic," *French Colonial History* 6 (2005): 17–32.

well suited for the colonial environment or colonial circumstances. "It was unable to respond to the variety of demands made upon it. Widely differing local conditions, whether geographic, demographic, social, or economic, proved too much for the rigidity and control it sought but could not achieve."[43]

This becomes evident, too, in France's inability to adequately provision its colonies, which were frequently in need of basic goods, including foods, supplies, fabrics, and even physicians and surgeons, as we saw in the introduction to this chapter. After all, it was a lack of supplies that in part influenced Feuquières and Bénard's resistance to burning the ship from Sète, even if they ultimately bowed to pressure. With its cargos of foods, spirits, and other necessities, *Les États de Languedoc* arrived in Martinique only days after the governor and intendant had informed Paris that "the island has not seen a vessel from the Mediterranean in over a year, which does inexpressible harm ... by the lack of provisions which these vessels have accustomed to bring."[44] It was thus not an easy decision to burn the vessel from Sète. And orders to burn any ships coming from the Mediterranean during the Plague of Provence – which were dispatched across the Atlantic world, and even in the Spanish colony of the Philippines – were neither easily nor frequently executed. Questions pertaining to the ships' ownership and compensation were significant, as were the needs of the colonies, which sometimes went for years without provisions. For all these reasons, then – the threat of local upheaval, lack of metropolitan oversight, and distinct colonial needs and concerns – plague-time regulations across the Atlantic colonies existed very differently on paper than they did in practice.

Economic Interests and Plague-Time Violence in the Caribbean

During the Plague of Provence, regulations to prevent the disease from entering French colonial ports came with various caveats that prioritized commerce and economic interests over public health. Among the

---

[43] Pritchard, *In Search of Empire*, 263.
[44] First quoted in the introduction to this chapter. Feuquières and Bénard to the *Conseil de Marine*, Fort Royal, April 6, 1721, Col. C8B 7, f. 42, ANOM.

most notable examples were the exceptions made for *négriers* or slave ships, which were to be given swift access to colonial ports even if they were carrying people infected with any of a number of diseases other than plague. Numerous documents from the *Conseil de Marine* warn officials in the colonies against excessive protective measures or lengthy quarantines against these vessels, including one letter from August 1721 on "precautions taken against the communication of the plague of Provence."[45] Here, the *Conseil* informed the governor-general and intendant of Saint-Domingue that the regent generally approved of protective measures taken on the island, including a recent twenty-one-day quarantine for a ship called *La Ville de Cette* in Le Cap.[46] However, they cautioned that colonial officials must avoid creating "mauvaises difficultés" for the entry of vessels from the *Ponant* where there was no suspicion of disease, and especially for the slave ships, which the Council claimed carried no suspicious merchandise "and do not arrive in the islands until nine or ten months after their departure."[47] The Council insisted that there was no reason to fear that these slave ships would be infected with any diseases other than those which exist on the coast of Guinea, "the most common of which are scurvy, ophthalmia or *mal de yeux* [eye infection], and smallpox. The first is communicated only on the vessels and is easily cured ... the second is not communicable, and the smallpox only requires some precautions."[48] The Marine Council maintained that if smallpox is

---

[45] "Lettre du Ministre à Messieurs de Sorel et Duclos sur la vente des nègres apportées de la côte d'Afrique," Paris, August 15, 1721, Col. F3 270, 39–42, ANOM. The same instructions were sent several more times for the duration of the Plague of Provence. For example: "Memoire du Roy pour servir d'instruction a M. de Montholon Intendant a S. Domingue," Paris, October 19, 1721, B 44, ff. 475–6, ANOM; "A Messieurs de Sorel et de Montholon," Paris, March 30, 1722, B 45, f. 683, ANOM.

[46] Léon, marquis de Sorel was governor-general of Saint-Domingue from 1719 to 1723. The acting intendant at this time was Jean-Baptiste Dubois Duclos, but he was not formally appointed until 1729 (until 1735). In 1720, modern-day Cap-Haïtien was known as Cap-Français (previously Cap-François), which was known to the Taíno peoples of the Caribbean as Guárico.

[47] The implication was that by the time the ships arrived in the islands, plague would no longer be present. "Lettre du Ministre à Messieurs de Sorel et Duclos ...," August 15, 1721, B 44, ff. 39–40, ANOM.

[48] Ibid.

the only disease present on a slave ship arriving in the islands, it will suffice for it simply to anchor offshore rather than be put through a quarantine. In this way, the healthy Africans can be brought on land, and the captain can decide whether to have the sick treated on board or on land in a designated area far from the towns until they are healed. Once cured, they could then be joined with the healthy ones "to be cleaned and refreshed for fifteen days" after which they can be sold.[49] Thus the Council cautioned Governor Sorel and the intendant, Duclos, of being too rigorous with the quarantining of slave ships, which could ruin the shipowners through the loss of "the greater part of the negroes in the cargo." Moreover, the Councilors warned, merchants already lost so many Africans to the long trans-Atlantic journey that any additional losses during a quarantine "could deter [them] from a trade so valuable to the colonies" that their commerce must be favored and preserved.[50] After all, "smallpox has never been regarded in the islands as a *maladie pestilentielle* [pestilential disease], and the disorders it can cause are not of too dangerous a consequence."[51]

The downplaying of smallpox to protect the lucrative trans-Atlantic commerce in human beings is striking. By the eighteenth century, the disease had become a leading cause of death in Europe killing as many as 400,000 Europeans per year.[52] At the time the Council wrote this letter, it was ravaging parts of England, the Boston colony, and even the Caribbean island of Barbados, where a "very mortal" outbreak was killing twenty to thirty people per day.[53] Five decades later, the same disease would kill a French king.[54] And yet, in the years leading up to the Plague of Provence, the economy of the Atlantic slave trade and the presence of enslaved persons in the French Circum-Caribbean had increased dramatically alongside the rapidly growing

---

[49] Ibid., 41.
[50] Ibid.
[51] A remarkable statement given the role of this disease in decimating the native populations of the very island to which this letter was addressed, i.e. Hispaniola. Ibid., 42.
[52] Donald R. Hopkins, *The Greatest Killer: Smallpox in History* (Chicago: University of Chicago Press, 2002), 42.
[53] Coss, *The Fever of 1721*, 62. Seth, *Difference and Disease*, 122.
[54] King Louis XV would succumb to the illness on May 10, 1774, leaving France in the hands of his young grandson, the ill-fated Louis XVI, and Marie Antoinette.

number of sugar works on the islands. Pritchard has pointed out that, "Between 1701 and 1715, the number of Africans in the French West Indies grew more rapidly than at any time during the previous thirty years."[55] In the years between 1714 and the start of the plague in 1720, 10,200 enslaved people arrived in Martinique and 19,349 arrived in Saint-Domingue.[56] In 1720 alone, 3,667 slaves disembarked in Saint-Domingue – 36 percent more than the previous four-year average, yet the supply of enslaved laborers could not satisfy the demand in these islands.[57] By 1719, there were 338 sugar plantations on Martinique (up from 186 in 1701) and 199 in Saint-Domingue (up from 35 in 1701). These numbers grew to 437 and 339, respectively, by 1730.[58] Other French colonial exports included indigo, cotton, coffee, cacao, among others, but no crop rivaled sugar "for export earnings, capital investment, or enslaved labor."[59] Profit margins and commercial gains, then, seemed to outstrip concerns about public health in the colonies.

This manifested itself in different ways during the plague years, and involved not only slave ships, but foreign merchant vessels, especially those of the Spanish Americas. Numerous encounters, some of them extremely violent, took place between the French and Spanish in the colonies, prompting French colonial officials to file complaints against the numerous "violences" committed against the French. Letters cited excessive leniency from the metropole in these matters and sought punishment for the wrongdoers. Officials in Paris, however, including the regent and the Marine Council, repeatedly responded not with calls or plans for justice, but with warnings against responding too harshly to the Spaniards of the Americas, lest they be deterred from visiting the French colonies.

---

[55] Pritchard, *In Search of Empire*, 12.

[56] Ibid., 222.

[57] Ibid., 222. "By 1715 the slave population [in the French Caribbean] numbered nearly 77,000—more than three times the white population in the French islands. In addition, between 1716 and 1730, more than 110,000 Africans were probably carried into the French colonies. An estimated 390,000 enslaved people were imported into the French Circum-Caribbean during the years before 1730." Pritchard, *In Search of Empire*, 12.

[58] Pritchard, *In Search of Empire*, 179; Gigi, "The Materiality of Empire," 89.

[59] Burnard and Garrigus, *The Plantation Machine*, 14.

Two incidents that unfolded in the summer of 1720 – one off the coast of Saint-Domingue, and the other off the coast of Venezuela – provide an instructive look at the kinds of confrontations that took place, and how both local and metropolitan officials responded.[60] On September 16, 1720, two of the men involved, both from the port town of Saint-Pierre, Martinique, sat down before Governor-General Feuquières in Fort Royal to give an official account of the terrible ordeal they had suffered at the hands of Spaniards two months earlier. The first, Artus Le Baube, captain of a schooner (*goélette*) named *La Forbanne*, recounted that on January 28, 1720, he departed Saint-Pierre with his crew and headed for the coasts of Pointe de Spade (Punta Cana) in Spanish Santo Domingo to fish for *carret*, or hawks-bill sea turtle (*Testudo imbricata*). They sojourned off the coasts of Hispaniola for months, fishing in several different spots without incident, that is, until July 27 when the crew spotted some Spaniards on land who appeared to have been hunting (for "boeufs marons") armed only with spears and accompanied by their dogs. It is unclear how, but one of the Spaniards soon came on board and asked the captain for wine under the pretext that their parish priest needed it to celebrate the mass. Although Le Baube had only one bottle, he handed it over, asking in return for the Spaniard to bring him and his crew some tobacco the next day.

On the afternoon of July 28, the same Spaniard, accompanied by another man, appeared on the coast and signaled from land, at which point Le Baube sent a canoe carrying four of his sailors armed with two rifles. As the men approached land, one of the Spaniards stepped into the canoe, quickly spun around, and "with a kind of cutlass with-out guard which they call a *manchette*" (a machete), fired a blow to the head of the first sailor and slit it open, then attacked a second sea-man with a blow to the stomach. The remaining two sailors quickly threw themselves to the sea in an effort to swim back to the vessel, but at that moment a number of other Spaniards appeared, perhaps as many as thirty. Armed with spears, they ran to the shore and attacked the fleeing men, who made it only halfway back to *La Forbanne* before succumbing to multiple spear wounds.

---

[60] Venezuela at this time was part of the Viceroyalty of New Granada (*Virreinato de Nueva Granada*) in the Spanish Empire.

Le Baube now found himself alone on board the schooner and seeing that nine of the Spaniards were headed toward him in his own
canoe with intent to seize his vessel, he took his rifle loaded with three
bullets and shot in the direction of the men, possibly killing at least
two of them. This made the men return to land, at which point Le
Baube, having cut the lines to his anchor and grapple, raised his sail as
best he could and in very bad weather made it to "La Monne" (Mona
Island, Puerto Rico, just southeast of Punta Cana) in three days.[61] At La
Monne, Le Baube encountered three sailors, "to whom he recounted
his sad adventures," and who accompanied him back to Martinique
where he arrived earlier on the day that he provided this testimony.[62]

In July 1720, around the same time as the episode near Hispaniola, Gervais Pertuson, boatswain of a small vessel named *La Marie*,
departed Saint-Pierre to fish for turtles in the Testigues off the coast of
Venezuela.[63] On August 3, he encountered a Spanish corsair from Margarita Island. The captain, named Palarme, invited Pertuson on board,
along with three other men who were fishing on the islands at the same
time: a man named Creuzet, master of the boat *l'Hirondelle* of Martinique; and two others named Charles and Perdurand, masters and
co-owners of *l'Henriette* of Guadeloupe. They were initially received
well on board, but the next day, August 4, the Spanish captain seized
the ships *La Marie* and *l'Henriette*, left the shipmasters and crew at
the Testigues, and headed back to Margarita Island with their vessels
(*l'Hirondelle* was left unharmed because of its small size). At this time,
Pertuson and Charles, masters of the two seized vessels, urged Creuzet
to take them and their crew to Margarita on *l'Hirondelle* to see what
could be done. Upon their arrival on August 6, however, the men were
promptly imprisoned where they remained nineteen days. In this time,
the two masters, along with two sailors of each crew, were questioned.
The interpreter, a Frenchman named Ollivier François, informed the
men that they might have already been released were it not for the fact

[61] To this day, the Mona Passage strait between the islands of Hispaniola
and Puerto Rico is considered among the most difficult to navigate in the
Caribbean.
[62] Declaration of Captain Artus Le Baube to Feuquières, Fort Royal, September
16, 1720, Col. C8A 27, f. 206–206v, ANOM.
[63] The small islands of the Testigues, known as *Islas Los Testigos*, are near
Venezuela's Margarita Island.

that the governor and *contador* of Margarita themselves owned the *corsaire* responsible for this unlawful seizure. François added that the governor of Margarita "had often mocked the docility of the French for not retaliating against the Spaniards who captured so many vessels from them, which led him to believe that [the French] were very weak."[64]

On September 18, 1720, Feuquières submitted the official accounts of both Le Baube and Pertuson to the *Conseil de Marine* in France with complaints about the "pillages et assassinats" that the Spaniards were inflicting upon the French and their vessels in the Americas. Hoping that something could be done to prevent further assaults, he requested that the formal declarations from Le Baube and Pertuson be transmitted to his Catholic Majesty in Madrid. From Feuquières' perspective, it was entirely possible that orders for the string of attacks against the French were coming from the Spanish king himself. Yet nearly three months later, Feuquières was disappointed by a response from Philippe d'Orléans in which he stressed that any reprisals must not risk jeopardizing trade with the Spanish colonies.[65] Officials in Paris insisted that Spanish governors in the colonies had no such orders from his Catholic Majesty to attack and seize French vessels. Ultimately, the regent gave Feuquières permission to retaliate against the Spaniards "as he deemed necessary," but there were some significant provisos. First, he must "use this permission moderately" in order to protect trade relations with the Spanish in the colonies. Nor should any reprisals be taken against Spanish vessels that seek to enter the ports of the French Antilles. On the contrary, "it is necessary to seek to attract them, because they can bring gold, silver, and prime merchandise [to the islands]."[66]

---

[64] This last line is of particular interest, because one of Feuquières' primary complaints in his letters to Paris about the assaults of the Spaniards against the French in the Americas was that the latter were not properly defending themselves. One wonders if this final anecdote was thus added for effect. Declaration of Gervais Pertuzon to Feuquières, Fort Royal, September 16, 1720, Col. C8A 27, f. 207–207v, ANOM.

[65] "Projet de mémoire du roi à M. de Feuquières," Paris, December 10, 1720, Col. C8A 27, f. 148, ANOM.

[66] "Décision du Régent au sujet des avanies faites par les Espagnols aux navires français depuis la suspension d'armes," Paris, July 15, 1721, Col. C8B 7, no. 72, ANOM.

This placed French colonial officials in a predicament. On the one hand, they were given permission to punish Spanish aggressors, but on the other, they were severely limited in their ability to effectively do anything. In other words, they could *not* act as they "deemed necessary," since doing so would mean potentially discouraging Spanish ships from going to the French islands. Feuquières' frustration is palpable in his letters to Paris at this time. "I do not see that I can make any use of the order that the Council sent me to use reprisals against [the Spaniards] given the restriction that is inserted therein for Spanish ships that may come to trade in these islands."[67] In his view, the Spaniards, "who commit the same kind of violence every day," would only be emboldened by France's failure to retaliate. As he wrote to the Council, "I cannot dispense with representing to the Council that it is in the interest of the King and of the nation in general not to leave unpunished all the cruelties exercised against the French on the coasts of Spain [including the colonies], both by the governments and by the subjects of his Catholic Majesty."[68] But the reprisals would not come. Instead, officials in Paris only doubled down on orders to appease the Spaniards in the Americas. The pursuit of Spanish silver and gold seemed to outweigh all other considerations.[69]

It is important to note that the desire on the part of officials in France to trade with the Spaniards did not extend to those of the mainland but was restricted specifically to the Spaniards of the Americas whose trade was deemed more valuable for its bullion. Numerous communications from Paris persistently reiterated the importance of restricting trade with all foreigners – including those in the Americas such as the British or Dutch – except the Spaniards of the Americas, whose trade must be preserved and expanded.[70] Essentially, under the terms of the 1717 *Lettres patentes* – intended to exclude foreign merchants,

---

[67] Feuquières to the *Conseil de Marine*, Fort Royal, April 17, 1721, Col. C8A 28, f. 206–206v, ANOM.

[68] Ibid., 207.

[69] And these efforts did pay off. France maintained the advantage even over Britain in the quest for Spanish precious metals. See Crouzet, "La rivalité commerciale franco-anglaise dans l'empire espagnol, 1713–1789."

[70] "Memoire du Roy au Bénard, Intendant des Isles du Vent," Paris, October 5, 1721, B 44, ff. 360v–361, ANOM.

and constantly referenced in these documents[71] – only vessels arriving from authorized port cities in France could trade in the French Antilles.[72] French-owned ships would handle all imports and exports, and these could only arrive in the colonies from a French port, even if the goods on board originated abroad.[73] Any vessels arriving from a foreign port, including those originating in France, but especially those of foreigners, were to be "confiscated upon arrival" – except those of Spaniards in the Americas.[74] Officials in Paris maintained that this trade "can only be advantageous to the nation, and it is in the interest of the colony to [take part] and to increase it as much as possible. Bénard must work as much to increase this commerce, as to *annihilate* trade with other foreigners."[75]

Nevertheless, the threat of confiscation deterred neither French nor foreign merchants arriving from unauthorized ports to trade in the French islands. Given the needs of the colonies, local officials often permitted the trade to take place, which drew frequent disapproval from Paris. Merchant vessels arriving in Martinique from Cádiz, for example – which was among the most recurrent points of origin – were a regular source of consternation for the Marine Council. In numerous letters, the Council reminded colonial officials that they "must not permit vessels from Martinique to travel to Cádiz in order

---

[71] Countless contemporary documents express this concern for excluding foreign trade, for example, "[The Council] advises you to adhere exactly to the Regulation of 1717 ... and to reanimate your attention to the prevention of foreign trade." *Conseil de Marine* to Bénard, Paris, October 5, 1721, B 44, f. 361v, ANOM.

[72] Mandelblatt, "How Feeding Slaves Shaped the French Atlantic," 202. These are the same *Lettres patentes* that helped instigate Le Gaoulé and other uprisings in the colonies.

[73] Silvia Marzagalli, "The French Atlantic World in the Seventeenth and Eighteenth Centuries," in *The Oxford Handbook of the Atlantic World, 1450–1850*, edited by Nicholas Canny and Philip Morgan (Oxford: Oxford University Press, 2011), 243.

[74] *Conseil de Marine* to Bénard, Paris, September 17, 1721, B 44, f. 340, ANOM.

[75] Emphasis added. "Memoire du Roy au Bénard, Intendant des Isles du Vent," Paris, October 5, 1721, B 44, f. 361, ANOM. Many other documents make the same point, for example: Feuquières and Bénard to Philippe II, Duke of Orléans, Regent of France, Saint-Pierre, February 7, 1722, Col. C8A 30, f. 20–20v, ANOM.

to return to Martinique."[76] Such communications also went to Pierre-Nicolas Partyet (the French consul in Cádiz), who was charged with informing the captains of all vessels from Martinique in Cádiz that "it is in their best interest to come to France before returning to the colony, otherwise the vessels will be confiscated."[77]

Frequent letters to the intendant of Martinique in particular reveal metropolitan officials' displeasure at the unauthorized trade, and emphasize the importance of observing the 1717 regulations. Their denunciation of commerce with the Spaniards of the mainland, however, was matched only by their eagerness for trade with those of the Americas. In September 1721, for example, they wrote:

You have extended the trade with the Spaniards too much, having led yourself to believe that it is permitted for the colonies to [trade] with the Spaniards of Europe. His Majesty [approves] of the trade with the Spaniards of America, and even recommends that you motivate the inhabitants [of the island to this end] since this trade is advantageous both to the kingdom and to the colonies. In exchange for our merchandise, these people give us gold [and] silver ... But you are forbidden from tolerating trade in any form with the Spaniards of Europe, because they only bring goods that the islands must receive from France, and not from Spain.[78]

A year later, in 1722, they wrote:

The commerce permitted to the Spanish is limited to those of the Americas only ... The Council believes it is again necessary to repeat that all commerce with foreigners is *absolument interdit*, including that with the Spanish, with the sole exception in all cases of those of the Americas ... Only French ships coming from France or other French colonies and those of the Spanish Americas are permitted.[79]

Communications like these went out to the colonies regularly during the plague years, as vessels from unauthorized ports continued to

---

[76] *Conseil de Marine* to Feuquières and Bénard, Paris, October 5, 1721, B 44, f. 359v, ANOM.

[77] *Conseil de Marine* to Pierre-Nicolas Partyet, consul of France in Cádiz, Paris, December 10, 1721, B 44, ANOM.

[78] Ibid., 340–1v.

[79] *Conseil de Marine* to Feuquières and Bénard, Paris, June 5, 1722, B 45, ff. 520v–521, ANOM.

make their way into the French colonies, often with approval from local officials, and the French remained keen on obtaining Spanish silver.

Although illicit trade and violent assaults like those discussed earlier took place throughout the history of the colonial Atlantic, they occurred with especially high frequency in both times of war and of disease. In war times, the increased insecurity of the Atlantic meant that crimes and piracy took place more frequently because of related hostilities. It also became more challenging for the metropoles to furnish their colonies with adequate stores and supplies, which meant that colonial administrators were compelled to authorize the entrance of foreign ships.[80] But why would *disease* drive up illicit trade and maritime violence? By the eighteenth century, the disaster centralism discussed in previous chapters meant that public health measures imposed by the capitals of Europe's emerging nation states extended, at least in theory, across their vast empires. Beginning most notably with the Plague of Provence, plague-time regulations from the metropoles of Europe were dispatched to port cities throughout the colonies in the Americas and Asia. And the prescribed practices – such as trade embargoes, extensive quarantining, and vessel searches and *fondeos* – were inherently aggressive. In the colonies, all these regulations essentially took the form of hostility against foreigners in the ports, especially the French, which helps to explain the string of assaults described earlier.

Anti-French Policy and the Plague of Provence in the Spanish Colonies

French interest in Spanish gold and silver was not lost on the Spaniards themselves. During the plague-time embargo placed on all French vessels in Spain and its colonies, Spanish officials regularly reported on the eagerness of French merchants to trade in their ports in search of bullion. In 1723, for example, the new governor of Spanish Pensacola, Don Alexandro Wauchop (also Alejandro Wauchope), wrote to the viceroy of New Spain, the marquess of Casafuerte, "It is appropriate to cut off communications [with the French], because their sole

---

[80] Marzagalli, "The French Atlantic World," 243.

guiding principle and policy is, under any pretext, to introduce their trade and take the silver."[81] This was a major source of frustration for the Spanish, who were as keen to keep the French out of their ports as the French were to access them. For years *before* plague emerged in Marseille, the Spanish Crown worked to curb illicit commerce and foreign presence in its domestic and colonial port cities. To limit the entry of foreign goods, for example, only foreigners who had been granted a *carta de naturaleza* (naturalization certificate) by the king were permitted to trade or reside in the Spanish colonies. For the most part, however, options were limited, as any major restrictions against foreign vessels stood in violation of recent treaties, including the Peace of Utrecht and the Treaty of The Hague. The public health emergency in Provence therefore presented an opportunity to address many of these challenges.

In response to news of plague in France, the Spanish Crown dispatched a series of *reales cédulas* (royal decrees) to prohibit the entry of French vessels – and later, all foreign vessels – across the colonies.[82] Much of what these orders prescribed was in line with pre-plague efforts to curb foreign commerce, but the Crown could now take several additional measures thanks to the threat of infection from Provence. Decrees sent to the *Audiencia de Quito* and the viceroy in New Spain (Mexico) in December 1720 began to lay out – on paper, if not in practice – how the Spanish colonies were to respond to the threat of plague from Provence.[83] The document begins with news of

[81] Alexandro Wauchop to the marqués de Casafuerte, composed aboard a *paquebot*, February 21, 1723, Audiencia de México 380, f. 17, AGI. Lieutenant Colonel Wauchop was a Scotsman who had served in Spain's Irish Brigade (the *Regimiento Hibernia* or O'Neill's Regiment), and as frigate captain (*capitán de fragata*). In 1722, he was chosen to reclaim Pensacola for Spain from the French as part of the treaty that ended the War of the Quadruple Alliance. His short governorship lasted from late 1722 to February 1723. See William B. Griffen, "Spanish Pensacola, 1700–1763," *The Florida Historical Quarterly* 37, no. 3/4 (1959): 255–57.

[82] See, for example: "Los Ofiz⁵ R⁵ de la Veracruz dan qᵗᵃ ...," Veracruz, November 30, 1721, Audiencia de México 858, AGI.

[83] One of the decrees, dated December 2, 1720, is enclosed in this response from Quito over a year later: "Orden de no admitir navíos franceses," Quito, April 29, 1722, Audiencia de Quito 129, N. 27, AGI. Three days later, the same

increased efforts by French merchants to trade in the Spanish Americas "in order to save their goods and themselves" from the plague that reigned in Provence, reports that must no doubt be accurate "given how notoriously the French already introduce their fraudulent *ropas* [clothes] in the [Spanish] Indies."[84] And with the trade of both Spain and Italy closed off to them because of the Plague of Provence, French merchants were now left with little recourse "outside of trading in the [Spanish] Indies, where there are so many poorly guarded ports."[85] In order to prevent the "grave damage that would result (may God forbid it) if infected merchandise were introduced in the [Spanish] Indies," the king resolved that all French vessels were now completely prohibited from entering Spanish colonial ports. Under no circumstances should these ships be admitted, "even if under the pretext of a temporary arrival, lack of supplies, or any other setback that may be presented, because this is a situation in which the health of the territory is of primary concern." French ships requesting entry in these ports were to be turned away even if they were from ports untouched by the plague, and any that insisted on entering were to be burned or sunk. Such a case happened weeks earlier when a French vessel that had suffered a collision off the coast of Spain requested to enter the local port. Having been turned away, the crew pleaded for help and insisted on entering, but they were soon fired upon causing the ship to sink offshore. "This

decree was sent elsewhere in the Spanish colonies, including New Spain, with only the names of the ports in question changed. For example: *Real cédula* ("El Rey, Por quanto se ha puesto en mi noticia que en Francia se disponian muchos ..."), Madrid, December 5, 1720, Audiencia de México 413, AGI.

[84] In August, a few weeks after learning that plague was in France, officials in Madrid wrote the secretary of Peru to stress the importance of curbing illicit commerce in the South Sea. Several ships on the coasts of Provence, allegedly destined for sparsely populated French Mississippi, were being loaded with so much merchandise that the Spanish consul in Marseille feared they must instead be headed for the Spanish Americas. "There is no doubt that if we do not impede this kind of trade, the entirety of the [Spanish] Indies will be filled with [foreign] goods, and the commerce of Spain will be entirely destroyed." See: *Consejo de Indias* to Don Francisco de Arana (*Secretario del Consejo y Cámara de Indias de la negociación del Perú*), Madrid, August 22, 1720, Indiferente General 276, AGI.

[85] "Orden de no admitir navíos franceses," Quito, April 29, 1722, Audiencia de Quito 129, N. 27, AGI; *Real cédula* ("El Rey ..."), Madrid, December 5, 1720, Audiencia de México 413, AGI.

cannot be attributed to impiety on my part," the Spanish king insisted, "for the severity was not in the damage that resulted to the ship, but in the attention that had to be paid to public health."[86] French *goods* that made their way inland were also burned across the Spanish, and other, colonies at this time. This occurred more frequently than the destruction of entire vessels. In 1722, the governor of Cuba ordered the burning of French clothes that had entered the island, "because of the suspicion that they could be carrying infection, despite having been assured that they had been stored in the port of Léogâne [Saint-Domingue] for more than three years."[87] Throughout the plague years, and for months thereafter, such orders were communicated across the Spanish Empire to some of its primary administrative centers, including Quito and Veracruz, from which they were further disseminated to cities such as Havana,[88] Cartagena, Manila,[89] and others.

By the summer of 1721, the decrees took on a new sense of urgency when Philip V learned that French products from Provence were being allowed to pass to the French Indies after quarantine and inspection. Suspecting that the French would inevitably attempt to introduce these goods in the Spanish colonies "on their ships or on those of other nations," he reaffirmed the orders of December 5, 1720:

And if any [of these goods] are somehow clandestinely introduced (which should not happen given the particular attention that would be directed to the public health), these must be seized and immediately burned, and all those involved in introducing the goods are to be punished according to the laws and orders against the practice of illicit commerce and those against

---

[86] Ibid.

[87] "En cumplimiento de lo que se mando gentilmente ...," Havana, February 24, 1722, Audiencia de Santo Domingo 379, no. 40, AGI.

[88] In July 1721, for example, Gregorio Guazo y Calderón, the governor of Cuba, confirmed receipt of the December 1720 decrees from Veracruz, ordering that "under no circumstances should French ships be admitted due to the grave damages that could result to public health." "Muy Señor mio, con la flotta del cargo de Don Fernando Chacon ...," Havana, July 8, 1721, Audiencia de Santo Domingo 378, AGI.

[89] In a letter dated June 15, 1725, Spanish officials in the Philippines confirmed receipt of a *Real cédula* with a date of May 1, 1723, in which they were still being ordered "to prohibit with utmost efficiency the entrance of vessels and goods from France in the ports of these islands so as to prevent the injuries that could otherwise result." And this *cédula* was only the most recent

the transporting of any goods from infected territories ... I have resolved to repeat again the strictest orders to the viceroys, presidents, and governors of the Indies so that they look after the [public] health, and under no circumstances or pretexts, nor previous communication ... even if it came from me [the king], can you admit any French ship or French clothing, unless it comes in the fleets and galleons and other ships dispatched and loaded in the Bay of Cádiz or in the Port of Sanlúcar de Barrameda. And any ... official who gives them entry will suffer pain of death.[90]

The success of orders like these depended almost entirely on the cooperation of the colonial officials who would need to enforce the measures in question. Part of the problem for the king, however, was that this proved highly difficult to ensure. Letters from Madrid to colonial governors and viceroys regularly told of the "great harms" of turning a blind eye to illicit trade. During the Plague of Provence, these communications revealed the king's frustration with colonial administrators who neglected his instructions, and included strict penalties for those who were found in violation of the orders. In a royal decree of 1721, the king protested his officials' apparent disregard for restrictions against foreign commerce, maintaining that if they had heeded the rules over the past several years, the "fraudsters" would not be as emboldened to enter Spanish ports during the plague. In order to operate in Spanish ports, he argued, these foreigners required the tolerance of the king's viceroys and governors on whom fell the responsibility of preventing the "prejudicial abuse of illicit trade."[91] But transgressions would no longer go unnoticed or unpunished. Colonial officials who were found in violation of their duties would no longer be granted formal processes to determine their guilt. Instead, all that was needed for them to "pass to their punishment" was for the king to receive word that they had failed to comply with their obligations:

reminder sent to the Philippines of the embargo as late as 1723, a year after the epidemic had ceased. See, among others: "Los Oficiales Reales de Filipinas a SM," Manila, June 15, 1725, Audiencia de Filipinas 191, no. 60, AGI; "Marqués de Torre Campo a V.M.," Manila, June 30, 1725, Audiencia de Filipinas 140, no. 31, AGI.

90 Such punishments included incarceration and death. *Real cédula* ("El Rey ..."), Madrid, August 23, 1721, Audiencia de México 414, AGI.

91 *Real cédula* ("El Rey, Por quanto teniendo presente el importante punto de impedir los comercios ilicitos en mis dominios de las Americas ..."), Madrid, 1721, Audiencia de México 414, AGI.

And in order that [the punishment] correspond to so grave and recurrent a crime, and that it serve as an example … I have resolved that transgressors will be punished according to those laws on illicit introductions and commerce … that impose the penalty of life and loss of property; and so that no one can claim ignorance of this, my Royal resolution … I command that it be disseminated via public proclamations without delay in all the provinces, cities, towns, and places of [the empire] … so that transgressors, not to exclude the viceroys, may be punished with the rigorous penalties that come forewarned.[92]

Yet even "severe resolutions" like this did little to change practices on the ground, and at least part of the reason was simple: the colonies had needs and wants that Spain was unable to supply. Much as we saw with the case in France at this time, Spain also at times struggled to supply its colonies with adequate provisions, especially *ropas*. During the Plague of Provence, the "falta de ropas," or lack of clothes and fabrics, in the Viceroyalty of Peru – which encompassed much of the western half of the South American continent – was a significant issue that required the attention of the Crown.[93] Not only was this shortage blamed for keeping Spanish ports open to illicit foreign commerce but the illicit *ropas* themselves – which could very well be infected with plague – were deemed a public health risk.[94] By 1720, numerous letters revealed concern about the dearth of supplies, lamenting that

---

[92] Ibid.
[93] Spanish documents that mention the issue of the *falta de ropas* at this time are abundant. For examples, see also: *Consejo de Indias* to Don Francisco de Arana, Madrid, August 22, 1720, Indiferente General 276, AGI; "El Virrey de Nueva España da quenta a V.Mag …," Mexico, November 4, 1721, Audiencia de México 488, AGI; "Orden de no admitir navíos franceses," Quito, April 29, 1722, Audiencia de Quito 129, N. 27, AGI; "El Virrey de Nueva España haze presente a V.M. …," Mexico, June 20, 1722, Audiencia de México 488, AGI.
[94] For these reasons, Spanish colonial plague-time orders included promises that the dearth of supplies would be addressed. For example: "Having been so many years that Spain has not sent goods to those domains [Viceroyalty of Peru], and [the territory] being so extensive, it follows that [the people] are very short of clothes and that they have used whatever means necessary to obtain them through foreigners … because they could not after all be forced to walk around naked, so this will be one of the main remedies to avoid foreign commerce, since by receiving their clothes from Spain, they will no longer need what is introduced by other means." *Consejo de Indias* to Don Francisco de Arana, Madrid, August 22, 1720, Indiferente General 276, AGI.

it had been months, sometimes over a decade, since the last Spanish vessel arrived in a given port with provisions.[95] Writing to the secretary of Peru in November 1720, for example, the Spanish Council of the Indies acknowledged that although fleets had more frequently been to New Spain, it had been thirteen years since the last galleons went to Peru, so that the commerce and "the consumption of that vast dominion has been [entirely] dependent on foreigners, especially the French."[96] Plague or no plague, when foreigners arrived in the ports of the Spanish colonies carrying much-needed goods, colonial officials felt compelled to look the other way. As elsewhere in the colonial world, local needs often outweighed allegiance to the rules of the metropole.

In the end, foreign encroachment on Spanish commerce in the decades leading up to 1720; significant losses in recent treaties; foreign, and especially French, ambitions to obtain Spanish silver and gold; the Bourbon King Philip V's reforms aimed at improving Spain's footing in the larger realm of international trade and influence; and a desire to protect public health – all joined together to influence how Spain would respond to the Plague of Provence in its colonies. Its focus on stamping out foreign commerce predated 1720, but the public health crisis allowed the Crown to impose stricter rules, including even the sinking or burning of "suspected" goods and vessels. The advantages of these plague-time regulations were not lost on Spanish officials. In 1723, a year after the epidemic had effectively ended in France, the viceroy of New Spain reported to Madrid on the French in neighboring Louisiana:

---

[95] The transport of clothes to the colonies was only part of the problem. More fundamental was the issue of production in the metropole, which these communications also promised to address. See, for example: *Real cédula*, Madrid, 1721, Audiencia de México 414, AGI.

[96] *Consejo de Indias* to Don Francisco de Arana (*Secretario del Consejo y Cámara de Indias de la negociación del Perú*), Madrid, November 26, 1720, Indiferente General 276, AGI. It is worth noting that from 1717 to 1722, the Andes region grappled with its own public health crisis. With similar virulence to the plague, though seemingly unrelated, the Great Andean Pandemic took as many as 200,000 lives, depopulating towns and villages over a period of 5 years. See: Kris Lane, *Pandemic in Potosí: Fear, Loathing and Public Piety in a Colonial Mining Metropolis* (University Park: The Pennsylvania State University Press, 2021), 15.

We have been avoiding trade and communications with the French on account of the plague, and even though there is no illness present in Louisiana, we find it convenient to abide by these precautions. It is advantageous for many reasons that this separation [from the French] endure, even if it is under the pretext of the plague, because through it we achieve that no French goods enter these areas.[97]

The Spanish Crown wanted the French out of its ports, both in the metropole and its colonies, and its wishes were made clear across the empire. It is no wonder then that Franco-Spanish encounters in the Caribbean during the plague of Provence – like those reported by Feuquières in Martinique – so often turned violent. The French and Spanish already had a decades-long history of antagonism. Remarking on the nature of the Franco-Spanish relationship in the 1690s, Pritchard wrote, "French-Spanish animus remained as harsh as ever. In Spanish eyes, all Frenchmen were murderous pirates to be dealt with as brutally as possible."[98] Like all major disasters, the Plague of Provence revealed underlying challenges, aggressions, and objectives that were already there.

…

On the surface, the centralization of disaster management in parts of Europe during the Plague of Provence extended to the colonies in the Americas and Asia. As news of the epidemic arrived in every corner of the European empires, so too did directives from the metropoles for protecting public health. In turn, colonial administrators kept officials in the capitals informed of any and all happenings on the ground. In fact, tracing the communication of news and regulations about the Plague of Provence reveals the extensive interconnectedness of the Atlantic world. As evidenced by accounts like that of the Sète affair or of the ship and cargo burnings that took place off coasts across the European colonies, the Great Plague Scare stretched across oceans. At times it caused disorder, as when vessels suspected of infection arrived in colonial ports. Yet it is worth noting that these episodes of panic during the plague years were not necessarily commonplace in the colonies.

---

[97] "El Virrey de Nueva España [marqués de Casafuerte] da quenta a V.M. delo que ocurre …," Mexico, May 24, 1723, Audiencia de México 380, AGI.
[98] Pritchard, *In Search of Empire*, 316.

Instead, unlike parts of Europe, life for most colonists – including administrators and merchants – went on as usual.

Effective disaster centralism requires more than merely monitoring or making demands of the Crown's representatives. Demands must also be carried out, and particularly in the colonies, this was not always the case. The needs and concerns of those in the far-flung corners of Europe's empires were not necessarily in line with the wishes of the metropoles. Attempts to introduce taxes or restrict foreign commerce in the French Indies, for example, were sometimes met with protests and revolts as in Guadeloupe in 1715 or Le Gaoulé of 1717 in Martinique. And despite efforts to restrict the entry of vessels from France's Mediterranean coasts in the French colonies, these ships – often carrying much-needed supplies – nevertheless continued to make their way into the ports of the Antilles, even if, as in the Sète affair, they were not always well received.

In the Spanish colonies, perhaps more so than anywhere else across the European empires, attempts to impose plague-time regulations were met with significant challenges. Part of the problem was that the Spanish Crown's restrictions were much more severe than even those of France. For example, the king prohibited trade with the French and banned the entry of all French – and later, all foreign – vessels across the empire on pain of death. But there were larger issues at work. By 1720, Spain's inability to provide the Viceroyalty of Peru with supplies resulted in a long-standing dependency on illicit foreign commerce in much of Spanish South America. During his plague-time embargo against French commerce, the Spanish king faced the challenge of breaking this dependency and making his colonial viceroys and governors adhere to the rules. Indeed, what emerges in contemporary documents is a Spain that struggled to control activities in the colonies and to enforce its directives. Plague-time policies were put in place and repeatedly dispatched from Madrid across the empire. Local governors and viceroys eventually acknowledged receipt and swore compliance, but in reality, it was often business as usual. Illicit commerce continued, French vessels made their way into Spanish ports, and foreigners went on living and trading in the Spanish Indies without the requisite *cartas de naturaleza*.

As we saw in previous chapters, the disregard of public health measures was not limited to the colonies. Personnel, merchants, and others in the port cities of Europe might have also snubbed public health regulations during the Plague of Provence or found ways to monetize or otherwise take advantage of the crisis. And demonstrations against the Quarantine Act of 1721 in London effectively led to the repeal of its most reviled clauses a year later. What is unique about the colonies is that violations of these policies were more widespread, more unchecked, and based on a more genuine need for provisions, which the metropole was not always able to effectively supply. In the French and Spanish colonies, then, economic interests and/or local needs, and even mere wants, overshadowed concerns about public health during the Plague of Provence.

Officials in both Paris and Madrid informed their representatives in the colonies of the plague in France and offered directions for protecting public health, but these differed largely in degree and severity. Whereas the Spanish king imposed severe plague-time regulations and sought to monitor activities in both Spain *and* the colonies, officials in Paris – who themselves imposed such strict and comprehensive measures *within* France – appeared to take a relatively more relaxed approach overseas. Unlike administrators in the Spanish colonies, who were given stringent orders on pain of death and dispossession, those of the French colonies saw no such threats. Officials in the French colonies were given much more freedom to act as they saw fit. During the Plague of Provence, this language was very common in correspondence from the *Conseil de Marine* to the governors and intendents of the islands. Feuquières and Bénard, for example, were often told to proceed based on what they judged to be appropriate, as when deciding how to deal with a ship from the Mediterranean, or how long of a quarantine to impose. The king of Spain, meanwhile, offered no such liberties, and carefully dictated every move his governors, viceroys, and other administrators should take to protect public health. Accordingly, French colonial administrators also received orders that were significantly less rigorous, and that came with notable exceptions. Slave ships were to be permitted into port with minimal inconveniences even if they were carrying people infected with any of a variety of diseases. And French restrictions against foreign commerce in the Antilles excluded trade with the Spanish Americas – and their gold and silver – which was considered far too valuable to prohibit. Essentially, while the Spanish Crown worked to ban all French, and then all foreign, commerce during the Plague of Provence, officials in Paris worked equally hard to *expand* it with the Spanish in the Americas.

Why these differences between French and Spanish plague-time policies in the colonies? Why were plague-time measures in the French colonies more relaxed than those in the Spanish colonies, and even those mainland in France, despite concerns that the islands would be "lost without resource" if plague were to spread overseas?[99] Part of the reason was sheer distance. French officials rationalized allowing potentially infected vessels to enter colonial ports on the grounds that they had been at sea for enough months that any presence of plague would have disappeared by the time it arrived. Spanish documents reveal no such considerations. Contemporary French sources also reveal a sense of indifference about public health in the colonies. In 1721, as we saw earlier, the French *Conseil de Marine* instructed administrators in Saint-Domingue to avoid inconveniencing slave ships with burdensome inspections or quarantines lest they be discouraged from returning to the islands. Among the diseases to which the colonists should not overreact was smallpox, which they insisted was "not of too dangerous a consequence." More than indifference, statements like this also betray contemporary understandings about disease environments or diseases of place, which is to say, the idea that different maladies were characteristic of different climates and could thus be expected to manifest themselves in particular ways depending on both geography and the acclimatization (or lack thereof) of a population.[100] By the eighteenth century, such notions at times influenced how officials might approach or manage public health crises in the colonies.

If we phrase the question another way, however – that is, why were Spain's policies in the colonies so much more severe that those of France? – the answer is perhaps much simpler, or more complex depending on one's perspective. As we saw in Chapter 4, the Spanish monarch at this time, Philip V – known as he is for his centralizing endeavors, which took the form of various new policies and initiatives known together as the Bourbon Reforms – used the Great Plague Scare as a means to help improve Spain's place in the competitive Indies market and the wider balance of Europe. What more effective

---

[99] See footnote 14.
[100] For more on these understandings in the case of Britain, see, Suman Seth's *Difference and Disease*; Mark Harrison, *Medicine in an Age of Commerce and Empire: Britain and Its Tropical Colonies 1660–1830* (Oxford: Oxford University Press, 2010).

way was there to achieve this than by cutting out all of Spain's foreign competitors in the Indies themselves? In times of peace and health, recent treaties made this difficult, but in times of crisis, everything was on the table.

In the age of COVID, none of this should come as a surprise. The COVID-19 pandemic, like the Plague of Provence three centuries earlier, has taught us that the motivations behind a society's responses to public health crises are not as simple as doing everything possible to save lives. Instead, they point to an extremely complex process that may be influenced by a myriad of factors including financial and/or diplomatic concerns, perceived violations of personal liberty, political partisanship, whether it is an election year, and so on. The considerations that come into play as leaders deliberate how to best manage an epidemic (or any other major disaster) vary from case to case, but the fact that saving lives is not the only – or, at times, even the primary – concern is unchanging.

Epilogue

But these ideas gave way to another that was then associated with every thought, entered at every sense, thrust itself even into the frivolous talk of the debauch, because it was easier to turn it into a joke than to pass it over in silence—the plague.

Alessandro Manzoni[1]

In 1975, philosopher and historian Michel Foucault wrote, "The plague-stricken town, traversed throughout with hierarchy, surveillance, observation, writing; the town immobilized by the functioning of an extensive power that bears in a distinct way over all individual bodies—this is the utopia of the perfectly governed city."[2] Indeed, during the Plague of Provence, authorities in Marseille and other infected Provençal and Languedocien towns exercised unlimited power – largely under centralized oversight – to help bring the crisis under control. Some of the mechanisms put in place during the disaster would remain long thereafter as a means to maintain added control over individuals, public health, trade, and smuggling. New apparatuses such as the *Conseil de la santé* in Paris – meant to safeguard the realm by "containing everybody in one rule"[3] – would help increase royal oversight in part through greater communication between the Crown and the provinces. Yet this was not only true of "the plague-stricken town." The emergency in 1720 – in this case, the mere *threat* of plague beyond the borders of France – presented rulers across Europe with opportunities to flex their centralizing muscles in the name of public health. Ruling from the capitals of Europe's emerging nation states,

---

[1] Alessandro Manzoni, *The Betrothed*, translated by Daniel J. Connor (New York: MacMillan, 1924), 562.
[2] Michel Foucault, *Discipline and Punish: The Birth of the Prison*, translated by Alan Sheridan (New York: Vintage Books, 1977), 198.
[3] Takeda, *Between Crown and Commerce*, 127.

leaders stepped in to oversee the management of plague prevention efforts – what I have referred to as disaster centralism throughout this study – and achieved various other objectives in the process. Parts of Europe emerged from the Provençal plague more centralized, bureaucratized, and interconnected.

This increased central oversight during the Provençal plague was in line with the concentration of state power that had most markedly been taking place for decades by the early eighteenth century. At least since the beginning of the second plague pandemic in the fourteenth century, the handling of crises in France and Europe consisted mostly of the localized implementation of sanitary, preventative, and relief mechanisms, with little or no central supervision or guidance – a product of the more regionalized organization of the European political landscape.[4] Writing about the Renaissance, for example, historian Matthew Vester has described how pandemics were managed "by a host of regional actors who formulated ad hoc policies … Pragmatism drove the decision-making of these local elites, whose actions were largely supported by the population, and not imposed by the sovereign."[5] By the late seventeenth and early eighteenth centuries, however, we see a monopolization of power and an expansion and intensification of state interference in previously regional or local matters. Gaining impetus after the Peace of Westphalia in 1648,[6] this shift coincided with what historian James B. Collins has recognized as the "transition from immature to mature monarchical state [that] happened roughly between 1690 and 1725."[7]

---

[4] Of course, there are always exceptions. See, for example, Chapter 2 on Genoa and Italy.

[5] Matthew Vester, "Pandemic Politics During the Renaissance," *History Workshop* (June 18, 2020), www.historyworkshop.org.uk/pandemic-politics-during-the-renaissance.

[6] In *Le Siècle de Louis XIV*, Voltaire referred to the Peace of Westphalia – which consists of the two treaties that brought the Thirty Years' War and the Eighty Years' War to an end – as "the basis for all future treaties." The documents recognized such concepts as national self-determination, co-existing sovereign states, and the balance of power, the latter of which was later a major cause in the War of the Spanish Succession and a major theme in the resulting Treaty of Utrecht. Voltaire, *The Age of Louis XIV*, translated by Martyn P. Pollack (New York: J.M. Dent & Sons, Limited, 1926), 50.

[7] Collins, *The State in Early Modern France*, xiii.

In the first years of the eighteenth century, France was seeing increases in population, production, and urbanization as more and more people left their villages and small towns for bigger ones in larger numbers. At the same time, people came to expect the government to expand its role in such areas as policing, poor relief, education, and sanitation and public works, and the state created a bureaucracy that "became steadily more professional, more intrusive, and more threatening to elites as the century wore on."[8] This was especially the case in times of crisis, as we see during the Plague of Provence, which the government used partly as an opportunity to showcase the integrity and value of the state by extending its reach into previously local matters.

Far from a mere repackaging of earlier plague prevention policies, then, the outbreak of 1720–22 signified a move toward disaster centralism – a more statist approach to disaster management – the likes of which we take for granted today. This is not to say that the process of centralization has unfolded in a linear progression, increasing over time from the eighteenth century to today. Instead, there have been fits and starts, and more recently, even shifts toward entirely new forms of disaster management.[9] All along the way, moreover, community responses and instances of what historian Jacob Remes has called "disaster citizenship" have remained, as they do today, critical.[10] Local individuals and organizations are not only first on the scene but possess an understanding of local communities and dynamics that is indispensable in times of crisis. Yet the centralization of disaster, public health, and risk management has come to represent an essential, and even distinguishing characteristic of the nation state.

---

[8] Ibid., 254 & 208.

[9] Consider, for example, the privatization or corporatization of disaster management today. Across the globe, most notably in the United States, private companies and corporations are assuming the responsibilities of disaster management and too often exploiting crises for financial gain. For more on this, see, for example: Kevin Fox Gotham and Miriam Greenberg, *Crisis Cities: Disaster and Redevelopment in New York and New Orleans* (New York: Oxford University Press, 2014); Kevin Fox Gotham, "Disaster, Inc.: Privatization and Post-Katrina Rebuilding in New Orleans," *Perspectives on Politics* 10, no. 3 (September 2012): 633–46; Naomi Klein, *The Shock Doctrine: The Rise of Disaster Capitalism* (New York: Picador, 2007).

[10] Jacob A. C. Remes, *Disaster Citizenship: Survivors, Solidarity, and Power in the Progressive Era* (Champaign: University of Illinois Press, 2015).

At least since the eighteenth century, people have increasingly come to expect their nation's leaders to step in and mitigate the damage in times of crisis – dispatching personnel, providing funding and aid, and even making an appearance, or at least delivering words about the matter at hand. Essentially, there has been a growing belief in the idea that, as sociologist Kevin Gotham has phrased it, "disaster victims have a democratic right to aid and recovery resources as members and citizens of a sovereign nation-state."[11] The Plague of Provence marks a significant moment in this process. It represents the largest, most notable early example of a concentrated, transnational effort by the heads of Europe's emerging nation states to oversee the handling of a major public health crisis or disaster.

...

More recently, the SARS-CoV-2 (COVID-19) pandemic has brought the question of disaster centralism to the fore. Conversations about the need for, or effectiveness of, big government in times of crisis have emerged across the globe. In the United States at least, opinions have largely fallen along party lines, but the fact that the discussions are taking place is telling.[12] Disasters, after all, are great revealers. Calamitous

---

[11] Gotham, "Disaster, Inc.," 642. Further down he adds that "there is no reason for having a state in the first place if it cannot protect and aid its citizens" in times of crisis.

[12] Countless editorials and opinion pieces have been published on this question since the beginning of the pandemic. Historian Naomi Oreskes appreciated as much during an interview for *The New Yorker*. In response to a question about the United States' handling of the pandemic under the Trump administration, she answered: "I've noticed that, just in the last week or so, increasingly I'm seeing people writing things like 'Coronavirus proves the need for big government.' Because it's really difficult to control a pandemic on the state or local level. The C.D.C. is a federal agency. The National Institutes of Health is a federal agency. All of the organizations we have that are set up to deal with a crisis of this type are federal agencies. And so for the Trump Administration to have acted briskly and promptly and in line with the scientific evidence on this would have been for it to embrace the role of the federal government and say, 'This is exactly why we have a powerful federal government. This is exactly why we have federal agencies of this sort.'" Early in the pandemic, Pamela Rendi-Wagner, chairwoman of the Austrian Social Democratic Party, argued that the coronavirus crisis confirms the need for a strong state: "The calls for a supportive, protecting state become louder as we reach the end of the crisis – even from parties that have repeatedly discredited

events such as epidemics expose power structures, political interests, economic or diplomatic concerns; they lay bare the strengths or weaknesses in a state, underlying divisions and tensions, and who among the populace is most valued, or deemed disposable and thus rendered vulnerable by targeted structural inequities.[13] The present study has demonstrated that they can be just as revealing about the social and political dynamics of regions far removed from the heart of the crisis.

This decentering, bird's-eye view approach to the study of the Plague of Provence has allowed us to trace the diplomatic, economic, and social ramifications of the event beyond French borders, into neighboring regions and across oceans. It has demonstrated the

such an idea in the past … The corona crisis shows that the neo-liberal concept has failed. A strong state and a good public health system were maintained in Austria thanks to social democratic governments … The state compensates for the disadvantages that arise in a society shaped by the free market. Therefore, an effective, resilient state is always of central importance, not only in times of crisis." Isaac Chotiner, "How to Talk to Coronavirus Skeptics," *The New Yorker* (March 23, 2020), www.newyorker.com/news/q-and-a/how-to-talk-to-coronavirus-skeptics; Pamela Rendi-Wagner, "Es braucht eine neue Solidarität für Österreich," *Die Presse* (April 30, 2020), www.diepresse.com/5807157/es-braucht-eine-neue-solidaritat-fur-osterreich. For other examples, see: Lindsay M. Chervinsky, "States Can't Fight Coronavirus on Their Own – And the Founding Fathers Knew It," *Time* (April 6, 2020), https://time.com/5815477/founders-constitution-pandemic; Clea Simon, "International forum cites strong government response as key in battle against COVID," *The Harvard Gazette* (October 7, 2020), https://news.harvard.edu/gazette/story/2020/10/strong-government-response-needed-in-covid-battle. The question has even attracted celebrities. See: Cate Blanchett, "Cate Blanchett: 'Covid-19 Has Ravaged the Whole Idea of Small Government,'" *The Guardian* (October 29, 2020), www.theguardian.com/books/2020/oct/29/cate-blanchett-covid-19-has-ravaged-the-whole-idea-of-small-government. Some of those who have argued *against* a strong centralized government during the COVID-19 pandemic include, for example: Ryan Bourne, "The COVID-19 Case for Bigger Government Is Weak," *Cato Institute* (September 9, 2021), www.cato.org/pandemics-policy/covid-19-case-bigger-government-weak; Michael Brendan Dougherty, "The Coronavirus Response Shows That Federalism Is Working," *National Review* (March 16, 2020), www.nationalreview.com/2020/03/coronavirus-response-shows-federalism-working; Nick Burns, "America's Response to the Coronavirus Crisis Proves Federalism Isn't Dead," *National Review* (April 2, 2020), www.nationalreview.com/2020/04/coronavirus-response-federalism-state-local-governments-take-lead/#slide-1.

[13] Elinor Accampo and Jeffrey H. Jackson, "Introduction," *French Historical Studies* 36, no. 2, Special Issue on Disaster in French History (Spring 2013): 165.

ways in which a calamitous event in one place could yet transgress national and geographic boundaries to influence the political objectives, economic policies, public health regulations, and thus quotidian life, in places far from the locus of disaster. Following these networks of influence in turn reveals the very complex nature of relationships between competing states in the increasingly interconnected world of the eighteenth century, and the ways in which these relations could inform and drive disaster management. An exploration of the many factors that have influenced state responses to disasters in the past can help us better understand the inherent complexity of managing catastrophe today, especially as we confront the more frequent occurrence of disasters – including disease epidemics and pandemics – as a result of human-caused climate change, globalization, population growth, and urbanization.[14] The COVID-19 pandemic, after all, will not be the last. And if history is any indication, it will certainly not be the worst.

---

[14] It is highly probable that pandemics will take place even more frequently than they did in the twentieth century. As Tong Wu and colleagues have observed: "Three interrelated world trends may be exacerbating emerging zoonotic risks: income growth, urbanization, and globalization. Income growth is associated with rising animal protein consumption in developing countries, which increases the conversion of wild lands to livestock production, and hence the probability of zoonotic emergence. Urbanization implies the greater concentration and connectedness of people, which increases the speed at which new infections are spread. Globalization—the closer integration of the world economy—has facilitated pathogen spread among countries through the growth of trade and travel. High-risk areas for the emergence and spread of infectious disease are where these three trends intersect with predisposing socioecological conditions including the presence of wild disease reservoirs, agricultural practices that increase contact between wildlife and livestock, and cultural practices that increase contact between humans, wildlife, and livestock." Tong Wu et al., "Economic Growth, Urbanization, Globalization, and the Risks of Emerging Infectious Diseases in China: A Review," *Ambio* 46, no. 1 (February 2017): 18.

Bibliography

ARCHIVAL COLLECTIONS CITED[1]

France

Archives départementales des Bouches-du-Rhône, Marseille (ADBRM)

Fonds Intendance Sanitaire de Marseille (série 200 E): 166, 287
Delta: 150, 2450
Family Papers: 24 E 11, 13 E 16
Other Series: 1F 80 (Guillaume de Nicolaï, 1629–1722)

Archives historiques de la Chambre de Commerce et d'Industrie Marseille-Provence, Marseille (ACCIM)

Police Sanitaire Maritime: G13, G14

Archives municipales de Marseille (AMM)

Police et justice, série FF: 182
Bureau de la santé, série GG (Peste 1720–22: 319–455): 325, 362, 426, 428

---

[1] Beyond this list, I consulted several archival collections that I did not ultimately cite in this book. Although these documents helped shape my understanding of the plague's influence abroad and the extent and nature of contemporary communications networks, they are not included in this list of cited collections.

Archives nationales de France, Paris (AN)

Consulats – Mémoires et documents. Affaires étrangères (AE) BIII: 42, 342, 361
Correspondance consulaire. Affaires étrangères (AE) BI: 224, 225, 226, 229, 233, 235, 238, 239, 246
Fonds de la Marine, Ancien (MAR): B3 275, B7 310

Archives nationales d'outre-mer, Aix-en-Provence (ANOM)

Fonds ministériels, Colonies:
Série B, Secrétariat d'Etat à la Marine, Correspondance au départ avec les colonies: 42, 44, 45
Sous-série C8, Correspondance à l'arrivée, Martinique: A 25, A 27, A 28, A 30, B 4, B 7, B 9
Sous-Série F3: Collection Moreau de Saint-Méry: 26, 252, 270
Dépôt des fortifications des colonies: 13 DFC (Martinique)

Bibliothèque nationale de France, Paris (BNF)

Manuscrit 18595, 1667

Italy

Archivio di Stato di Genova (ASG)

Fondo Senarega, Collegii Diversorum: 206

Archivio di Stato di Roma (ASR)

Bandi, Collezione 1: busta 57

Archivio di Stato di Venezia (ASV)

Antichi regimi, Provveditori e Sopraprovveditori alla sanità (Sanità): filze 90, 644, 651, 665
Ambasciata in Spagna: 79 (segnatura precedente 87)

Portugal

Arquivo Nacional Torre do Tombo (TdT)

Ministério dos Negócios Estrangeiros (MNE): Livro 789

Biblioteca Nacional de Portugal (BNP)

Gazeta de Lisboa

Spain

Archivo General de Indias, Seville (AGI)

Audiencia de Filipinas: legajos 140, 191
Audiencia de México: legajos 380, 413, 414, 488, 858
Audiencia de Santo Domingo: legajos 378, 379
Audiencia de Quito: legajo 129
Indiferente General: legajo 276

Archivo General del Reino de Valencia (ARV)

Sección de Audiencia: Libro del Acuerdo de la Real Audiencia, 1721

Archivo Histórico Nacional de España (AHN)

Sección de Consejos: legajos 1476, 10145
Sección de Estado: legajos 506, 4837

Archivo Municipal de Cádiz (AMC)

Actas Capitulares (AC): Cavildos del año de 1720, libro no. 76

Archivo Municipal de Murcia (AMU)

Actas Capitulares (AC): 338 (folio 190)

United Kingdom

British Library, London (BL)

816. m. 13, No. 91
816. m. 13, No. 93
816. m. 13, No. 94

The National Archives of the United Kingdom, London (TNA)

State Papers Foreign (SP)
France: 78/166, 78/168, 78/169, 78/170
Genoa: 79/12, 79/13, 79/14
Portugal: 89/29
Savoy and Sardinia: 92/30
Spain: 94/92
Tuscany: 98/24
Venice: 99/62

Historical Newspapers

Applebee's Original Weekly Journal (London)
Daily Courant (London)
Daily Journal (London)
Daily Post (London)
Evening Post (London)
Gaceta de Madrid (Madrid)
Gazeta de Lisboa (Lisbon)
London Gazette (London)
London Journal (London)
Post Boy (London)
Post Man and the Historical Account (London)
The Weekly Journal or Saturday's Post (London)
Weekly Journal or British Gazetteer (London)
Weekly Packet (London)

Published Primary Sources

[Anonymous]. *By the Lords Justices, A Proclamation, Requiring Quarentine to Be Performed by Ships Coming from the Mediterranean, Bourdeaux, or Any of the Ports or Places on the Coast of France in the Bay of Biscay, or from the Isles of Guernsey, Jersey, Alderney, Sarke, or Man, 27 Octob. 1720.* London: John Baskett, 1720.

[Anonymous]. *By the Lords Justices, A Proclamation Requiring Quarentine to Be Performed by Ships Coming from Bourdeaux, or Any of the Ports or Places on the Coast of France in the Bay of Biscay, 14 Oct. 1720.* London: John Baskett, 1720.

[Anonymous]. *Discours sur ce qui s'est passé de plus considérable à Marseille pendant la Contagion.* Marseille: Chez Jean-Antoine Mallard, 1721.

[Anonymous]. *La Fête séculaire de la peste de 1720, ou Éloge de Belsunce.* Marseille: Rouchon, 1820.

[Anonymous]. *La Foire de Beaucaire: Nouvelle Historique et Galante.* Amsterdam: Paul Marret, 1708.

[Anonymous]. *Medicina Flagellata: or, The Doctor Scarify'd.* London: Printed for J. Bateman, 1721.

Argüelles, José Canga. *Diccionario de hacienda con aplicación a España*, tomo 2. Madrid: Imprenta de Don Marcelino Calero y Portocarrero, 1834.

Bacallar y Sanna, Vicente, Marqués de San Felipe. *Comentarios de la Guerra de España, e Historia de su Rey Phelipe V El Animoso, desde el principio de su reynado, hasta la Paz General del año 1725*, tomo 1. Genoa: Matheo Garvizza, 1725.

Bertrand, Jean-Baptiste. *Relation Historique de la Peste de Marseille en 1720.* Cologne: Chez Pierre Marteau, 1721.

Blackmore, Richard. *A Discourse Upon the Plague with a Preparatory Account of Malignant Fevers.* London: Printed for John Clark, 1721.

Blanchett, Cate. "Cate Blanchett: 'Covid-19 Has Ravaged the Whole Idea of Small Government.'" *The Guardian.* October 29, 2020. www.theguardian.com/books/2020/oct/29/cate-blanchett-covid-19-has-ravaged-the-whole-idea-of-small-government.

Boulter, Bishop Hugh. *A Sermon Preach'd Before the Lords Spiritual and Temporal in Parliament Assembled at the Collegiate Church of St. Peter's Westminster, on Friday, December the 16th, 1720.* London: Printed for Timothy Childe, 1720.

Bourne, Ryan. "The COVID-19 Case for Bigger Government Is Weak." *Cato Institute.* September 9, 2021. www.cato.org/pandemics-policy/covid-19-case-bigger-government-weak.

Boyle, John, 5th earl of Cork and Orrery. "Letter VI from Bologna, Oct. 24, 1754." In *Letters from Italy in the Years 1754 and 1755, by the Late Right Honourable John Earl of Corke and Orrery*, edited by John Duncombe, 59–72. London: B. White, 1773.

Bradley, Richard. *The Plague at Marseilles Consider'd: With Remarks Upon the Plague in General, Shewing Its Cause and Nature of Infection, with Necessary Precautions to Prevent the Spreading of That Direful Distemper, Publish'd for the Preservation of the People of Great-Britain.* London: Printed for W. Mears, 1721.

Browne, Joseph. *A Practical Treatise of the Plague and All Pestilential Infections That Have Happen'd in This Island for the Last Century.* London: Printed for J. Wilcox, 1720.

Burns, Nick. "America's Response to the Coronavirus Crisis Proves Federalism Isn't Dead." *National Review.* April 2, 2020. www.nationalreview.com/2020/04/coronavirus-response-federalism-state-local-governments-take-lead/#slide-1.

Byrd II, William. *Discourse Concerning the Plague.* London: Printed for J. Roberts, 1721.

Chervinsky, Lindsay M. "States Can't Fight Coronavirus on Their Own—And the Founding Fathers Knew It." *Time.* April 6, 2020. https://time.com/5815477/founders-constitution-pandemic.

Chicoyneau, François. *A Succinct Account of the Plague at Marseilles, Its Symptoms, and the Methods and Medicines Used for Curing It.* Dublin: George Grierson, 1721.

Chicoyneau, François, François Verni, and Jean Soulier. *Beknopt verhaal, raakende de toevallen van de pest te Marseille: neevens deszelfs voorzegging en geneezing.* Leyden: Johannes du Vivié, 1721.

Chicoyneau, François, François Verny, and Jean Soulier. *Observations et Reflexions, Touchant la Nature, les Evenemens, et le Traitment de la Peste de Marseille, Pour Confirmer ce qui est avancé dans la Relation touchant les accidens de la Peste, son Prognostic, & sa Curation, du 10 Decembre 1720.* Lyon: Chez les Freres Bruyset, 1721.

Chotiner, Isaac. "How to Talk to Coronavirus Skeptics." *The New Yorker.* March 23, 2020. www.newyorker.com/news/q-and-a/how-to-talk-to-coronavirus-skeptics.

Comisión de Salud Pública. *Proyecto de ley orgánica de sanidad pública de la Monarquía Española.* Madrid: Imprenta de Alban y Compañía, 1822.

Croissainte, Nicolas Pichatty de. *Journal abregé de ce qui s'est passé en la ville de Marseille, depuis qu'elle est affligée de la contagion, tiré du Mémorial de la Chambre du Conseil de l'Hôtel de Ville; tenu par le Sieur Pichatty de Croissainte Conseil & Orateur de la Communauté, et Procureur du Roy de la Police.* Paris: Jacques Josse, 1721.

d'Antrechaus, Jean. *Relation de la peste dont la ville de Toulon fut affligée en 1721, Avec des observations instructives pour la postérité.* Paris: Frères Estienne, 1726.

Davies, Edward. *A Sermon Preach'd on Friday Decemb. 16th 1720, Being the Day of Publick Fasting and Humiliation for the Averting God's Judgments, Particularly the Plague.* London: Printed for T. Hurt in Coventry, 1720.

Defoe, Daniel. *Due Preparations for the Plague, as Well as Soul and Body, Being Some Seasonable Thoughts Upon the Visible Approach of the Present Dreadful Contagion in France; the Properest Measures to Prevent It, and the Great Work of Submitting to it.* London: Bible and Dove, 1722.

Deidier, Antoine. *Dissertation, Où l'on établi un sentiment particulier sur la contagion de la peste, Le Latin à côté.* Paris: Chez Charles-Maurice d'Houry, 1726.

Dougherty, Michael Brendan. "The Coronavirus Response Shows That Federalism Is Working." *National Review.* March 16, 2020. www.nationalreview.com/2020/03/coronavirus-response-shows-federalism-working.

Durand-Molard, M. *"Ordonnance sur la peste." Code de la Martinique, nouvelle edition,*tome 1. Saint-Pierre, Martinique: Imprimerie de Jean-Baptiste Thounens, 1807.

Expilly, l'Abbé Jean-Joseph Expilly. *Tableau de la population de la France.* Paris: 1780.

Explainer. *Distinct Notions of the Plague with the Rise and Fall of Pestilential Contagion.* London: Printed for J. Peele, 1722.

Gagliardi, Domenico. *Consigli Preservativi, e curativi in tempo di contagio, Dati in luce in forma di Dialogo da Domenico Gagliardi, Protomedico Generale di Roma, e Stato Ecclesiastico.* Rome: Stamperia di S. Michele a Ripa Grande, 1720.

Gibson, Edmund. *The Causes of the Discontents in Relations to the Plague and the Provisions Against it, Fairly Stated and Consider'd.* London: Printed for J. Roberts, 1721.

Girardot, M. le baron de, ed. *Correspondance de Louis XIV avec M. Amelot, son Ambassadeur en Espagne, 1705–1709,* vol. 2. Nantes: Imprimerie Merson, 1864.

Heath, John Benjamin. *Some Account of the Worshipful Company of Grocers of the City of London.* London: W. Marchant, 1829.

Helvetius. *Remèdes contre la peste.* Paris: Pierre-Auguste Lemercier, 1721.

Hughes, Obadiah. *The Good Man's Security in Times of Publick Calamity: A Sermon Preach'd in Maid-Lane, Southwark, on Occasion of the Plague in France, Published at the Request of Many That Heard It.* London: Printed for John Clark, 1722.

Hutcheson, Archibald. *A Collection of Calculations and Remarks Relating to the South Sea Scheme & Stock, Which Have Been Already Published, with the Addition of Some Others, Which Have Not Been Made Publick 'Till Now*. London, 1720.

Jauffret, Louis-François, ed. Pièces historiques sur la peste de Marseille et d'une partie de la Provence, *en 1720, 1721 et 1722, trouvées dans les archives de l'hôtel de ville, dans celles de la préfecture, au bureau de l'administration sanitaire et dans le cabinet des manuscrits de la bibliothèque de Marseille, publiées en 1820 à l'occasion de l'année séculaire de la peste; avec le Portrait de Mr. de Belsunce et un fac simile de son écriture*, tome 1. Marseille: Chez les principaux libraires, 1820.

Jennings, David. *Behold the Desolations in the Earth! A Sermon Preach'd at Crosby-Square, Nov. 30, 1721, a Time of Solemn Prayer on Occasion of the Plague in France*. London: Printed for John Clark, 1721.

Journal of the House of Lords. London: His Majesty's Stationery Office, 1721. British History Online.

Lassels, Richard. *The Voyage of Italy, or a Compleat Journey Through Italy in Two Parts: With the Characters of the People, and the Description of the Chief Towns, Churches, Monasteries, Tombs, Libraries, Pallaces, Villas, Gardens, Pictures, Statues, and Antiquities: as Also of the Interest, Government, Riches, Force, &c. of All the Princes: with Instructions Concerning Travel*. Paris: Vincent du Moutier, 1670.

Machiavelli, Nicolo. *The Prince*, translated by George Bull. London: Penguin Books, 2003.

Manget, Jean-Jacques. *Traité de la Peste Recueilli, des meilleurs auteurs*. Geneva: Chez Philippe Planche, 1721.

Manget, Jean-Jacques. *Traité de la peste, et de moyens de s'en preserver, tome premier*. Lyon: les freres Bruyset, 1722.

Manzoni, Alessandro. *The Betrothed*, translated by Daniel J. Connor. New York: MacMillan, 1924.

Mead, Richard. *A Discourse on the Plague*. London: Printed for A. Millar, 1720.

Mead, Richard. *A Short Discourse Concerning Pestilential Contagion and the Methods to Be Used to Prevent It*. London: Printed for Sam. Buckley, 1720.

Muratori, Lodovico Antonio. *Del governo della peste, e delle manière di guardarsene*. Modena: Bartolomeo Soliani Stamperia Ducale, 1714.

Muratori, Lodovico Antonio. *Relazione della peste di Marsiglia, pubblicata da i medici, che hanno operato in essa, con alcune osservazioni di Lodovico Antonio Muratori*. Brescia: Gian-Maria Rizzardi, 1721.

Newlin, Thomas. *God's Gracious Design in Inflicting National Judgments: A Sermon Preach'd Before the University of Oxford at St. Mary's on Friday, Dec. 16th 1720*. Oxford: Printed at the Theatre, 1721.

Parliament of Great Britain. *A Compleat Collection of the Protests of the Lords During This Last Session of Parliament*. London: Booksellers of London and Westminster, 1722.

Parliament of Great Britain. *A Compleat History of the Late Septennial Parliament*. London: Printed for J. Peele at Locke's-Head in Paternoster-Row, 1722.

Parliament of Great Britain. *Parliamentary History of England: From the Earliest Period to the Year 1803*, vol. 7. London: T. C. Hansard, 1811.

Parliament of Great Britain. *The History and Proceedings of the House of Commons from the Restoration to the Present Time*, vol. 8. London: Printed for Richard Chandler, 1742.

Parliament of Great Britain. *The History and Proceedings of the House of Commons from the Restoration to the Present Time*, vol. 6. London: Printed for Richard Chandler, 1742.

Parliament of Great Britain, House of Commons. *"The Humble Petition of the Bailiffs, Town-Clerk, Capital Burgesses, and Other the Inhabitants of the Ancient Town of Tamworth, in the Counties of Warwick and Stafford." A Collection of the Several Petitions of the Counties, Boroughs, & c. Presented to the House of Commons, Complaining of the Great Miseries the Nation Labours Under, by the Great Decay of Trade, Manufactures, and Publick Credit, Occasion'd by the Mismanagements of the Late Directors of the South-Sea Company, their Aiders, Abettors, and Confederates, &c.* London: E. Morphew, 1721.

Paterson, James. *A Warning to Great-Britain in a Sermon Preach'd at Several Churches in and about London, Upon the Spreading of the Plague in France, and Now Publish'd for the Benefit of Others*. London: Printed for the Author, s.a.

Pestalozzi, Jérôme-Jean. *Avis de Precaution Contre La Maladie Contagieuse de Marseille, Qui contient une idée complette de la Peste, & de ses accidens*. Turin: Chez Pierre Joseph Zappate, 1721.

Pickering, Danby. *The Statutes at Large, from the Fifth to the Ninth Year of King George I*, vol. 14. Cambridge: Joseph Bentham, 1765.

Pye, George. *A Discourse of the Plague; Wherein Dr. Mead's Notions Are Consider'd and Refuted*. London: J. Darby, 1721.

Rendi-Wagner, Pamela. "Es braucht eine neue Solidarität für Österreich." *Die Presse*. April 30, 2020. www.diepresse.com/5807157/es-braucht-eine-neue-solidaritat-fur-osterreich.

Rose, Philip. *A Theorico-Practical, Miscellaneous, and Succinct Treatise of the Plague, Shewing Its Nature, Signs, Causes, Prevention and Cure.* London: Printed for T. Jauncy, 1721.

Saint-Simon, Louis de Rouvroy, duc de. *Mémoires XI,* edited by A. de Boislisle. Paris: Hachette et cie, 1895.

Scarborough, Charles. *A Practical Method as Used for the Cure of the Plague in London, in 1665.* London: Printed for B. Lintot, 1722.

Scheuchzer, Johann Jacob. Λοιμογραφια *Massiliensis: Die in Marseille und Provence Eingerissene Pest-Seuche.* Zurich: Bodmer, 1720.

Sharp, Samuel. *Letters from Italy, Describing the Customs and Manners of That Country in the Years 1765, and 1766.* London: R. Cave, 1767.

Simon, Clea. "International Forum Cites Strong Government Response as Key in Battle Against COVID." *The Harvard Gazette.* October 7, 2020. https://news.harvard.edu/gazette/story/2020/10/strong-government-response-needed-in-covid-battle.

Sloane, Hans. *The First Part of the Treatise of the Late Dreadful Plague in France, Compared with That Terrible Plague in London, in the Year 1665, in Which Died Near a Hundred Thousand Persons.* London: H. Parker, 1722.

Strother, Edward. *Experience'd Measures How to Manage the Smallpox; to Which Is Added, the Proper Method to Be Used in the Plague.* London: Printed for Charles Rivington, 1721.

Sydenham, Thomas. *The Works of Thomas Sydenham, M.D., on Acute and Chronic Diseases: with Their Histories and Modes of Cure.* Philadelphia: Benjamin & Thomas Kite, 1809.

Tolon, Maurice de. *Le capucin charitable, enseignant la méthode pour remedier aux grandes miseres que la peste a coûtume de causer parmi les peuples.* Lyon: Les Freres Bruyset, 1721 (originally published 1662).

Voltaire. *Candide, ou l'Optimisme.* Paris: Larousse, 1991.

Voltaire. *The Age of Louis XIV,* translated by Martyn P. Pollack. New York: J. M. Dent & Sons, Limited, 1926.

Wilcocks, Bishop Joseph. *A Sermon Preach'd Before the Honourable House of Commons, at St. Margaret's Westminster, on Friday, Decemb. 16th 1720.* London: Printed for Timothy Childe, 1720.

Secondary Sources

Accampo, Elinor and Jeffrey H. Jackson. "Introduction." *French Historical Studies* 36, no. 2. Special Issue on Disaster in French History (Spring 2013): 165–74.

Alberola Romá, Armando. "Centralismo Borbónico y pervivencias forales: La reforma del gobierno municipal de la ciudad de Alicante (1747)." *Estudis: Revista de historia moderna* 18 (1992): 147–72.

Alberola Romá, Armando. "La pugna por el control de la administración local en la primera mitad del siglo XVIII: El proyecto de reforma del ayuntamiento de Alicante (1747)." In *Política y hacienda el el Antiguo Régimen*, edited by José Ignacio Fortea Pérez and Carmen Maria Cremades Griñán. Murcia: Universidad de Murcia, 1992, 145–54.

Alberola Romá, Armando. "Riadas, inundaciones y desastres en el sur Valenciano a finales del siglo XVIII." *Papeles de geografía* 51–2 (2010): 23–32.

Alberola Romá, Armando. "Una enfermedad de carácter endémico en el Alicante del XVIII: Las fiebres tercianas." *Revista de historia moderna: Anales de la Universidad de Alicante* 5 (1985): 127–40.

Alberola Romá, Armando and David Bernabé Gil. "Tercianas y calenturas en tierras meridionales valencianas: Una aproximación a la realidad médica y social del siglo XVIII." *Revista de historia moderna* 17 (1998–9): 95–112.

Alimento, Antonella and Koen Stapelbroek, eds. *The Politics of Commercial Treaties in the Eighteenth Century: Balance of Power, Balance of Trade*. Basingstoke: Palgrave Macmillan, 2017.

Alonso-Fernández, Francisco. *Felipe V: El rey fantasma*. Cordova: Editorial Almuzara, 2020.

[Anonymous]. "Musée d'Histoire de Marseille—Chroniques de la peste: 1720." *Musées Méditerranée: Association pour la conservation et la valorisation des collections publiques de France, Région Sud Provence-Alpes-Côte d'Azur* (2019). www.musees-mediterranee.org/portail/index .php?menu=1&num_musee=68.

Arquiola, Elvira, Jose Luis Peset, Mariano Peset, and Santiago La Parra. "Madrid, villa y corte, ante la peste de Valencia de 1647–1648." *Estudis: Revista de historia moderna* 5 (1976): 29–46.

Assereto, Giovanni. *"Per la comune salvezza dal morbo contagioso": I controlli di sanità nella Repubblica di Genova*. Genoa: Città del silenzio, 2011.

Assereto, Giovanni. "Polizia sanitaria e sviluppo delle istituzioni statali nella Repubblica di Genova." In *Controllare il territorio. Norme, corpi e conflitti tra medioevo e prima guerra mondiale*, edited by Livio Antonielli and Stefano Levati, 167–87. Soveria Mannelli: Rubbettino, 2013.

Bamji, Alexandra. "Health Passes, Print and Public Health in Early Modern Europe." *Social History of Medicine* 32, no. 3 (August 2019): 441–64.

Banks, Kenneth. *Chasing Empire Across the Sea: Communications and the State in the French Atlantic, 1713–1763*. Montreal: McGill-Queen's University Press, 2006.

Banks, Kenneth. "Communications and 'Imperial Overstretch': Lessons from the Eighteenth-Century French Atlantic." *French Colonial History* 6 (2005): 17–32.

Barona, Josep, and Josep Bernabeu-Mestre. *La salud y el Estado: El movimiento sanitario internacional y la administración española, 1851–1945*. Valencia: Universitat de València, 2008.

Bérenger, D. Théophile, O. S. B. *Journal du maitre d'hotel Mgr de Belsunce durant la peste de Marseille, 1720–1722*. Paris: Mairie de Victor Palmé, 1878.

Bertrand, Régis. "L'iconographie de la peste de Marseille, ou la longue memoire d'une catastrophe." In *Images de la Provence: Les représentations iconographiques de la fin du Moyen Age au milieu du XXe siècle, edited by Centre méridional d'histoire sociale des mentalités et des cultures (collectif)*, 75–90. Aix-en-Provence: Presses universitaires de Provence, 1992.

Béthencourt Massieu, Antonio de, ed. *Felipe V y el Atlántico: III centenario del advenimiento de los Borbones*. Gran Canaria: Ediciones del Cabildo de Gran Canaria, 2002.

Betrán Moya, José Luis. "Sociedad y peste en la Barcelona de 1651." *Manuscrits: Revista d'història moderna* 8 (January 1990): 255–82.

Betrán Moya, José Luis. "La peste como problema historiográfico." *Manuscrits: Revista d'història moderna*, no. 12 (1994): 283–319.

Betrán Moya, José Luis. *La peste en la Barcelona de los Austrias*. Lleida: Editorial Milenio, 1996.

Biraben, Jean-Noël Biraben. *Les hommes et la peste en France et dans les pays européens et méditerranéens, tomes 1 & 2*. Paris: Mouton & Co., 1975.

Black, Jeremy. *The British Abroad: The Grand Tour in the Eighteenth Century*. Stroud: Sutton Publishing, 2003.

Blake, John B. *Public Health in the Town of Boston, 1630–1822*. London: Oxford University Press, 1959.

Booker, John. *Maritime Quarantine: The British Experience, c. 1650–1900*. Aldershot: Ashgate Publishing, 2007.

Boran, Elizabethanne. "The 1720 Marseille Plague." *Edward Worth Library* (2020). https://edwardworthlibrary.ie/exhibitions-at-the-worth/smaller-exhibitions/1720-at-the-edward-worth-library.

Bos, Kirsten I., Alexander Herbig, Jason Sahl et al. "Eighteenth-Century *Yersinia pestis* Genomes Reveal the Long-Term Persistence of an Historical Plague Focus." *eLife* (2016), doi: 10.7554/eLife.12994.

Bourde, André. "La Provence au grand siècle." In *Histoire de la Provence*, edited by Édouard Baratier. Paris: Privat, 1987, 305–41.

Bowers, Kristy Wilson. *Plague and Public Health in Early Modern Seville*. Rochester: University of Rochester Press, 2013.

Bramanti, Barbara, Yarong Wu, Ruifu Yang, Yujun Cui, Nils Christian Stenseth. "Assessing the Origins of the European Plagues Following the Black Death: A Synthesis of Genomic, Historical, and Ecological Information." *Proceedings of the National Academy of Sciences* 118, no. 36 (August 2021): 1–6.

Brilli, Catia. *Genoese Trade and Migration in the Spanish Atlantic, 1700–1830*. Cambridge: Cambridge University Press, 2016.

Brockliss, Laurence, and Colin Jones. *The Medical World of Early Modern France*. Oxford: Clarendon Press, 1997.

Burnard, Trevor, and John Garrigus. *The Plantation Machine: Atlantic Capitalism in French Saint-Domingue and British Jamaica*. Philadelphia: University of Pennsylvania Press, 2016.

Bustos Rodríguez, Manuel. "Les associations de commerce autour de la 'Carrera de Indias' au XVIIIe siècle." In *Le commerce atlantique franco-espagnol: acteurs, négoces et ports, XVe–XVIIIe siècle*, edited by Jean-Philippe Priotti and Guy Saupin. Rennes: Presses universitaires de Rennes, 2008, 275–84.

Buti, Gilbert. "L'Intendance de la Santé de Marseille au XVIIIe siècle: service sanitaire ou bureau de renseignements?" In *La quotidiana emergenza: I molteplici impieghi delle istituzioni sanitarie nel Mediterraneo moderno*, edited by Paolo Calcagno and Daniele Palermo, 43–61. Palermo: New Digital Frontiers, 2017.

Campbell, Peter R. *Power and Politics in Old Regime France, 1720–1745*. London: Routledge, 1996.

Cañizares-Esguerra, Jorge, ed. *Entangled Empires: The Anglo-Iberian Atlantic, 1500–1830*. Philadelphia: University of Pennsylvania Press, 2018.

Carmichael, Ann G. "Plague Persistence in Western Europe: A Hypothesis." *The Medieval Globe* 1, no. 1 (2014): 157–91.

Carmichael, Ann G. "Registering Deaths and Causes of Death in Late Medieval Milan." In *Death in Medieval Europe: Death Scripted and Death Choreographed*, edited by Joëlle Rollo-Koster, 209–36. London: Routledge, 2017.

Carmona García, Juan Ignacio. *La Peste en Sevilla*. Seville: Ayuntamiento de Sevilla, 2005.

Carrière, Charles, Marcel Courdurié, and Ferréol Rebuffat. *Marseille ville morte: la peste de 1720*. Marseille: M. Garçon, 1968.

Casey, James. *Early Modern Spain: A Social History*. London: Routledge, 1999.

Casey, James. *España en la Edad Moderna: Una historia social*. Madrid: Editorial Biblioteca Nueva, 2001.

Castro, Concepción de. "Le Conseil et les premiers ministres des Finances sous Philippe V: conflits et intégration (XVIIIe siècle)." In *Les finances royales dans la monarchie espagnole, XVIe–XIXe siècles*, edited by Anne Dubet. Rennes: Presses universitaires de Rennes, 2008, 89–102.

Caylux, Odile. *Arles et la peste, 1720–1721*. Aix-en-Provence: Presses universitaires de Provence, 2009.

Chase-Levenson, Alex. *The Yellow Flag Quarantine and the British Mediterranean World, 1780–1860*. Cambridge: Cambridge University Press, 2020.

Cheney, Paul. "The Political Economy of Colonization: From Composite Monarchy to Nation." In *The Economic Turn: Recasting Political Economy in Enlightenment Europe*, edited by Steven Kaplan and Sophus Reinert, 71–87. London: Anthem Press, 2019.

Cheney, Paul. *Revolutionary Commerce: Globalization and the French Monarchy*. Cambridge, MA: Harvard University Press, 2010.

Christelow, Allan. "French Interest in the Spanish Empire during the Ministry of the Duc de Choiseul, 1759–1771." *The Hispanic American Review* 21, no. 4 (November 1941): 515–37.

Cipolla, Carlo M. *Public Health and the Medical Profession in the Renaissance*. Cambridge: Cambridge University Press, 1976.

Cipolla, Carlo M. *Fighting the Plague in Seventeenth-Century Italy*. Madison: University of Wisconsin Press, 1981.

Cohn, Jr., Samuel K. *Cultures of Plague: Medical Thinking at the End of the Renaissance*. Oxford: Oxford University Press, 2010.

Collingridge, William. "On Quarantine." *British Medical Journal* 1 (1897): 646–9.

Collins, James B. *The State in Early Modern France*. New York: Cambridge University Press, 2009.

Coss, Stephen. *The Fever of 1721: The Epidemic That Revolutionized Medicine and American Politics*. New York: Simon & Schuster, 2017.

Crawshaw, Jane L. Stevens. *Plague Hospitals: Public Health for the City in Early Modern Venice*. New York: Routledge, 2016.

Crawshaw, Jane L. Stevens. "The Places and Spaces of Early Modern Quarantine." In *Quarantine: Local and Global Histories*, edited by Alison Bashford, 15–34. New York: Palgrave, 2016.

Crespo Solana, Ana. "La acción de José Patiño en Cádiz y los proyectos navales de la Corona del siglo XVIII." *Trocadero: Revista de historia moderna y contemporanea*, no. 6–7 (1994–5): 35–50.

Crespo Solana, Ana. *La Casa de Contratación y la Intendencia General de la Marina en Cádiz, 1717–1730.* Cádiz: Universidad de Cádiz, 1996.

Crespo Solana, Ana. *El Comercio marítimo entre Amsterdam y Cádiz, 1713–1778.* Madrid: Banco de España – Servicio de Estudios, 2000.

Crespo Solana, Ana. "El Comercio y la armada de la monarquía: La Casa de Contratación y la Intendencia General de la Marina de Cádiz, 1717–1750." *Jornadas de Historia Marítima* xxiv, no. 39 (2001): 63–78.

Crespo Solana, Ana. "El comercio holandés y la integración de espacios económicos entre Cádiz y el Báltico en tiempos de guerra (1699–1723)." *Investigaciones de Historia Económica* 3, no. 8 (2007): 45–76.

Crespo Solana, Ana. "Merchants and Observers: The Dutch Republic's Commercial Interests in Spain and the Merchant Community in Cádiz in the Eighteenth Century." *Dieciocho: Hispanic Enlightenment* 32, no. 2 (Fall 2009): 193–224.

Crouzet, François. "La rivalité commerciale franco-anglaise dans l'empire espagnol, 1713–1789." *Histoire: Economie et Société* 31 (2012/13): 19–29.

Dadson, Trevor J., and J. H. Elliott, eds. *Britain, Spain, and the Treaty of Utrecht 1713–2013.* New York: Routledge, 2014.

Dale, Richard. *The First Crash: Lessons from the South Sea Bubble.* Princeton: Princeton University Press, 2004.

Dauverd, Céline. *Imperial Ambition in the Early Modern Mediterranean: Genoese Merchants and the Spanish Crown.* New York: Cambridge University Press, 2015.

Dean, Katharine R., Fabienne Krauer, and Lars Walløe et al. "Human Ectoparasites and the Spread of Plague in Europe During the Second Pandemic." *Proceedings of the National Academy of Sciences* 115, no. 6 (2018): 1304–9.

Dean, Katharine R., Fabienne Krauer, and Lars Walløe et al. "Reply to Park et al.: Human Ectoparasite Transmission of Plague During the Second Pandemic Is Still Plausible." *Proceedings of the National Academy of Sciences* 115, no. 34 (2018): E7894–5.

DeLacy, Margaret. *The Germ of an Idea: Contagionism, Religion, and Society in Britain, 1660–1730.* London: Palgrave Macmillan, 2016.

den Hond, Bas. "Plague Bug May Have Lurked in Medieval England Between Outbreaks." *Earth & Space Science News* 98 (May 8, 2017). https://doi.org/10.1029/2017EO073063.

Désos, Catherine. *Les Français de Philippe V: Un modèle nouveau pour gouverner l'Espagne, 1700–1724.* Strasbourg: Presses universitaires de Strasbourg, 2009.

Domínguez Ortiz, Antonio. *Historia de Sevilla: La Sevilla del siglo XVII*. Seville: Universidad de Sevilla Secretariado de Publicaciones, 1986.

Domínguez Ortiz, Antonio. *La Sociedad Española en el Siglo XVII: El Estamento nobiliario*, vol. 1. Granada: Universidad de Granada, 1992.

Dubet, Anne. *Jean Orry et la réforme du gouvernement de l'Espagne (1701–1706)*. Clermont-Ferrand: Presses Universitaires Blaise-Pascal, 2009.

El Hadj, Jamel. "Les chirurgiens et l'organisation sanitaire contre la peste à Marseille, 17e–18e siècles." PhD diss., EHESS, 2014.

Elliott, J. H. *Empires of the Atlantic World: Britain and Spain in America 1492–1830*. New Haven: Yale University Press, 2006.

Ermus, Cindy. "Memory and the Representation of Public Health Crises: Remembering the Plague of Provence in the Tricentennial." *Environmental History* 26, no. 4 (October 2021): 776–88.

Filippini, Jean-Pierre. *Il Porto di Livorno e la Toscana, 1676–1814*, vol. 2. Naples: Edizioni Scientifiche Italiane, 1998.

Fitzpatrick, Brian. *Catholic Royalism in the Department of the Gard, 1814–1852*. Cambridge: Cambridge University Press, 1983.

Foucault, Michel. *Discipline and Punish: The Birth of the Prison*, translated by Alan Sheridan. New York: Vintage Books, 1977.

Fresquet Febrer, José Luis. "Los medicos frente a la enfermedad en la Valencia del siglo XVIII." In *Estudios sobre la profesión médica en la sociedad valenciana, 1329–1898*, edited by José María López Piñero. Valencia: Ajuntament de València, 1998.

Frostin, Charles. "Les Pontchartrain et la pénétration commerciale française en Amérique espagnole (1690–1715)." *Revue Historique* 245, no. 498 (April–June 1971): 307–36.

Gaffarel, Paul, and the marquis de Duranty. *La Peste de 1720 a Marseille et en France, d'après des documents inédits*. Paris: Perrin et Cie, 1911.

García Cárcel, Ricardo. "La opinión de los españoles sobre Felipe V después de la Guerra de Sucesión." *Cuadernos de Historia Moderna Anejos* 1 (2002): 103–25.

García Cárcel, Ricardo. *Felipe V y los españoles: Una vision periférica del problema de España*. Barcelona: Plaza & Janés Editores, 2002.

García-Baquero González, Antonio. *Cádiz y el Atlantico (1717–1778): El comercio colonial español bajo el monopolio gaditano*. Seville: Imprenta C.S.I.C., 1976.

García-Baquero González, Antonio. "El comercio colonial en la época de Felipe V: El reformismo continuista." In *Felipe V y su tiempo: congreso internacional*, vol. 1, edited by Eliseo Serrano Martín. Zaragoza: Institución "Fernando el Católico," 2004, 75–102.

García-Baquero González, Antonio, and Pedro Collado Villalta. "Les Français à Cadix au XVIIIe siècle: La colonie marchande." In *Les Français en Espagne à l'époque modern, XVIe–XVIIIe siècles, ouvrage collectif*, edited by Centre national de la recherche scientifique. Paris: Éditions du Centre national de la recherche scientifique, 1990, 173–96.

García-Mauriño Mundi, Margarita. *La pugna entre el Consulado de Cádiz y los jenízaros por las exportaciones a Indias, 1720–1765*. Seville: Universidad de Sevilla, 1999.

Geltner, Guy. *Roads to Health: Infrastructure and Urban Wellbeing in Later Medieval Italy*. Philadelphia: University of Pennsylvania Press, 2019.

Ghachem, Malick W. "'No Body to be Kicked?' Monopoly, Financial Crisis, and Popular Revolt in 18th-Century Haiti and America." *Law & Literature* 28, no. 3 (2016): 403–31.

Giffin, Karen, Aditya Kumar Lankapalli, Susanna Sabin et al. "A Treponemal Genome from an Historic Plague Victim Supports a Recent Emergence of Yaws and its Presence in 15th-century Europe." *Scientific Reports* 10, no. 9499 (2020): 1–13.

Gigi, Arad. "The Materiality of Empire: Forts, Labor, and the Colonial State in the French Lesser Antilles, 1661–1776." PhD diss., Florida State University, 2018.

Girard, Albert. *El comercio francés en Sevilla y Cádiz en tiempo de los Habsburgo*. Seville: Editorial Renacimiento, 2006.

González Enciso, Agustín. *Felipe V: La renovación de España: Sociedad y economía en el reinado del primer Borbón*. Pamplona: EUNSA, 2003.

González Enciso, Agustín. "La industria en el reinado de Felipe V." In *Felipe V y su tiempo: congreso internacional*, vol. 1, edited by Eliseo Serrano Martín, 49–73. Zaragoza: Institución "Fernando el Católico," 2004.

Goodman, Dena. *The Republic of Letters: A Cultural History of the French Enlightenment*. Ithaca: Cornell University Press, 1994.

Gordon, Daniel. "Confrontations with the Plague in Eighteenth-Century France." In *Dreadful Visitations: Confronting Natural Catastrophe in the Age of Enlightenment*, edited by Alessa Johns. New York: Routledge, 1999.

Goodman, Dena. *Becoming a Woman in the Age of Letters*. Ithaca: Cornell University Press, 2009.

Gotham, Kevin Fox. "Disaster, Inc.: Privatization and Post-Katrina Rebuilding in New Orleans." *Perspectives on Politics* 10, no. 3 (September 2012): 633–46.

Gotham, Kevin Fox, and Miriam Greenberg. *Crisis Cities: Disaster and Redevelopment in New York and New Orleans*. New York: Oxford University Press, 2014.

Green, Monica. "The Four Black Deaths." *American Historical Review* 125, no. 5 (December 2020): 1601–31.

Griffen, William B. "Spanish Pensacola, 1700–1763." *The Florida Historical Quarterly* 37, no. 3/4 (1959): 242–62.

Guellil, Meriam, Oliver Kersten, Amine Namouchi, Stefania Luciani, Isolina Marota, Caroline A. Arcini, Elisabeth Iregren, Robert A. Lindemann, Gunnar Warfvinge, Lela Bakanidze, Lia Bitadze, Mauro Rubin, Paola Zaio, Monica Zaio, Damiano Neri, Nils Christian Stenseth, and Barbara Bramanti. "A Genomic and Historical Synthesis of Plague in 18th-Century Eurasia." *Proceedings of the National Academy of Sciences* 117, no. 45 (November 2020): 28328–35.

Guey, Jean-Louis. *Mémoires ou livre de raison d'un bourgeois de Marseille, 1674–1724.* Montpellier: Bureau des Publications de la Société pour l'étude des Langues Romanes, 1881.

Hanotin, Guillaume. *Jean Orry: Un homme des finances royales entre France et Espagne, 1701–1705.* Cordova: Universidad de Córdoba, 2009.

Harkness, Deborah E. "Maps, Spiders, and Tulips: the Cole-Ortelius-L'Obel family and the Practice of Science in Early Modern London." In *From Strangers to Citizens: The Integration of Immigrant Communities in Britain, Ireland and Colonial America, 1550–1750,* edited by Randolph Vigne and Charles Littleton, 184–96. Brighton: Sussex Academic Press, 2001.

Harrison, Mark. *Medicine in an Age of Commerce and Empire: Britain and Its Tropical Colonies 1660–1830.* Oxford: Oxford University Press, 2010.

Harrison, Mark. *Contagion: How Commerce has Spread Disease.* New Haven: Yale University Press, 2013.

Haydon, Daniel T., S. Cleaveland, L. H. Taylor, and M. K. Laurenson. "Identifying Reservoirs of Infection: A Conceptual and Practical Challenge." *Emerging Infectious Diseases* 8, no. 12 (December 2002): 1468–73.

Heagerty, John J. *Four Centuries of Medical History in Canada,* vol. 2. Toronto: Macmillan Company of Canada Limited, 1928.

Henderson, John. *Florence Under Siege: Surviving Plague in an Early Modern City.* New Haven: Yale University Press, 2019.

Henderson, John. "The Invisible Enemy: Fighting the Plague in Early Modern Italy." *Centaurus* 62, no. 2 (May 2020): 263–74.

Hildesheimer, Françoise. *Le Bureau de la santé de Marseille sous l'ancien régime.* Marseille: Fédération historique de Provence, 1980.

Hildesheimer, Françoise. *La terreur et la pitié: L'Ancien Régime à l'épreuve de la peste.* Paris: Éditions Publisud, 1990.

Hilton, Ronald. "Spaniards in Marseilles in the XVIIIth Century." *Bulletin Hispanique* 40, no. 2 (1938): 176–85.

Hopkins, Donald R. *The Greatest Killer: Smallpox in History*. Chicago: The University of Chicago Press, 2002.

Horowitz, Andy. *Katrina: A History, 1915–2015*. Cambridge, MA: Harvard University Press, 2020.

Hunt, Lynn, and Jack R. Censer. "Think Globally, Act Historically: Teaching the French Revolution and Napoleon." *Age of Revolutions* (December 11, 2017). https://ageofrevolutions.com/2017/12/11/think-globally-act-historically-teaching-the-french-revolution-and-napoleon.

Jonas, Raymond. *France and the Cult of the Sacred Heart*. Berkeley: University of California Press, 2000.

Kamen, Henry. *The War of Succession in Spain, 1700–15*. Bloomington: Indiana University Press, 1969.

Kamen, Henry. *Empire: How Spain Became a World Power, 1492–1763*. New York: Harper Collins, 2003.

Kierner, Cynthia A. *Inventing Disaster: The Culture of Calamity from the Jamestown Colony to the Johnstown Flood*. Chapel Hill: University of North Caroline Press, 2019.

Kirk, Thomas Allison. *Genoa and the Sea: Policy and Power in an Early Modern Maritime Republic, 1559–1684*. Baltimore: Johns Hopkins University Press, 2005.

Klein, Naomi. *The Shock Doctrine: The Rise of Disaster Capitalism*. New York: Picador, 2007.

Klooster, Wim. "Inter-Imperial Smuggling in the Americas, 1600–1800." In *Soundings in Atlantic History: Latent Structures and Intellectual Currents, 1500–1830*, edited by Bernard Bailyn and Patricia L. Denault. Cambridge, MA: Harvard University Press, 2009.

Klooster, Wim, and Gert Oostindie. *Realm Between Empires: The Second Dutch Atlantic, 1680–1815*. Ithaca: Cornell University Press, 2018.

Krekić, Bariša. *Dubrovnik in the Fourteenth and Fifteenth Centuries: A City Between East and West*. Norman: University of Oklahoma Press, 1972.

Kuethe, Allan J. "La política colonial de Felipe V y el proyecto de 1720." In *Orbis incognitvs: avisos y legajos del Nuevo Mundo, Homenaje al profesor Luis Navarro García*, vol. 1., edited by Fernando Navarro Antolín. Huelva: Universidad de Huelva, 2007: 233–41.

Kuethe, Allan J., and Kenneth J. Andrien. *The Spanish Atlantic World in the Eighteenth Century: War and the Bourbon Reforms, 1713–1796*. New York: Cambridge University Press, 2014.

Lane, Kris. *Pandemic in Potosí: Fear, Loathing and Public Piety in a Colonial Mining Metropolis*. University Park: The Pennsylvania State University Press, 2021.

Larcena, Danièle, Jean-Marc Azorin, and Yvette Coutant et al. *La Muraille de la peste*. Vaucluse: Les Alpes de Lumière, 1993.

Le Gouic, Olivier. "Des négociants français aux portes des Indes: les Lyonnais à Cadix au XVIIIe siècle." In *Le commerce atlantique franco-espagnol: acteurs, négoces et ports, XVe-XVIIIe siècle,* edited by Jean-Philippe Priotti and Guy Saupin. Rennes: Presses universitaires de Rennes, 2008, 285–317.

Lee, William, ed. *Daniel Defoe: His Life, and Recently Discovered Writings, Extending from 1716 to 1729*, vol. 2. London: John Camden Hotten, 1869.

León Sanz, Virginia. "Felipe V y la sociedad catalana al finalizar la guerra de sucesión." *Pedralbes: Revista d'història moderna* 23 (2003): 271–94.

Levenson, Thomas. *Money for Nothing: The Scientists, Fraudsters, and Corrupt Politicians Who Reinvented Money, Panicked a Nation, and Made the World Rich*. New York: Random House, 2020.

Liss, Peggy K. *Atlantic Empires: The Network of Trade and Revolution, 1713–1826*. Baltimore: The Johns Hopkins University Press, 1983.

López García, José Miguel. "Sobrevivir en la corte: Las condiciones de vida del pueblo llano en el Madrid de Felipe V." In *Felipe V y su tiempo: congreso internacional*, vol. 1, edited by Eliseo Serrano Martín. Zaragoza: Institución "Fernando el Católico," 2004, 133–66.

Lucenet, Monique. *Les grandes pestes en France*. Paris: Aubier, 1985.

Lucenet, Monique. "La peste, fléau majeur." *Bibliothèques d'Université de Paris*. www.biusante.parisdescartes.fr/histoire/medica/presentations/peste.php.

Lynch, John. *Bourbon Spain, 1700–1808*. Cambridge: Basil Blackwell, 1989.

Mandelblatt, Bertie. "How Feeding Slaves Shaped the French Atlantic: Mercantilism and the Crisis of Food Provisioning in the Franco-Caribbean During the Seventeenth and Eighteenth Centuries." In *The Political Economy of Empire in the Early Modern World*, edited by Sophus A. Reinert and Pernille Røge. Basingstoke: Palgrave Macmillan, 2013, 192–220.

Mapp, Paul W. *The Elusive West and the Contest for Empire, 1713–1763*. Chapel Hill: University of North Carolina Press, 2011.

Martín Corrales, Eloy. *Comercio de Cataluña con el Mediterráneo musulmán, siglos XVI–XVIII: El comercio con los "enemigos de la fe."* Barcelona: Edicions Bellaterra, 2001.

Martin, Meredith, and Gillian Weiss. "The Art of Plague and Panic: Marseille, 1720." *Platform*, April 27, 2020. www.platformspace.net/home/the-art-of-plague-and-panic-marseille-1720.

Martin, Meredith and Gillian Weiss. *The Sun King at Sea: Maritime Art and Galley Slavery in Louis XIV's France*. Los Angeles: Getty Publications, 2022.

Marzagalli, Silvia. "The French Atlantic World in the Seventeenth and Eighteenth Centuries." In *The Oxford Handbook of the Atlantic World, 1450–1850*, edited by Nicholas Canny and Philip Morgan, 235–51. Oxford: Oxford University Press, 2011.

McCloy, Shelby T. "Government Assistance During the Plague of 1720–22 in Southeastern France." *The Social Service Review* 12, no. 2 (June 1938): 298–318.

McLachlan, Jean O. *Trade and Peace with Old Spain 1667–1750: A Study of the Influence of Commerce on Anglo-Spanish Diplomacy in the First Half of the Eighteenth Century*. Cambridge: Cambridge University Press, 1940.

McNeill, John Robert. *Atlantic Empires of France and Spain: Louisbourg and Havana, 1700–1763*. Chapel Hill: University of North Carolina Press, 1985.

Mézin, Anne. *Les consuls de France au siécle des lumières, 1715–1792*. Paris: Ministère des Affaires étrangèrs, 1997.

Moitt, Bernard. *Women and Slavery in the French Antilles, 1635–1848*. Bloomington: Indiana University Press, 2001.

Monteano, Peio J. *Ira de Dios: Los Navarros en la era de la peste, 1348–1723*. Pamplona: Gráfica Ona, 2002.

Moral Ruiz, Joaquín del, Juan Pro Ruiz, and Fernando Suárez Bilbao. *Estado y territorio en España, 1820–1930: La formación del paisaje nacional*. Madrid: Libros de la Catarata, 2007.

Morel-Deledalle, Myriame, and Claude Badet. "Marseille aux XVIIe & XVIIIe siècles." In *Vivre en quarantaine dans les ports de Marseille aux XVIIe et XVIIIe siècles*, edited by Myriame Morel-Deladalle. Marseille: Musée d'Histoire de Marseille, 1987.

Morineau, Michel. *Incroyables gazettes et fabuleux métaux: Les retours des trésors américains d'après les gazettes hollandaises, XVIe–XVIII^esiècles*. Cambridge: Cambridge University Press, 1985.

Mullett, Charles. "A Century of English Quarantine, 1709–1825." *Bulletin of the History of Medicine* 23, no. 6 (November–December 1949): 527–45.

Mullett, Charles. *The Bubonic Plague and England: An Essay in the History of Preventive Medicine*. Lexington: University of Kentucky Press, 1956.

Mullett, Charles. "The English Plague Scare of 1720–23." *Osiris* 2 (1936): 484–516.

Muñoz Machado, Santiago. *La sanidad pública en España: Evolución histórica y situación actual*. Madrid: Instituto de Estudios Administrativos, 1975.

Namouchi, Amine, Meriam Guellil, and Oliver Kersten et al. "Integrative approach using *Yersinia pestis* genomes to revisit the historical landscape of plague during the Medieval Period." *Proceedings of the National Academy of Sciences* 115, no. 50 (December 2018): E11790–7.

Núñez de Prado, Sara. "De la Gaceta de Madrid al Boletín Oficial del Estado." *Historia y Comunicación Social* 7 (2002): 147–60.

O'Flanagan, Patrick. *Port Cities of Atlantic Iberia, c. 1500–1900*. Aldershot: Ashgate Publishing Limited, 2008.

Ozanam, Didier. "La colonie française de Cadix au XVIIIe siècle, d'après un document inédit (1777)." In *Melanges de la Casa de Velazquez,* tome 4, edited by Centre National de la recherche scientifique. Paris: Éditions E. de Boccard, 1968, 259–347.

Panzac, Daniel. *Quarantaines et lazarets: l'Europe et la peste d'Orient, XVIIe–XXe siècles*. Aix-en-Provence: Édisud, 1986.

Park, Sang Woo, Jonathan Dushoff, David J. D. Earn, Hendrik Poinar, and Benjamin M. Bolker. "Human Ectoparasite Transmission of the Plague During the Second Pandemic Is Only Weakly Supported by Proposed Mathematical Models." *Proceedings of the National Academy of Sciences* 115, no. 34 (2018): E7892–3.

Pastore, Alessandro. *Crimine e giustizia in tempo di peste nell'Europa moderna*. Rome: Editori Laterza, 1991.

Pearce, Adrian J. *The Origins of Bourbon Reform in Spanish South America, 1700–1763*. New York: Palgrave Macmillan, 2014.

Pedemonte, Danilo. "Quando il nemico è visibile: il magistrato di sanità genovese come strumento di controllo del territorio e di politica economica." *Storia Urbana* 147 (2015): 33–54.

Pedemonte, Danilo. "La 'pubblica salute' dello Stato genovese: il Magistrato di Sanità della Repubblica come strumento di governo delle informazioni, controllo del territorio e politica economica." In *La quotidiana emergenza: I molteplici impieghi delle istituzioni sanitarie nel Mediterraneo moderno*, edited by Paolo Calcagno and Daniele Palermo, 99–120. Palermo: New Digital Frontiers, 2017.

Peñafiel Ramón, Antonio, and Concepción Peñafiel Ramón. "Repercusión de la epidemia de peste marsellesa de 1720 en la ciudad de Murcia : Realidad de un gran miedo." *Contrastes: Revista de Historia Moderna* 3–4 (1987–8): 53–70.

Perdiguero Gil, Enrique. "Con medios humanos y divinos" : La lucha contra la enfermedad y la muerte en Alicante en el siglo XVIII." *Dynamis: Acta Hispanica ad Medicinae Scientiarumque Historiam Illustrandam* 22 (2002): 121–50.

Peset Reig, Mariano, and María Pilar Mancebo Alonso. "Valencia y la peste de Marsella de 1720." In *Primer Congreso de Historia del País Valenciano: celebrado en Valencia del 14 al 18 de abril de 1971*, vol. III. Valencia: Universidad de Valencia, 1973, 567–78.

Peset, Mariano, and José L. Peset. *Muerte en España: Politica y sociedad entre la peste y el colera*. Madrid: Seminarios y Ediciones, 1976.

Peset, Mariano, Pilar Mancebo, and José L. Peset. "Temores y defensa de España frente a la peste de Marsella de 1720." *Asclepio: Archivo Iberoamericano de Historia de la Medicina y Antropología Médica* 23 (1971): 131–89.

Petitjean Roget, Jacques. *Le Gaoulé: La révolte de la Martinique en 1717.* Fort-de-France: Société d'histoire de la Martinique, 1966.

Phillips, Carla Rahn. "The Growth and Composition of Trade in the Iberian Empires, 1450–1740." In *Rise of Merchant Empires: Long-Distance Trade in the Early Modern World, 1350–1750,* edited by James D. Tracy, 34–101. Cambridge: Cambridge University Press, 1990.

Plank, Geoffrey. *Atlantic Wars from the Fifteenth Century to the Age of Revolution.* New York: Oxford University Press, 2020.

Porter, Stephen. *The Great Plague.* Stroud: Sutton Publishing, 1999.

Pradells Nadal, Jesús. *Del foralismo al centralismo: Alicante 1700–1725.* Alicante: Universidad de Alicante, 1984.

Pritchard, James. *In Search of Empire: The French in the Americas.* Cambridge: Cambridge University Press, 2004.

Rambert, Gaston. *Histoire du commerce de Marseille,* tome 5, *De 1660 à 1789.* Paris: Librairie Plon, 1957.

Rambert, Gaston. "La France et la politique commercial de l'Espagne au XVIIIe siècle." *Revue d'histoire modern et contemporaine* 6e, no. 4 (October–December 1959): 269–88.

Remes, Jacob. *Disaster Citizenship: Survivors, Solidarity, and Power in the Progressive Era.* Champaign: University of Illinois Press, 2015.

Ringrose, David R. *Spain, Europe, and the "Spanish Miracle," 1700–1900.* New York: Cambridge University Press, 1996.

Rivoire, Hector. "Notice sur la Foire de Beaucaire." In *Mémoires de l'Académie Royale du Gard.* Nîmes: C. Durand-Belle, 1844.

Rodríguez Ocaña, Esteban. "El resguardo de la salud: Organización sanitaria española en el siglo XVIII." *Dynamis: Acta Hispanica ad Medicinae Scientiarumque Historiam Illustrandam* 7–8 (1987–8): 145–70.

Rowlands, Guy. *The Financial Decline of a Great Power: War, Influence, and Money in Louis XIV's France.* Oxford: Oxford University Press, 2012.

Sahm, Wilhelm. *Geschichte der Pest in Ostpreussen.* Leipzig: Verlag von Duncker & Humblot, 1905.

Sala, Raymond. *Le Visage de la mort dans les Pyrénées catalanes: Sensibilités et mentalités religieuses en Haut-Vallespir, XVIIe, XVIIIe et XIXe siècles.* Paris: Economica, 1991.

Santer, Melvin. *Confronting Contagion: Our Evolving Understanding of Disease.* Oxford: Oxford University Press, 2015.

Schmid, Boris V., Ulf Büntgen, W. Ryan Easterday et al. "Climate-Driven Introduction of the Black Death and Successive Plague Reintroductions into Europe." *Proceedings of the National Academy of Sciences* 112, no. 10 (March 2015): 3020–5.

Sée, H. "Esquisse de l'histoire du commerce français à Cadix et dans l'amérique espagnole au XVIIIe siècle." *Revue d'histoire modern* 3e, no. 13 (January–February 1928): 13–31.

Seguin-Orlando, Andaine, Caroline Costedoat, Clio Der Sarkissian, Stéfan Tzortzis, Célia Kamel, Norbert Telmon, Love Dalén, Catherine Thèves, Michel Signoli, and Ludovic Orlando. "No Particular Genomic Features Underpin the Dramatic Economic Consequences of 17th-Century Plague Epidemics in Italy." *iScience* 24 (April 23, 2021): 1–14.

Serrano Martín, Eliseo, ed. *Felipe V y su tiempo: congreso internacional*, vol. 1. Zaragoza: Institución "Fernando el Católico," 2004.

Seth, Suman. *Difference and Disease Medicine, Race, and the Eighteenth-Century British Empire*. Cambridge: Cambridge University Press, 2018.

Shaw, Christine. "Genoa." In *The Italian Renaissance State*, edited by Andrea Gamberini and Isabella Lazzarini, 220–36. Cambridge: Cambridge University Press, 2012.

Shovlin, John. *Trading with the Enemy: Britain, France, and the 18th-Century Quest for a Peaceful World Order*. New Haven: Yale University Press, 2021.

Slack, Paul. *The Impact of Plague in Tudor and Stuart England*. London: Routledge & Kegan Paul, 1985.

Slack, Paul. "Plague, Population and Political Economy in England 1550–1730." *Le Interazioni fra economia e ambiente biologico nell'Europa preindustriale secc. XII–XVIII*, edited by Simonetta Cavaciocchi, 383–98. Florence: Firenze University Press, 2010.

Slack, Paul. "Responses to Plague in Early Modern Europe: The Implications of Public Health." *Social Research: An International Quarterly* 87, no. 2 (Summer 2020): 409–28.

Slack, Paul. "Perceptions of Plague in Eighteenth-Century Europe." *Economic History Review* (April 2021): 1–19.

Slavin, Philip. "Out of the West: Formation of a Permanent Plague Reservoir in South-Central Germany (1349–1356) and Its Implications." *Past & Present* 252, no. 1 (August 2021): 3–51.

Snowden, Frank M. *Epidemics and Society: From the Black Death to the Present*. New Haven: Yale University Press, 2019.

Soons, Alfred H. A., ed. *The 1713 Peace of Utrecht and Its Enduring Effects*. Leiden: Brill, 2019.

Spyrou, Maria A., Marcel Keller, and Rezeda I. Tukhbatova et al. "A Phylogeography of the Second Plague Pandemic Revealed Through the Analysis of Historical *Y. pestis* Genomes." *Nature Communications* 10, no. 4470 (2019), doi: 10.1038/s41467-019-12154-0.

Stein, Stanley J., and Barbara H. Stein. *Silver, Trade, and War*. Baltimore: Johns Hopkins University Press, 2003.

Steinberg, Ted. *Acts of God: The Unnatural History of Natural Disaster in America*. New York: Oxford University Press, 2000.

Storrs, Christopher. *The Spanish Resurgence, 1713–1748*. New Haven: Yale University Press, 2016.

Strocchia, Sharon T. "Introduction: Women and Healthcare in Early Modern Europe." *Renaissance Studies* 28, no. 4 (September 2014): 496–514.

Sweet, Rosemary. *Cities and the Grand Tour: The British in Italy, c.1690–1820*. Cambridge: Cambridge University Press, 2012.

Takeda, Junko Thérèse. "Between Conquest and Plague: Marseillais Civic Humanism in the Age of Absolutism, 1660–1725." PhD diss., Stanford University, 2006.

Takeda, Junko Thérèse. *Between Crown and Commerce: Marseille and the Early Modern Mediterranean*. Baltimore: Johns Hopkins University Press, 2011.

Thomson, J. K. J. *Clermont-de-Lodève, 1633–1789: Fluctuations in the Prosperity of a Languedocian Cloth-Making Town*. Cambridge: Cambridge University Press, 1982.

Tomić, Zlata Blažina, and Vesna Blažina. *Expelling the Plague: The Health Office and the Implementation of Quarantine in Dubrovnik, 1377–1533*. Montreal: McGill-Queen's University Press, 2015.

Uekötter, Frank. "It's the Entanglements, Stupid." *Journal for the History of Environment and Society* 5. Special issue on "COVID-19 and Environmental History" (2020): 103–11.

United Nations Office for Disaster Risk Reduction. "Terminology." www.undrr.org/terminology.

Varela Peris, Fernando. "El papel de la Junta Suprema de Sanidad en la política sanitaria Española del siglo XVIII." *Dynamis: Acta Hispanica ad Medicinae Scientiarumque Historiam Illustrandam* 18 (1998): 315–40.

Varlık, Nükhet. "New Science and Old Sources: Why the Ottoman Experience of Plague Matters." *The Medieval Globe* 1, no. 1 (2014): 193–227.

Varlık, Nükhet. "Introduction." In *Plague and Contagion in the Islamic Mediterranean: New Histories of Disease in Ottoman Society*, edited by Nükhet Varlık, ix–xix. Kalamazoo: ARC Humanities Press, 2017.

Varlık, Nükhet. "'Oriental Plague' or Epidemiological Orientalism? Revisiting the Plague Episteme of the Early Modern Mediterranean." In *Plague and Contagion in the Islamic Mediterranean: New Histories of Disease in Ottoman Society*, edited by Nükhet Varlık, 57–87. Kalamazoo: ARC Humanities Press, 2017.

Varlık, Nükhet. "Rethinking the History of Plague in the Time of COVID-19." *Centaurus* 62, no. 2 (May 2020): 285–93.

Varlık, Nükhet. "New Questions for Studying Plague in Ottoman History." *TRAFO – Blog for Transregional Research*. June 29, 2021. https://trafo.hypotheses.org/29284.

Vázquez Gestal, Pablo. *Una nueva majestad: Felipe V, Isabel de Farnesio y la identidad de la monarquía (1700–1729)*. Madrid: Marcial Pons Historia, 2013.

Vester, Matthew. "Pandemic Politics During the Renaissance." *History Workshop* (June 18, 2020). www.historyworkshop.org.uk/pandemic-politics-during-the-renaissance.

Viñes Rueda, José Javier. *La Sanidad española en el siglo XIX*. Navarre: Departamento de Salud, 2006.

Walker, Geoffrey J. *Spanish Politics and Imperial Trade, 1700–1789*. Bloomington: Indiana University Press, 1979.

Warner, Jessica. *Craze: Gin and Debauchery in an Age of Reason*. New York: Basic Books, 2002.

Weber, Klaus, and Torsten dos Santos Arnold. "Ports to 'New Worlds': Lisbon, Seville, Cádiz (15th–18th Centuries)." In *The Power of Cities: The Iberian Peninsula from Late Antiquity to the Early Modern Period*, edited by Sabine Panzram. Leiden: Brill, 2019, 321–61.

Weinreich, Spencer J. "Unaccountable Subjects: Contracting Legal and Medical Authority in the Newgate Smallpox Experiment (1721)." *History Workshop Journal* 89 (Spring 2020): 22–44.

Wilson, Adrian. "The Politics of Medical Improvement in Early Hanoverian London." In *The Medical Enlightenment of the Eighteenth Century*, edited by A. Cunningham and R. French, 4–39. Cambridge: Cambridge University Press, 1990.

Wood, Laurie Marie. "Îles de France: Law and Empire in the French Atlantic and Indian Oceans, 1680–1780." PhD Diss., University of Texas at Austin, 2013.

Wu, Tong, Charles Perrings, Ann Kinzig, James P. Collins, Ben A. Minteer, and Peter Daszak. "Economic Growth, Urbanization, Globalization, and the Risks of Emerging Infectious Diseases in China: A Review." *Ambio* 46, no. 1 (February 2017): 18–29.

Zarzoso, Alfonso. "Protomedicato y boticarios en la Barcelona del siglo XVIII." *Dynamis: Acta Hispanica ad Medicinae Scientiarumque Historiam Illustrandam* 16 (1996): 151–71.

Zarzoso, Alfonso. "¿Obligación moral o responsabilidad política?: Las autoridades Borbónicas en tiempo de epidemias en la Cataluña del siglo XVIII." *Revista de historia moderna* 17 (1998–9): 73–94.

Ziegler, Michelle. "The Black Death and the Future of Plague." *The Medieval Globe* 1, no. 1 (2014): 259–83.

Zuckerman, Arnold. "Plague and Contagionism in Eighteenth-Century England: The Role of Richard Mead." *Bulletin of the History of Medicine* 78, no. 2 (Summer 2004): 273–308.

Index

Printed in the United States
by Baker & Taylor Publisher Services